TREATMENT OPTIONS IN UROLOGICAL CANCER

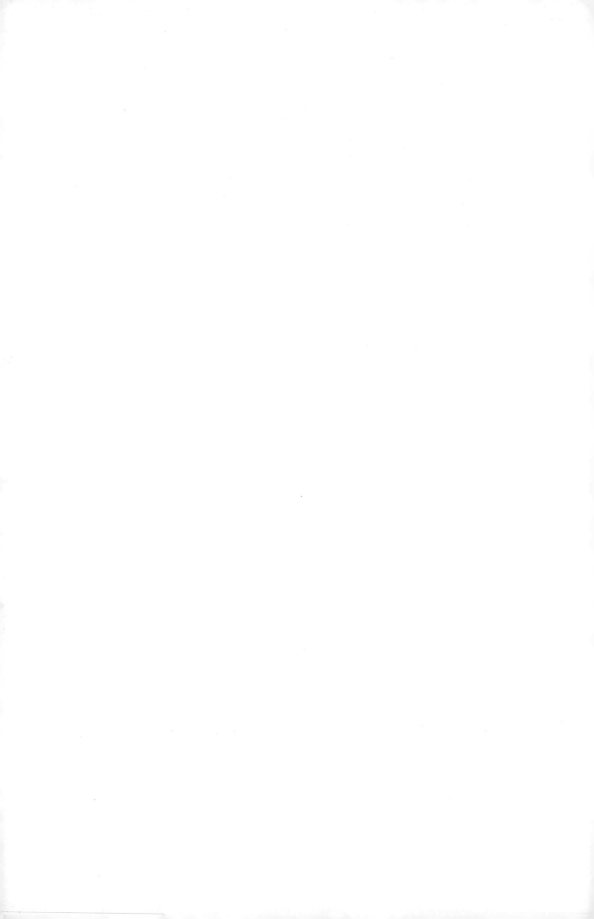

TREATMENT OPTIONS IN UROLOGICAL CANCER

EDITED BY

Jonathan Waxman BSc, MD, MBBS, FRCP
Department of Cancer Medicine, Imperial College of Science,
Technology and Medicine, London

Blackwell
Science

© 2002 by Blackwell Science Ltd
a Blackwell Publishing company
Editorial Offices:
Osney Mead, Oxford OX2 0EL, UK
   Tel: +44(0)1865 206206
108 Cowley Road, Oxford OX4 1JF, UK
   Tel: +44(0)1865 791100
Blackwell Publishing USA, 350 Main Street, Malden, MA 02148-5018, USA
   Tel: +1 781 388 8250
Iowa State Press, a Blackwell Publishing Company, 2121 State Avenue, Ames, Iowa 50014-
   8300, USA
   Tel: +1 515 292 0140
Blackwell Munksgaard, Nørre Søgade 35, PO Box 2148, Copenhagen, DK-1016, Denmark
   Tel: +45 77 33 33 33
Blackwell Publishing Asia, 54 University Street, Carlton, Victoria 3053, Australia
   Tel: +61 (0)3 9347 0300
Blackwell Verlag, Kurfürstendamm 57, 10707 Berlin, Germany
   Tel: +49 (0)30 32 79 060
Blackwell Publishing, 10 rue Casimir Delavigne, 75006 Paris, France
   Tel: +33 1 53 10 33 10

Contents

Contributors, ix

Preface, xiii

Part 1 Kidney Cancer

1   The Molecular Biology of Kidney Cancer, 3
    E. P. Castle, G. S. Hallman & J. B. Thrasher

2   Cytokines and Angiogenesis Inhibitor Treatments, 31
    S. Chowdhury & M. Gore

3   Surgical Management of Metastatic Renal Cancer, 49
    D. F. Badenoch

    Kidney Cancer: Commentary, 55
    J. Waxman

Part 2 Bladder Cancer

4   The Molecular Biology of Bladder Cancer, 59
    P. E. Keegan, D. E. Neal & J. Lunec

5   Surgery for Advanced Bladder Cancer, 84
    D. W. W. Newling

6   Chemotherapy and Bladder Cancer, 98
    F. Calabrò & C. N. Sternberg

7   Treatment Options in Superficial (pTa/pT1/CIS) Bladder Cancer, 118
    J. L. Ockrim & P. D. Abel

    Bladder Cancer: Commentary, 137
    J. Waxman

Part 3 Prostate Cancer

8   The Molecular Biology of Prostate Cancer, 141
    J. Wang & J. Waxman

9   Surgical Pathology of Prostate Cancer, 160
     C. S. Foster

10   Prostate Radiotherapy, 189
     C. R. Lewanski & S. Stewart

11   Prostate Cancer: Immediate vs. Deferred Treatment, 206
     D. Kirk

12   Hormone Therapy of Prostate Cancer, 220
     R. Agarwal & J. Waxman

13   Chemotherapy in Hormone Refractory Prostate Cancer, 237
     J. J. Knox & M. J. Moore

14   Radical Prostatectomy, 253
     T. J. Christmas & A. P. Doherty

15   The Case against Radical Surgery for Early Prostate Cancer, 264
     Leslie E. F. Moffat

     Prostate Cancer: Commentary, 275
     J. Waxman

Part 4 Testicular Cancer

16   Genetics of Adult Male Germ Cell Tumours, 279
     J. Houldsworth, G. J. Bosl & R. S. K. Chaganti

17   Surveillance, Chemotherapy, and Radiotherapy for Stage 1 Testicular
     Germ Cell Tumours, 293
     D. H. Palmer & M. H. Cullen

18   Chemotherapy of Testicular Cancer, 305
     I. A. Burney & G. M. Mead

19   Salvage Chemotherapy Regimens for Relapsing Germ Cell Cancer, 317
     M. L. Harvey & G. M. Mead

20   Surgery for Testicular Cancer, 328
     W. F. Hendry

     Testicular Cancer: Commentary, 350
     J. Waxman

Part 5 Penile Cancer

21   Viral Agents in the Development of Penile Cancer, 353
     P. H. Rajjayabun, T. R. L. Griffiths & J. K. Mellon

22   Current Concepts in the Management of Penile Cancer, 366
     R. Sarin & H. B. Tongaonkar

     Penile Cancer: Commentary, 382
     J. Waxman

Index, 383

Colour plates fall between pp. 178 and 179

Contributors

Mr Paul D. Abel
Department of Surgical Oncology
    and Technology
Faculty of Medicine
Imperial College of Science,
    Technology and Medicine
Hammersmith Campus
Du Cane Road
London W12 0NN
UK

Dr Roshan Agarwal
Department of Medical Oncology
Chelsea and Westminster Hospital
Fulham Road
London
UK

Mr David F. Badenoch
123 Harley Street
London W1G 6AY

Dr George J. Bosl
Department of Medicine
The Patrick M Byrne Chair in
    Clinical Oncology
Memorial Sloan-Kettering Cancer
    Center
1275 York Avenue
New York, New York 10021
U.S.A.

Dr Ikram A. Burney
Department of Medicine
The Aga Khan University
Stadium Road
Karachi 74800
Pakistan

Dr Fabio Calabro
Department of Medical Oncology
Vincenzo Pansadoro Foundation
Clinic Pio XI
Via Aurelia 559
Rome
Italy 00165

Dr Erik P. Castle
Section of Urology
University of Kansas Medical
    Center
3901 Rainbow Boulevard
Kansas City
KS 66160-7390
USA

Dr R. S. K. Chaganti
Department of Medicine
Memorial Sloan-Kettering Cancer
    Center
1275 York Avenue
New York
New York 10021
USA

Dr Simon Chowdhury
Department of Medicine
Royal Marsden Hospital
Fulham Road
London SW3 6JJ
UK

Mr Timothy J. Christmas
Department of Urology
Imperial College School of Medicine
Charing Cross Hospital
Fulham Palace Road
London W6 8RF
UK

Dr Michael H. Cullen
Cancer Centre at the Queen
    Elizabeth Hospital
University Hospital Birmingham
    NHS Trust
Birmingham B15 2TH
UK

Mr A. P. Doherty
Consultant Urologist
Queen Elizabeth Hospital
Edgbaston
Birmingham B15 2TH
UK

Professor Christopher S. Foster
Department of Cellular and
    Molecular Pathology
University of Liverpool
Daulby Street
Liverpool L69 3GA
UK

Dr Martin Gore
Department of Medicine
Royal Marsden Hospital
Fulham Road
London SW3 6JJ
UK

Mr T. R. L. Griffiths
University Department of Urology
Freeman Hospital
Newcastle-upon-Tyne NE7 7DN
UK

Dr Gregg S. Hallman
Cape Girardeau Urology Associates
3 Doctors Park
Cape Girardeau
MO 63701
USA

Dr M. L. Harvey
The Wessex Medical Oncology Unit
Royal South Hants Hospital
Southampton SO14 0YG
UK

Mr William F. Hendry (retired)
Department of Urology
St Bartholomew's Hospital
West Smithfield
London EC1A 7BE
UK

Dr Jane Houldsworth
Department of Medicine
Memorial Sloan-Kettering Cancer
    Center
1275 York Avenue
New York
New York 10021
USA

Mr Phil E. Keegan
Department of Surgery and the
    Cancer Research Unit
The Medical School
University of Newcastle
Newcastle upon Tyne
NE2 4HH
UK

Professor David Kirk
Department of Urology
Gartnavel General Hospital
1053 Great Western Road
Glasgow G12 0YN
UK

Dr Jennifer J. Knox
Department of Medical Oncology
Princess Margaret Hospital
University Health Network
610 University Avenue
Toronto, Ontario
Canada M5G 2M9

Dr Conrad R. Lewanski
Department of Radiotherapy
Charing Cross Hospital
Fulham Palace Road
London W6 8RF
UK

Dr J. Lunec
Cancer Research Unit
The Medical School
University of Newcastle
Newcastle upon Tyne NE2 4HH
UK

Dr G. M. Mead
The Wessex Medical Oncology Unit
Royal South Hants Hospital
Southampton SO14 0YG
UK

Professor Kilian Mellon
University of Leicester
Leicester
UK

Mr Leslie E. F. Moffat
Department of Urology
Aberdeen Royal Infirmary
Aberdeen AB25 2ZN
UK

Professor Malcolm J. Moore
Department of Medicine and
    Pharmacology
Princess Margaret Hospital
University Health Network
University of Toronto
610 University Avenue
Toronto, Ontario
Canada M5G 2M9

Professor D. E. Neal
Department of Surgery
The Medical School
University of Newcastle
Newcastle upon Tyne NE2 4HH
UK

Professor Don W. W. Newling
Department of Urology
Free University Medical Centre
De Boelelaan 1117
1007 MB Amsterdam
The Netherlands

Mr Jeremy L. Ockrim
Imperial College School of Medicine
Department of Urology
Charing Cross Hospital
Fulham Palace Road
London W6 8RF
UK

Dr Daniel H. Palmer
CRC Institute for Cancer Studies
The Medical School
University of Birmingham
Birmingham B15 2TA
UK

Mr Paul H. Rajjayabun
Department of Surgery
The Medical School
University of Newcastle
Newcastle upon Tyne NE2 4HH
UK

Dr Rajiv Sarin
Tata Memorial hospital
Parel
Mumbai
400 012
India

Dr Cora N. Sternberg
Department of Medical Oncology
Vincenzo Pansadoro Foundation
Clinic Pio XI
Via Aurelia 559
Rome
Italy 00165

Dr Simon Stewart
Department of Radiotherapy
Charing Cross Hospital
Fulham Palace Road
London W6 8RF
UK

Professor J. Brantley Thrasher
Section of Urology
University of Kansas Medical Center
3901 Rainbow Boulevard
Kansas City
KS 66160-7390
USA

Professor Herman B. Tongaonkar
Professor and Surgeon
Department of Urologic Oncology
Tata Memorial Hospital
Parel
Mumbai 400 012
India

Dr Jayson Wang
Imperial Cancer Research Fund
44 Lincoln's Inn Fields
London WC2A 3PX
UK

Professor Jonathan Waxman
Department of Cancer Medicine
Faculty of Medicine
Imperial College School of Science,
    Technology and Medicine
Hammersmith Campus
Du Cane Road
London W12 0NN
UK

Preface

Urological malignancies are a significant part of both urological and oncological practice. There have been changes in the epidemiology of urological malignancy so that these diseases have become important for all of us and our government.

There have been significant changes in our understanding of the biology of this group of tumours, and these changes are very much at the forefront of molecular biology. This science has been applied to urological tumours, and we are at a point where we are close to understanding the chromosomal change in testicular and renal cancers and the causes for androgen independence in prostate cancer.

There have also been significant changes in the treatment of urological malignancies. New hormonal therapies have become available for prostate cancer, cytokines have been developed for the treatment of renal tumours and new chemotherapy programmes have become available for testicular and bladder cancer.

A combined approach to the management of malignancy is never more important than in urological oncology, where oncologists, radiotherapists and surgeons together have brought forward practice and improved upon survival. But this is an area where we need to do better—an area where the multidisciplinary approach really does have to kick in in order to facilitate advances in research and survival. This ambition is, I hope, signposted in this book, which brings together the science and treatment of urological cancer.

Part 1
Kidney Cancer

1: The Molecular Biology of Kidney Cancer

E. P. Castle, G. S. Hallman & J. B. Thrasher

Introduction

Renal cell carcinoma (RCC) accounts for approximately 3% of adult malignancies [1]. It is the most common primary renal malignancy, accounting for 30 000 cases annually in the United States [2,3]. RCC affects males twice as frequently as females, is more common in those from urban settings and most commonly affects individuals between the ages of 50 and 70. The aetiology of this disease has been studied extensively, and the strongest candidate that has been identified is cigarette smoking [2,4–6]. In addition, obesity, prescription diuretic use and occupational exposures such as leather finishing products and asbestos may lead to RCC [2,4,5,7–10]. An increased incidence is found in patients with end-stage renal disease, especially in those with acquired renal cystic disease, and in individuals with congenital disorders such as von Hippel–Lindau disease, tuberous sclerosis or autosomal dominant polycystic kidney disease [2,4,11–15]. The clear cell histopathological type (Fig. 1.1) is the most common, accounting for 80–85% of RCC, while papillary histopathology is seen in 5–10% of tumours [4,16].

RCC occurs in sporadic and familial forms. The familial forms of disease are typified by the tendency for development of multifocal and bilateral tumours and earlier age of onset [4,17]. Four different types of familial RCC have been identified: RCC in von Hippel–Lindau disease, hereditary clear cell renal carcinoma, hereditary papillary renal carcinoma and hereditary renal oncocytoma [4]. With the identification of the familial nature of some renal carcinomas, intense investigation into the genetic alterations leading to tumour formation has ensued. Promising genetic loci have been identified and characterized in each of the familial forms of RCC, and investigation continues in order to further delineate the specific functions of these genes. Herein, we will discuss in detail the molecular genetics of renal carcinomas as well as molecular markers that may play an important role in the future with respect to the diagnosis and management of these tumours.

Von Hippel–Lindau disease

Von Hippel–Lindau (VHL) disease is a hereditary cancer syndrome character-

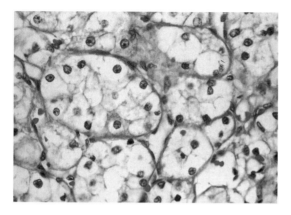

Figure 1.1 Renal cell
carcinoma—clear cell variant.

ized by the presence of benign and malignant tumour development in multiple
organ systems, including the eyes, cerebellum, spine, inner ear, pancreas,
adrenal gland and kidneys [4]. Retinal angiomas, cerebellar and spinal haem-
angioblastomas and renal cell carcinomas are the hallmark lesions of this
disease. Renal cysts, pancreatic cysts and carcinomas, phaeochromocytomas,
epididymal and broad ligament cystadenomas and endolymphatic sac
tumours may also manifest in affected individuals. The incidence of VHL is
estimated to be 1/36 000 live births [18,19]. It is inherited in an autosomal
dominant fashion and has an estimated penetrance of 80–90% by the age of
65 [18,19]. RCC eventually develops in 28–45% of those affected with VHL
[4]. These tumours are frequently multicentric and bilateral and are predominantly of the clear cell variety [4,20–24] (Fig. 1.2). The management of RCC
in these patients involves nephron-sparing surgery to help maintain renal
function as long as possible and to reduce the risk of metastatic disease
[4,20,25–29].

Epidemiological data suggest that tumour-suppressor gene inactivation is
responsible for the development of VHL [18,30]. According to Knudson's
'two-hit' hypothesis, the carriers of mutations in a tumour-suppressor gene
have a germline mutation in one allele of the gene, and a somatic mutation
occurs in the homologous normal allele, which leads to tumour formation
[18,31]. The germline mutation is transmitted in an autosomal dominant
fashion with each offspring having a 50% risk of inheriting the mutated allele.
These genes normally inhibit tumour development through regulation of
cell proliferation and differentiation, and their inactivation predisposes an
individual to cancer through loss of these regulatory processes.

Researchers sought to confirm that the VHL gene was indeed a tumour-
suppressor gene. Tory *et al.* [32] used restriction fragment length polymorphism (RFLP) analysis to evaluate RCC from VHL patients and showed that
the wild-type chromosome 3p allele, which was inherited from the unaffected

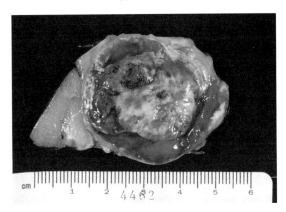

Figure 1.2 VHL tumour —
gross specimen.

parent, was lost. Thus, these patients retained only the abnormal germline copy of the gene inherited from the affected parent. Lubensky *et al.* [33] subsequently demonstrated loss of the wild-type 3p allele with maintenance of the inherited, mutated allele in 25 of 26 renal lesions from individuals with VHL. This loss of heterozygosity (LOH) was detectable in atypical renal cysts and cysts with RCC *in situ*. Therefore, the VHL gene was indeed believed to be a tumour-suppressor gene, and loss of function of both gene copies appeared to be an important early step towards tumour formation.

The VHL gene was mapped to the short arm of chromosome 3, sub-band 25 (3p25) [20,34,35]. Seizinger *et al.* [34] used genetic linkage analysis to study nine families with VHL disease, which included 71 affected individuals, and found that the VHL gene linked to the RAF1 oncogene at 3p25. The linkage to RAF1 was confirmed by Hosoe *et al.* [36], who also reported linkage of the VHL gene to D3S18, a polymorphic DNA marker located at 3p26. Richards *et al.* [37] then demonstrated tight linkage of the VHL gene to the DNA probe D3S601, which was located in the region between RAF1 and D3S18. The VHL gene was subsequently identified by Latif *et al.* in 1993 through the use of yeast artificial chromosomes and cosmid-phage contigs [35]. It was found to be a single-copy gene with evolutionary conservation across several species, thus pointing to a role in essential cellular processes [2].

The VHL gene contains three exons with an open reading frame of 852 nucleotides that encode a protein of 213 amino acids [2,4]. Several hundred germline mutations have been recognized in VHL kindreds. These include microdeletions/insertions, large deletions and mis-sense and nonsense mutations. Chen *et al.* [38] studied 114 VHL families and identified mutations throughout the coding region, but clustering occurred at the 3′ end of exon 1 and the 5′ end of exon 3 with a paucity of mutations in exon 2. Specific mutations have since been correlated with certain phenotypic characteristics in

VHL patients. VHL type I families (without phaeochromocytoma) most frequently have large deletions, microdeletions/insertions or nonsense mutations, whereas in VHL type II families (with phaeochromocytoma) 96% of the
mutations are mis-sense [18,38,39]. Gnarra *et al.* [40] evaluated sporadic
clear cell renal carcinoma and found VHL gene mutations in 57% of the cancers with LOH of the gene in 98%. The mutations clustered at the 3′ end of
exon 1 and at the 5′ end of exon 3; however, exon 2 also had a high frequency
of mutations (45%). The high number of mutations as well as splice site mutations that would eliminate its translation suggested that exon 2 may have a
role in the function of the protein product.

The functions of the VHL gene protein product have been difficult to predict as there is no important homology to other proteins [18,35]. Further
characterization has been performed through cellular localization studies.
Immunofluorescence microscopy demonstrated that the protein product is
located primarily in the cytoplasm but can also be found in the nucleus
[4,18,20,41–44]. Co-immunoprecipitation of the VHL protein with two proteins of 9 and 16 kDa was also identified. These two proteins were subsequently identified as Elongin C and Elongin B, respectively [4,45–47]. This
protein interaction was very weak or nonexistent when certain mis-sense
mutations of the VHL gene occurred [4,44]. This relationship of the normal
VHL protein and loss of this association with certain mutations has led
several investigators to study protein–protein interactions. Many important
interactions have subsequently been identified.

The VHL protein product normally binds tightly to elongin B and C, which
are regulatory subunits of elongin (SIII), while it does not bind to elongin A
[4,45,48–50]. Elongin (SIII) is known to hasten DNA transcriptional elongation by RNA polymerase II by inhibiting temporary pausing of polymerase at
certain DNA sites and by controlling its release from DNA [4,18,51,52]. With
binding of elongin B and C, the VHL protein is able to abort the formation
of the active heterotrimeric protein elongin (SIII) [4,45]. The transcription of
certain genes may be downregulated as a result of these binding sequences
[18,49]. As mentioned previously, a number of VHL proteins with mis-sense
gene mutations have been found to complex minimally or not at all with the
Elongin regulatory subunits [4,44]. This inability to inhibit the formation of
elongin may lead to the loss of regulation of transcription rates of genes important in tumour suppression [18,44,50].

The association of VHL with elongin B and C may function to promote
tumour suppression in ways other than by influencing transcription rates by
RNA polymerase. Cullin-2 (Cul-2), a member of the Cdc53 family of proteins,
has been found to bind to VHL–elongin B/C, forming a stable tetrameric complex [4,53]. Cul-2 is involved in targeting specific proteins for ubiquitination
and proteasome degradation. After being tagged with ubiquitin, proteins are

destroyed by a proteasome [42,48]. VHL may therefore play a crucial role in this process by helping direct specific cellular proteins to proteasomes for degradation [48,54]. For example, HIF1-alpha, a transcription factor which enhances the transcription of hypoxia-inducible genes, undergoes ubiquitination and degradation under normoxic conditions [20,55,56]. Wild-type VHL appears to be critical for the series of steps leading to HIF1-alpha destruction [20,55]. Mutant forms of VHL theoretically could alter this relationship and cause enhanced hypoxia-inducible gene expression in normoxic conditions with neovascularization and resultant malignant growth.

Renal cancers associated with VHL are typically hypervascular. Several stimuli are believed to induce neoangiogenesis in tumours, including hypoxia and polypeptide growth factors [18,57]. Vascular endothelial growth factor (VEGF) is a polypeptide growth factor that assists in the migration, proliferation and differentiation of vascular endothelial cells [2]. This protein is normally expressed in the brain and kidney as well as other tissues, and it is markedly overexpressed in sporadic and VHL-associated RCC [2,58–61]. The VHL gene is believed to regulate VEGF [2,58,62–65]. Cell lines that lack wild-type VHL produce increased levels of hypoxia-inducible messenger RNAs such as VEGF mRNA under both hypoxic and normoxic conditions [18,58,62,63]. The restoration of the hypoxia-inducible profile of these mRNAs is possible with the reintroduction of the wild-type VHL protein into these VHL (–/–) cells, and VEGF production under normoxic conditions is prevented [2,58,62,63]. Evidence suggests that the VHL protein may regulate stabilization of these hypoxia-inducible mRNAs: VEGF mRNA stability is prolonged four times in cells without wild-type VHL compared with those in which wild-type VHL is reintroduced [2,66]. Therefore, it seems that regulation of VEGF mRNA stabilization is another important function of the VHL protein product.

Mukhopadhyay *et al.* [67] have shown that a direct interaction between the VHL gene product and the ubiquitous transcriptional activator Sp1 leads to transcriptional repression of the VEGF promoter. They found that Sp1 interacts with a specific isoform of protein kinase C in RCC causing transcriptional promotion of VEGF [64]. In the presence of the wild-type VHL protein product, Sp1 and protein kinase C interaction is inhibited, resulting in lower levels of VEGF. There may also be direct complexation of protein kinase C by the wild-type VHL protein leading to inhibited VEGF expression. Also, the VEGF receptors KDR and Flt-1 are overexpressed in sporadic and VHL-associated RCC [2,68]. The VHL protein may therefore have an important role in the control of these proteins' genes.

Another polypeptide growth factor, transforming growth factor β1 (TGF-β1), appears to be regulated by the VHL protein. This factor seems to function in a proliferative fashion through a paracrine mechanism to promote RCC formation [2,20,69,70]. Tumour development is suppressed with reintroduction of the wild-type VHL protein product which inhibits TGF-β1 production or through administration of anti-TGF-β1 antibodies [20,69].

In recent investigations, Ivanov and colleagues [4,71] have shown that the VHL gene downregulates the cell membrane spanning proteins carbonic anhydrases 9 and 12. They identified increased expression of these two proteins in two RCC cell lines which were without the wild-type VHL gene. These enzymes regulate extracellular pH and cell membrane ion channels, and evidence suggests that extracellular pH may affect invasiveness of cancer cells [20].

The VHL protein product has also been found to bind to fibronectin, an extracellular glycoprotein involved in extracellular matrix cell signalling through integrins [48,72–74]. Extracellular fibronectin matrix assembly is altered in VHL (–/–) cells, and this alteration is corrected with the reintroduction of the wild-type VHL protein [20,72]. In mutated cells, neovascularity parallels the changes in the extracellular matrix [20,75]. Tumour suppression may therefore be a result of appropriate fibronectin matrix assembly with regulation of neoangiogenesis.

VHL disease has provided investigators with a large framework to expand our knowledge of the basic molecular abnormalities leading to the development of RCC. The VHL gene and its general function as a tumour-suppressor gene have been identified, and several functions of the VHL protein product have been delineated. Mutations of the gene leading to inactivation have also been characterized and associated with specific clinical phenotypic results. Intense research continues in this disease to further understand the gene's multiple functions so that therapeutic targets might be established.

Sporadic clear cell renal carcinoma

Researchers have extensively evaluated chromosome 3 in sporadic RCC. Cytogenetic evaluation identified abnormalities of 3p in as many as 95% of renal tumours [2,76–80]. RFLP analysis for loss of heterozygosity showed consistent segmental loss on the short arm of chromosome 3 [4]. Subsequently, an area of deletion in the 3p21–26 region in clear cell renal carcinomas was described by Anglard *et al.* [81]. As this genetic locus for RCC was being further investigated and defined, Seizinger *et al.* mapped VHL disease to the short arm of chromosome 3 in the same genetic region [34]. With the identification of the VHL gene in 1993 by Latif *et al.* [35] its role in sporadic RCC formation was questioned.

Strong evidence accumulated suggesting that a single tumour-suppressor gene, the VHL gene, was responsible for both VHL-associated and sporadic clear cell RCC. Latif *et al.* showed VHL gene mutations in five sporadic RCC cell lines [35]. Gnarra *et al.* [40], through tumour evaluation from 108 patients, detected LOH at the VHL gene locus in 98% of clear cell RCC and found mutations of the remaining copy of the VHL gene in 57%. As was discussed earlier, mutations were identified in all three exons, but the majority involved exon 2 (45%), indicating that this coding region may impart an important function to the protein. No VHL gene mutations were found in 12 papillary renal carcinomas. Furthermore, Shuin *et al.* [2,82] analysed 47 sporadic RCCs and identified VHL mutations in 56% and LOH at the VHL locus in 84% of clear cell carcinomas. The same team also found no VHL gene mutations in eight non-clear cell carcinomas.

The finding that VHL gene mutation is associated with sporadic clear cell renal carcinoma provided further evidence that this gene plays a critical role in the development of clear cell renal carcinoma in general. Other genetic loci such as 3p13–14, 17p, and the p53 tumour-suppressor gene may be involved in the pathogenesis of sporadic clear cell renal carcinoma, but the data are much more convincing for the VHL gene in the development of this disease [2,83–85].

Hereditary clear cell renal carcinoma

Early studies attempting to identify the location of a gene responsible for renal carcinoma involved the analysis of families with multiple affected members. In 1979, Cohen *et al.* [86] published data on 10 family members with clear cell renal carcinoma from three generations. There was an autosomal dominant inheritance pattern present, and 8 of the 10 individuals had a balanced constitutional translocation of 3p to 8q. None of the family members with a normal karyotype developed RCC. Other investigators subsequently reported familial clear cell RCC with the development of early onset, multiple, bilateral tumours. Karyotypic analyses in these families consistently revealed translocations involving chromosome 3p and either chromosomes 2 or 6 [4,87,88].

Studies of these familial tumours has provided further evidence of the importance of VHL gene mutations in clear cell tumours. The tumours from family members with the balanced translocations t(3;8) and t(3;2) revealed deletion of one VHL allele in the chromosomal product [4,88,89]. Somatic mutations of the remaining VHL gene were identified in the majority of tumours (6/9) from these families [88,90]. Thus, the inactivation of both VHL alleles occurred leading to the development of RCC. Hereditary clear cell renal carcinomas appear to form as a result of a variation of the events leading to sporadic clear cell RCC [4,91].

Tuberous sclerosis

Tuberous sclerosis (TS) is an autosomal dominant inherited disease in 15–25% of cases, while 60–70% of cases result from *de novo* germline mutations [92,93]. The disease has been classically described as a triad of epilepsy, mental retardation and adenoma sebaceum. The birth incidence varies between 1 in 9000 and 1 in 170 000 [92,94]. Multiple hamartomas typically form in patients, including facial angiofibromas, periungual fibromas, calcified retinal hamartomas, multiple cortical tubers and renal angiomyolipomas [20]. RCC may also form in TS and can be found in approximately 2% of afflicted individuals [92]. TS-associated RCC may be single or multiple and unilateral or bilateral, and clear cell histology is the predominant type [95,96]. Two genes, tuberous sclerosis complex 1 (TSC1) on chromosome 9 and tuberous sclerosis complex 2 (TSC2) on chromosome 16, have been identified as being responsible for TS development [97].

TSC1 maps to 9q34 and contains 23 exons, and TSC2 maps to 16p13 and has 42 exons [20,98,99]. Mutations that have been reported to date in TSC1 are predicted to lead to a truncated protein product and are found mostly in familial forms of the disease [100]. Germline mutations of TSC2 include deletions, nonsense mutations and mis-sense mutations [101]. Tumours associated with TS have LOH at the TSC1 or TSC2 genetic locus as a result of inactivation of the wild-type allele [20,102,103]. This suggests that these genes are tumour-suppressor genes.

The TSC2 gene encodes a protein of 1807 amino acids [98]. With loss of the wild-type TSC2 allele, the functional protein (tuberin) is lost and tumour formation occurs. Tumour growth is suppressed *in vitro* through the introduction of wild-type TSC2 protein in TSC2 –/– RCC [20,104]. The TSC2 protein has significant homology to the catalytic domain of human guanosine triphosphatase (GTPase) activating protein 3 (GAP3) [98]. GAP proteins stimulate GTPases, and this interaction has negative regulatory effects on Ras/Ras-like protein GTP complexes [105]. Loss of function of tuberin may lead to activation of Rap1a and Rab5, which are Ras-like proteins involved in cellular signalling via growth factor receptors [20]. Hamartin is the 1164 amino acid protein product of the TSC1 gene, and it interacts with tuberin *in vivo* [106]. It may function by helping to control the same pathway as tuberin.

Papillary renal carcinoma

Papillary carcinoma is the second most common malignant tumour of the kidney. It is responsible for 10–15% of renal carcinomas [107,108]. It has a male predominance of 5–8:1. It has a better prognosis associated with it than clear cell carcinoma as the 5-year survival rate may be as high as 87–100% for stage I disease [109]. It also appears to be more common in patients on chronic dialysis for end-stage renal disease. The tumours tend to be multifocal and arise independently of one another [4,20,110] (Fig. 1.3). There are two broad classifications of this tumour: sporadic and hereditary. Papillary carcinoma is not associated with 3p mutations as found in clear cell carcinomas. Instead it is associated with a proto-oncogene, MET, found on chromosome 7. Studies have shown that the MET allele and the c-MET receptor have tumorigenic properties consisting of increased proliferation, motility, extracellular invasion and tubule formation [20,111]. Selective studies that have provided insight into the cytogenetic function of this tumour and its associated oncogene are discussed below.

Sporadic papillary carcinoma of the kidney is associated with more than one chromosomal abnormality. Roughly 80% of sporadic papillary tumours possess polysomies [110]. Tumour tissue from patients with this tumour has revealed trisomies of chromosomes 7, 16 and 17 [4,20,110,112]. Kovacs *et al.* [113] proposed that papillary carcinomas arise from papillary adenomas. Papillary adenomas are characterized by polysomies of chromosomes 7 and 17. They reported trisomy 17 in all adenomas and 80% in grade I, 50% in grade II and none in grade III carcinomas. Other chromosomal abnormalities reported include LOH and somatic translocation. Thrash-Bingham *et al.* [114] detected LOH on chromosomes 9q, 11q, 14q, 21q and 6p. Somatic translocation of chromosomes 1 and X [t(X;1)(p11;q21)] has been reported [115–117]. The transcription factor TEF3 at the breakpoint Xp11.2 has been considered to play a role in the development of this subgroup of papillary neoplasms. Fusion of the gene at 1q21.2 with the TEF3 gene seems to result in loss of transcriptional control in these tumours [117,118]. Loss of the Y chromosome in 80–90% of males with papillary renal carcinoma has also been found [113,119–121].

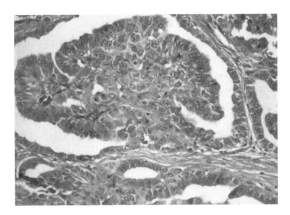

Figure 1.3 Renal cell carcinoma—papillary variant.

The high association of sporadic papillary renal carcinomas with abnormalities of chromosome 7 has led to the finding of the MET proto-oncogene, which is strongly associated with the hereditary form of this neoplasm. The gene was localized to 7q31.1–34 and is in the same supergene family (receptor tyrosine kinase) as RET, a proto-oncogene found in MEN II [4]. The MET gene is found in a high percentage of hereditary papillary renal carcinoma family members and in a subset of sporadic papillary renal carcinomas. The gene contains 21 exons spanning a 100-kb genomic region [20,122]. The gene is found in several different tissues, including neuronal tissue, endothelial cells, haematopoietic precursors, adult epithelial cells and the kidney [20,111]. Hereditary papillary renal cell carcinoma (HPRCC) is characterized by an autosomal dominant inheritance pattern and is associated with bilateral and multifocal renal tumours [4,122]. Zbar *et al.* [123–125] performed multigenerational studies of HPRCC. HPRCC family members were found to have germline mis-sense mutations of the tyrosine kinase portion of the MET gene. Another study by Schmidt *et al.* [126,127] evaluated two North American families with HPRCC. Both families possessed identical mutations in the MET region which were reportedly associated with a low penetrance: 19% at 40 years. HPRCC is clearly linked to genotypic mutations of the MET gene on chromosome 7.

Additional studies of the MET gene and c-MET receptor support its role as a proto-oncogene and not as a tumour suppressor. MET mutations studied by fluorescence *in situ* hybridization (FISH) reveal a non-random duplication of chromosome 7 [128,129]. Oncogenic properties of this gene come from studies of its amplification and mutations that result in the activation of its encoded protein. Function of the c-MET receptor is of special interest. It is a tyrosine kinase receptor involved in motility, proliferation and morphogenic signals [20]. Hepatocyte growth factor/scatter factor (HGF/SF) is its ligand [130]. Normal organogenesis is dependent on the MET receptor–HGF/SF pathway. Activation of cells possessing HGF/SF causes increased proliferation, increased motility, extracellular invasion and polarization and tubule formation [111]. Studies performed on mice with increased levels of tyrosine phosphorylation and enhanced kinase activity revealed a correlation between tumorigenesis and biological activity of this pathway [131]. Furthermore, 'knock-out' mice lacking HGF/SF die *in utero* associated with faulty organogenesis [20]. The C-terminal is the docking site of this receptor. Once activated by ligand binding, the receptor is upregulated by autocatalytic pathways ultimately increasing enzymatic and biological activity of the receptor [132,133]. It is this upregulation of the c-MET receptor that is suspected to result in the development of papillary renal cell carcinoma of patients with both the sporadic and the hereditary forms of this neoplasm.

The identification of the MET proto-oncogene and the receptor it encodes, c-MET, has given researchers some understanding of the formation of papillary renal carcinoma. These tumours can be either sporadic or familial. Although the exact function of the c-MET receptor has not been delineated, it clearly is important in normal organogenesis and possesses tumorigenic properties if amplified. In addition to the MET gene, other chromosomal abnormalities have been reported. Consequently, additional studies need to be performed in order to obtain a genuine understanding of the development of papillary renal carcinoma.

Wilms' tumour

Wilms' tumour is the most common malignant neoplasm of the urinary tract in children and one of the most common solid tumours of children. First described in 1814 by Rance and subsequently characterized by Max Wilms in 1899, Wilms' tumour has become an excellent model for the link between cancer and development [1]. The tumour occurs with a frequency of about 1 in 10 000 live births and approximately 350 new cases occur per year in the United States [1,134]. The peak incidence is between the third and fourth years of life, with 90% of patients presenting before the age of seven. There does not appear to be a sex predominance. Several other congenital abnormalities have been found in patients with Wilms' tumour, including aniridia, hemihypertrophy, musculoskeletal abnormalities, neurofibromatosis and second malignant neoplasms (sarcomas, adenocarcinomas and leukaemias). Wilms' tumour has also been associated with other congenital syndromes including Beckwith–Wiedemann, Denys–Drash, WAGR, Perlman and Bloom syndrome [1,135].

The biology of this tumour has been studied extensively and it is thought that its formation is due to aberrant expression of the normal developmental programme. Abnormal proliferation of metanephric blastemal tissue that lacks maturation and normal differentiation is felt to be the source of this tumour. Normal nephrogenesis is the product of controlled proliferation, differentiation and apoptosis. Wilms' tumour is likely to be due to the interruption of normal signalling, proliferation and controlled apoptosis during development [135]. Multiple chromosomal regions have been identified as playing a role in the development of Wilms' tumours; however, only the Wilms' tumour gene, WT1, has been clearly proven to play a significant role. Studies of normal gene function of WT1 suggest that its roles as a tumour suppressor and developmental regulator are crucial to normal nephrogenic development [134]. Furthermore, the presence of nephrogenic rests in Wilms' tumours supports the association of this tumour with immature blastemal tissue [135].

The WT1 gene maps to 11p13 and is expressed in normal developing nephrogenic tissue. Point mutations and LOH for alleles on 11p have been found in Wilms' tumours. Approximately 40% of cases of Wilms' tumour have been found to have LOH at the 11p alleles. The two-hit model by Knudson and Strong was based on studies of Wilms' tumour [136,137]. This model was also applied to retinoblastoma. Although the clinical observations associated with retinoblastoma fit the two-hit model appropriately, the development of Wilms' tumour appears to be more complex. The rarity of familial Wilms' tumour suggests that multiple gene abnormalities are involved [135].

The WT1 locus encodes four different proteins. It contains 10 exons and spans nearly 50 kb [134,138–141]. The gene has a zinc finger in which mutations are found. Alternative RNA splicing results in inclusion or exclusion of different exons resulting in as many as 16 WT1 isoforms [134]. It is the complex functions of these multiple splice variants that are involved in cellular development. Expression of the WT1 gene and function of its encoded proteins have been studied in the attempt to determine how WT1 regulates cellular maturation.

The exact function of WT1 is unknown but it is felt that its expression results in coordinated apoptosis, differentiation and proliferation. Haber *et al.* [142] have shown that wild-type WT1 can induce apoptosis in embryonal tumour cell lines. Englert *et al.* [143] created cell lines with WT1 expression which resulted in EGF-receptor downregulation and cell apoptosis. Studies such as these support the role of WT1 as a tumour suppressor. In addition, the development by Kreidberg *et al.* [144] of knock-out mice with a WT1 null mutation resulted in the failure of normal kidney development, suggesting WT1's role as a regulator of cell proliferation and differentiation. *In vitro* studies by Menke *et al.* [134] looked at the function of WT1 splice variants. They found that multiple WT1 isoforms may act as post-transcriptional regulators, with each having different functions and likely to be cell dependent. The specific role of WT1 as a transcriptional regulator is not clear as the physiologic ratio of splice variants and necessary cellular environment are all unknown. In all, one can conclude that the WT1 locus encodes data required by nephrogenic tissue to achieve normal developmental maturation.

Nephrogenic rests in kidneys removed for Wilms' tumour have been found to have mutations at WT1. Nephrogenic rests are microscopic residues of renal blastemal tissue, found in about 1 in 200–300 infant autopsies [135]. This immature blastemal tissue is rarely found after infancy except in kidneys removed for Wilms' tumour. It is felt that these rests are precursors for Wilms' tumour. Nephrogenic rests also occur in other syndromes associated with an increased incidence of Wilms' tumour. There are two broad classifications of rests: perilobar and intralobar. Both may be multi-focal and occasionally diffuse within the renal cortex. Grundy *et al.* [145] studied the association of LOH at WT1 and nephrogenic rests. In the 286 Wilms' tumours analysed, 40% of the nephrogenic rests had LOH for the alleles at 11p. Intralobar rests were found to have LOH at both 11p13 and 11p15. By contrast, perilobar rests had LOH only at 11p13. The alleles at 11p15 have been implicated in other types of childhood cancers, such as Beckwith–Weidemann syndrome, and are also felt to play a pathogenic role in the development of Wilms' tumour. Consequently, this locus has been named WT2 [135]. Other genes found at this locus include insulin-like growth factor-2 (ILGF-2), which is involved in the pathogenesis of childhood cancers.

In summary, studies of Wilms' tumour have been able to provide some insight into the links between cancer and development. It is known that normal renal development is dependent on controlled proliferation, differentiation and apoptosis. Although several models have been suggested for the genetic predisposition for Wilms' tumour it is clear that it is more complex than the two-hit model that can be applied to retinoblastoma. The association with immature blastemal tissue is still being clarified. Many chromosomal abnormalities are likely involved in its formation. The WT1 locus is certainly a very important regulator of cell formation and apoptosis in nephrogenesis. Although WT1 has been shown to act as a transcriptional factor regulating kidney development, its exact role has still to be determined. The role of WT2 and proteins encoded in or near this locus has also been an area of significant interest. Mutations at WT1 and WT2 have clearly been implicated in the formation of Wilms' tumour as well as in childhood syndromes associated with this tumour.

Renal oncocytoma

Renal oncocytoma is a neoplasm that occurs in 3–5% of renal tumours [110,146]. Although in a large number of these tumours no recurrent chromosomal changes are found, three genetic subgroups of tumours can be distinguished with numerical anomalies. In one group, loss of chromosomes Y and 1 has been observed [110,147–153]; in a second group, translocations involving the breakpoint region 11q13 ([t(5;11)(q35;q13)] and [t(9;11)(p23;q13)]) [152,154–158]. The third group includes a variety of genetic anomalies ranging from several monosomies, trisomies (chromosomes 1, 7, 12 and 14) [147,152,159] and LOH of chromosomes 17p, 17q, 10q and 3p. No p53 mutations have been reported [160,161]. There have been hereditary forms of renal oncocytoma reported. These hereditary forms lack von Hippel–Lindau germline mutations.

Papillary adenoma

Papillary adenoma is a tumour that occurs in as many as 20% of patients and is one of the most common renal neoplasms [110,162,163]. Genetic associations include trisomy or tetrasomy 7, trisomy 17 and the loss of chromosome Y [164,165]. There is a significant similarity between this tumour and papillary renal cell carcinoma. It is this similarity that suggests papillary adenoma may be a precursor to its malignant counterpart [110].

Metanephric adenoma

Metanephric adenoma is thought to be a benign neoplasm [110]. It has only recently been reported that these tumours possess chromosomal abnormalities. Brown *et al.* [166] published alterations including chromosomes 47, X, Y, 7 and 17. Prior to this report, cytogenetic and FISH analyses revealed no chromosomal abnormalities [110,167–169].

A summary of kidney tumours and associated genetic mutations is given in Table 1.1.

Molecular markers

The last decade has seen an explosion of research into the use of molecular markers as potential prognosticators in various malignancies. Authors have evaluated the use of various prognostic factors in renal cell carcinoma, such as tumour size, histological pattern, nuclear morphometry and DNA content, but none of these has proved to supply information independent of stage and grade [170–173]. Therefore, several studies have focused on the evaluation of new molecular markers. The prognostic value of cell proliferation markers, p53 mutations, growth factor expression and intratumoral microvessel density have been investigated [174–178]. However, to date, none of these parameters appears to be better predictive prognostic factors than stage and grade.

One molecular marker that has recently been studied is CD44. CD44 represents a large family of adhesion molecules that differ mainly in primary structure, with a predominant or standard form (CD44S, as it is referred to below) and various isoforms resulting from alternative splicing of 10 exons (CD44v1–v10) of a single gene mapped to chromosome 11 [179]. These adhesion molecules are involved in cell–extracellular matrix interactions. CD44 recognizes and bonds hyaluronan, a widely distributed component of extracellular matrix. Initially described as a molecule involved in lymphocyte homing, it has been shown *in vitro* to be involved in tumour cell interactions with the extracellular matrix during invasion and metastases. CD44S has been

Table 1.1 Summary of kidney tumours and associated genetic mutations. For abbreviations see text

Kidney tumour	Chromosomal alterations
Clear cell carcinoma	
Von Hippel–Lindau disease	3p (3p25.5)
Sporadic clear cell RCC	3p (3p13–14 and 3p21–26)
	17p
	p53
Hereditary clear cell RCC	3p, 8q, 2, 6
Tuberous sclerosis	TSC1 (9q34)
	TSC2 (16p13)
Papillary renal cell carcinoma	
Sporadic papillary RCC	1, 6p, 7 (MET), 9q, 11q, 14q, 16, 17, 21q
	X (TEF3)
	Y
Hereditary papillary RCC	7 (7q31.1–34) (MET)
Wilms' tumour	WT1 (11p13)
	WT2 (11p15)
Benign neoplasms	
Renal oncocytoma	1, 11q13, Y
	[t(5;11)(q35;q13)] and [t(9,11)(p23;q13)]
	Monosomies 1, 7, 12, 14
	LOH 3p, 17p, 17q, 10q
Papillary adenoma	Trisomy and tetrasomy 7
	Trisomy 17
	Loss of Y
Metanephric adenoma	7, 17, X, Y, 47

shown to enhance the growth and metastatic capacities of several tumour cell lines [180], and the expression of the standard form and certain variants has been reported to correlate with tumour progression in various malignancies. Past studies reported differential expression of CD44 molecules according to the histological type of renal cell carcinoma, and recently two studies have reported the correlation of CD44 expression and tumour progression or recurrence.

One study, by Gilcrease *et al.* [181], reported that CD44S staining with one type of monoclonal antibody (Mab2137) correlated with the progression and recurrence of 5 out of 43 tumours. Correlation was not found with statistical significance in papillary carcinomas. The authors also noted that CD44 expression is probably not an independent prognosticator for clear cell carcinomas because the staining with the antibody used correlated closely with Fuhrman nuclear grade. The second study, by Paradis *et al.* [182], reported results of immunohistochemical staining for CD44 standard form in 66 cases of conventional clear cell carcinoma composed of clear cells with or without a granular component. The authors concluded that CD44H positivity correlated significantly with patient survival. Furthermore, the authors stated that multivariate analysis revealed that stage, CD44 expression and nuclear grade emerged as independent prognostic factors.

These authors conclude with a discussion of where they feel CD44 immunostaining in renal cell carcinoma may eventually be incorporated into everyday practice. They state that in the group of clear cell carcinomas of low or intermediate grade and stage, CD44 immunostaining would be useful in determining prognostic subgroups among these tumours. However, they noted that this hypothesis needed to be confirmed in a larger study.

The discrepancies between these two studies highlight several inherent problems with the use of molecular markers to evaluate renal cell carcinoma. First, the studies to date that have evaluated molecular markers have generally been small, single-institution studies. Furthermore, the vast majority of studies have failed to show that these markers offer prognostic information independent of the two well-known prognostic factors in renal cell carcinoma, stage and grade. Multi-institutional trials with large numbers will be required to validate or refute the authors' findings.

Second, different immunohistochemical staining results have been reported with different monoclonal antibodies. Gilcrease *et al.* reported very different results for two antibodies. Paradis *et al.* used a different commercially available antibody to CD44, obtained from the United Kingdom, and reported for the first time that CD44 staining offered independent prognostic information in clear cell RCC. Differences in staining techniques, monoclonal antibodies used, tissue preparation and quantification of immunohistochemical staining are confounding factors that must be standardized in larger trials to eliminate potential bias.

Finally, interobserver variability in the assessment of CD44 expression is a potential confounding factor. Immunohistochemical staining is difficult to quantify. The scales used to quantify are usually arbitrarily chosen and interobserver variability is rarely tested. Eliminating this variability in further studies will be required to standardize testing for CD44 expression.

Molecular markers will likely play an increasingly important role in diagnosing, staging and predicting recurrences and directing the treatment of patients with many different malignancies. However, until larger trials without discrepancies, confounding factors and interobserver variability are completed, the use of molecular markers such as CD44 is limited.

Clinical implications

The role of molecular genetics in the diagnosis, prevention and treatment of kidney tumours is becoming increasingly important. The ability to characterize tumours based on genetic characteristics will help guide diagnostic and treatment strategies. Clinicians must be aware of the hereditary components and obtain a detailed family history in patients with renal tumours. Early diagnosis is crucial in treating renal tumours because of the resistance to radiation therapy and standard chemotherapeutic agents. Survival of patients who present with stage IV as compared with stage I disease is significantly decreased. If one can identify an inherited disorder early in a family, morbidity and mortality may be decreased in affected members. This has been the case with VHL disease. Early diagnosis of patients with VHL-associated renal tumours has led to prompt surgical treatment, hopefully minimizing metastatic development. Early diagnosis has also made nephron-sparing surgery in these patients a treatment option, decreasing morbidity associated with this disease. In addition, morbidity due to central nervous system disorders or ophthalmological disease in VHL patients has been decreased with early diagnosis.

With growing research interests in gene therapy and immunotherapy, understanding of the genotypic and phenotypic correlations of renal tumours is crucial to the development of new treatment modalities. The utility of gene-based therapy may soon be a reality. The ability to turn off an activated oncogene such as MET in papillary tumours or to replace an inactivated tumour-suppressor gene such as VHL may result in these becoming the future treatment of choice. Clearly, understanding molecular genetics should be a part of the urologist's armamentarium in the twenty-first century.

Acknowledgements

We thank the numerous investigators whose studies have contributed to the current understanding of the molecular biology of kidney tumours. In addition, we thank Dr Ivan Damjanov and the Pathology Department at the University of Kansas Medical Center for their assistance with the photographs used in this chapter.

References

1 Belldegrun A, deKernion JB. Renal tumors. In: Walsh P, Retik AB, Vaughan ED Jr, Wein AJ, eds. *Campbell's Urology*. Philadelphia: W.B. Saunders, 1996: 2283–92.

2 Walther MM, Enquist EG, Jennings SB, Gnarra JR, Zbar B, Linehan WM. Molecular genetics of renal cell carcinoma. In: Vogelzang NJ, Scardino PT, Shipley WU, Coffey DS, eds. *Comprehensive Textbook of Genitourinary Oncology*. Baltimore: Williams & Wilkins, 1996: 116–28.

3 Landis SH, Murray T, Bolden S, Wingo PA. Cancer statistics 1999. *CA Cancer J Clin* 1999; 48: 8–31.

4 Linehan WM, Zbar B, Klausner RD. Renal carcinoma. In: Scriver CR, Beaudet AL, Sly WS, Valle D, Vogelstein B, eds. *Metabolic and Molecular Basis of Inherited Disease*. 2000.

5   Yu MC, Mack TM, Hannish R, Cicioni C, Henderson BE. Cigarette smoking, obesity, diuretic use, and coffee consumption as risk factors for renal cell carcinoma. *J Natl Cancer Inst* 1986; **77**: 351–6.

6   McCredie M, Stewart JH. Risk factors for kidney cancer in New South Wales. *Eur J Cancer* 1992; **28A**: 2050–4.

7   Finkle WD, McLaughlin JK, Rasgon SA, Yeoh HH, Low JE. Increased risk of renal cell cancer among women using diuretics in the United States. *Cancer Causes Control* 1993; **4**: 555–8.

8   Malker HR, Malker BK, McLaughlin JK, Blot WJ. Kidney cancer among leather workers. *Lancet* 1984; **1**: 56–7.

9   Maclure M. Asbestos and renal adenocarcinoma: a case–control study. *Environ Res* 1987; **42**: 353–61.

10 Maclure M, Willett W. A case–control study of diet and risk of renal adenocarcinoma. *Epidemiology* 1990; **1**: 430–40.

11 Chung-Park M, Parveen T, Lam M. Acquired cystic disease of the kidneys and renal cell carcinoma in chronic renal insufficiency without dialysis treatment. *Nephron* 1989; **53**: 157–61.

12 Kovacs G, Ishikawa I. High incidence of papillary renal cell tumours in patients on chronic haemodialysis. *Histopathology* 1993; **22**: 135–9.

13 Gatalica Z, Schwarting R, Petersen RO. Renal cell carcinoma in the presence of adult polycystic kidney disease. *Urology* 1994; **43**: 102–5.

14 Levine E. Renal cell carcinoma in uremic acquired renal cystic disease: incidence, detection, and management. *Urol Radiol* 1992; **13**: 203–10.

15 Washecka R, Hanna M. Malignant renal tumors in tuberous sclerosis. *Urology* 1991; **37**: 340–3.

16 Bard RH, Lord B, Fromowitz F. Papillary adenocarcinoma of the kidney. *Urology* 1982; **19**: 16–20.

17 Linehan WM, Lerman MI, Zbar B. Identification of the VHL gene: its role in renal carcinoma. *JAMA* 1995; **273**: 564–70.

18 Couch V, Lindor NM, Karnes PS, Michels VV. Von Hippel–Lindau disease. *Mayo Clin Proc* 2000; **75**: 265–72.

19 Maher ER, Iselius L, Yates JR *et al.* Von Hippel–Lindau disease: a genetic study. *J Med Genet* 1991; **28**: 443–7.

20 Iliopoulos O, Eng C. Genetic and clinical aspects of familial renal neoplasms. *Semin Oncol* 2000; **27**: 138–49.

21 Lamiell J, Salazar F, Hsia Y. Von Hippel–Lindau disease affecting 43 members of a single kindred. *Medicine* 1989; **68**: 1–29.

22 Maher ER, Yates JR, Harries R *et al.* Clinical features and natural history of von Hippel–Lindau disease. *Q J Med* 1990; **77**: 1151–63.

23 Choyke P, Glenn G, Walther MM *et al.* The natural history of renal lesions in von Hippel–Lindau disease: a serial CT study in 28 patients. *Am J Radiol* 1992; **159**: 1229–34.

24 Poston CD, Jaffe GS, Lubensky IA *et al.* Characterization of the renal pathology of a familial form of renal cell carcinoma associated with von Hippel–Lindau disease: clinical and molecular genetic implications. *J Urol* 1995; **153**: 22–6.

25 Walther MM, Choyke P, Weiss G *et al.* Parenchymal sparing surgery in patients with hereditary renal cell carcinoma. *J Urol* 1995; **153**: 913–16.

26 Pearson JC, Weiss J, Tanagho EA. A plea for conservation of kidney in renal adenocarcinoma associated with von Hippel–Lindau disease. *J Urol* 1980; **124**: 910–12.

27 Palmer JN, Swanson BA. Conservative surgery in solitary and bilateral renal carcinoma: indications and technical considerations. *J Urol* 1987; **120**: 113–17.

28 Frydenberg M, Malek RS, Zincke H. Conservative renal surgery for renal cell carcinoma in von Hippel–Lindau's disease. *J Urol* 1993; **194**: 461–4.

29 Walther MM, Thompson N, Linehan WM. Enucleation procedures in patients with multiple hereditary renal tumors. *World J Urol* 1995; **13**: 248–50.

30 Maher ER, Yates JR, Ferguson-Smith MA. Statistical analysis of the two stage mutation model in von Hippel–Lindau disease, and in sporadic cerebellar haemangioblastoma and renal cell carcinoma. *Med Genet* 1990; **27**: 311–14.

31 Knudson AG Jr. Mutation and cancer: statistical study of retinoblastoma. *Proc Natl Acad Sci USA* 1971; **68**: 820–3.

32 Tory K, Brauch H, Linehan WM *et al*. Specific genetic change in tumors associated with von Hippel–Lindau disease. *J Natl Cancer Inst* 1989; **81**: 1097–101.

33 Lubensky IA, Gnarra JR, Bertheau P, Walther MM, Linehan WM, Zhuang Z. Allelic deletions of the VHL gene detected in multiple microscopic clear cell renal lesions in von Hippel–Lindau disease patients. *Am J Pathol* 1996; **149**: 2089–94.

34 Seizinger BR, Rouleau GA, Ozelius LJ *et al*. Von Hippel–Lindau disease maps to the region of chromosome 3 associated with renal cell carcinoma. *Nature* 1988; **332**: 268–9.

35 Latif F, Tory K, Gnarra J *et al*. Identification of the von Hippel–Lindau disease tumor suppressor gene. *Science* 1993; **260**: 1317–20.

36 Hosoe S, Brauch H, Latif F *et al*. Localization of the von Hippel–Lindau disease gene to a small region of chromosome 3. *Genomics* 1990; **8**: 634–40.

37 Richards FM, Maher ER, Latif F *et al*. Detailed genetic mapping of the von Hippel–Lindau disease tumour suppressor gene. *J Med Genet* 1993; **30**: 104–7.

38 Chen F, Kishida T, Yao M *et al*. Germline mutations in the von Hippel–Lindau disease tumor suppressor gene: correlations with phenotype. *Hum Mutat* 1995; **5**: 66–75.

39 Zbar B, Kishida T, Chen F *et al*. Germline mutations in the von Hippel–Lindau disease (VHL) gene in families from North America, Europe, and Japan. *Hum Mutat* 1996; **8**: 348–57.

40 Gnarra J, Tory K, Weng Y *et al*. Mutation of the VHL tumour suppressor gene in renal carcinoma. *Nature Genet* 1994; **7**: 85–90.

41 Corless CL, Kiebel A, Iliopoulos O, Kaelin WG Jr. Immunostaining of the von Hippel–Lindau gene product (pVHL) in normal and neoplastic human tissues. *Hum Pathol* 1997; **28**: 459–64.

42 Lee S, Neumann M, Stearman R *et al*. Transcription-dependent nuclear-cytoplasmic trafficking is required for the function of the von Hippel–Lindau tumor suppressor protein. *Mol Cell Biol* 1999; **19**: 1486–97.

43 Lee S, Chen DY, Humphrey JS, Gnarra JR, Linehan WM, Klausner RD. Nuclear/cytoplasmic localization of the von Hippel–Lindau tumor suppressor gene product is determined by cell density. *Proc Natl Acad Sci USA* 1996; **93**: 1770–5.

44 Duan DR, Humphrey JS, Chen DY *et al*. Characterization of the VHL tumor suppressor gene product: localization, complex formation, and the effect of natural inactivating mutations. *Proc Natl Acad Sci USA* 1995; **92**: 6459–63.

45 Duan DR, Pause A, Burgess WH *et al*. Inhibition of transcription elongation by the VHL tumor suppressor protein. *Science* 1995; **269**: 1402–6.

46 Garrett KP, Tan S, Bradsher JN, Lane WS, Conaway JW, Conaway RC. Molecular cloning of an essential subunit of RNA polymerase II elongation factor SIII. *Proc Natl Acad Sci USA* 1994; **91**: 5237–41.

47 Garrett KP, Aso T, Bradsher JN *et al*. Positive regulation of general transcription factor SIII by a tailed ubiquitin homolog. *Proc Natl Acad Sci USA* 1995; **92**: 7172–6.

48 Turner KJ. Inherited renal cancer. *BJU Int* 2000; **86**: 155–64.

49 Kibel A, Iliopoulos O, DeCaprio JD, Kaelin WG. Binding of the von Hippel–Lindau tumour suppressor protein to elongin B and C. *Science* 1995; **269**: 1444–6.

50 Kishida T, Stackhouse TM, Chen F, Lerman MI, Zbar B. Cellular proteins that bind the von Hippel–Lindau gene product: mapping of binding domains and the effect of missense mutations. *Cancer Res* 1995; **55**: 4544–8.

51 Decker HJ, Weidt EJ, Brieger J. The von Hippel–Lindau tumor suppressor gene: a rare and intriguing disease opening new insight into basic mechanisms of carcinogenesis. *Cancer Genet Cytogenet* 1997; **93**: 74–83.

52 Aso T, Lane WS, Conaway JW, Conaway RC. Elongin (SIII): a multisubunit regulator of elongation by RNA polymerase II. *Science* 1995; **269**: 1439–43.

53 Pause A, Lee S, Worrell RA *et al*. The von Hippel–Lindau tumor-suppressor gene product forms a stable complex with human CUL-2, a member of the Cdc53 family of proteins. *Proc Natl Acad Sci USA* 1997; **94**: 2156–61.

54 Salceda S, Caro J. Hypoxia-inducible factor 1α (HIF-1α) protein is rapidly degraded by the ubiquitin–proteasome system under normoxic conditions: its stabilization by hypoxia depends upon redox-induced changes. *J Biol Chem* 1997; **272**: 22642–7.

55 Maxwell PH, Wiesener RMS, Chang GW *et al*. The tumour suppressor protein VHL targets hypoxia-inducible factors for oxygen-dependent proteolysis. *Nature* 1999; **399**: 271–5.

56 Semenza GL. Hypoxia-inducible factor 1: master regulator of O_2 homeostasis. *Curr Opin Genet Dev* 1998; **8**: 588–94.

57 Kolch W, Martiny-Baron G, Kieser A, Marme D. Regulation of the expression of the VEGF/VPS and its receptors: role in tumor angiogenesis. *Breast Cancer Res Treat* 1995; **36**: 139–55.

58 Siemeister G, Weindel K, Mohrs K, Barleon B, Martiny-Baron G, Marme D. Reversion of deregulated expression of vascular endothelial growth factor in human renal carcinoma cells by von Hippel–Lindau tumor suppressor protein. *Cancer Res* 1996; **56**: 2299–301.

59 Berger DP, Herbstritt L, Dengler WA, Marme D, Mertelsmann R, Fiebig HH. Vascular endothelial growth factor (VEGF) mRNA expression in human tumor models of different histologies. *Ann Oncol* 1995; **6**: 817–25.

60 Takahashi A, Sasaki H, Kim SJ *et al*. Markedly increased amounts of messenger RNAs for vascular endothelial growth factor and placenta growth factor in renal cell carcinoma associated with angiogenesis. *Cancer Res* 1994; **54**: 4233–7.

61 Sato K, Terada K, Sugiama T *et al*. Frequent overexpression of vascular endothelial growth factor gene in human renal cell carcinoma. *Tohoku J Exp Med* 1994; **173**: 355–60.

62 Gnarra JR, Zhou S, Merrill MJ *et al*. Post-transcriptional regulation of vascular endothelial growth factor mRNA by the product of the VHL tumor suppressor gene. *Proc Natl Acad Sci USA* 1996; **93**: 10589–94.

63 Iliopoulos O, Levy AP, Jiang C, Kaelin WGJ, Goldberg MA. Negative regulation of hypoxia-inducible genes by the von Hippel–Lindau protein. *Proc Natl Acad Sci USA* 1996; **93**: 10595–9.

64 Pal S, Claffey KP, Dvorac HF, Mukhopadhyay D. The von Hippel–Lindau gene product inhibits vascular permeability factor/vascular endothelial growth factor expression in renal cell carcinoma by blocking protein kinase C pathways. *J Biol Chem* 1997; **272**: 27509–12.

65 Levy AP, Levy NS, Goldberg MA. Hypoxia-inducible protein binding to vascular endothelial growth factor mRNA and its modulation by the von Hippel–Lindau protein. *J Biol Chem* 1996; **271**: 25492–7.

66 Levy AP, Levy NS, Iliopoulos O, Jiang C, Kaplin WGJ, Goldberg MA. Regulation of vascular endothelial growth factor by hypoxia and its modulation by the von Hippel–Lindau tumor suppressor gene. *Kidney Int* 1997; **51**: 575–8.

67 Mukhopadhyay D, Knebelmann B, Cohen HT, Ananth S, Sukhatme VP. The von Hippel–Lindau tumor suppressor gene product interacts with Sp1 to repress vascular endothelial growth factor promoter activity. *Mol Cell Biol* 1997; **17**: 5629–39.

68 Wizigmann-Voos S, Breier G, Risau W, Plate KH. Up-regulation of vascular endothelial growth factor and its receptors in von Hippel–Lindau disease-associated and sporadic hemangioblastomas. *Cancer Res* 1995; **55**: 1358–64.

69 Ananth S, Knebelmann B, Gruning W *et al.* Transforming growth factor beta1 is a target for the von Hippel–Lindau tumor suppressor and a critical growth factor for clear cell renal carcinoma. *Cancer Res* 1999; **59**: 2210–16.

70 Gomella LG, Sargent ER, Wade TP, Anglard P, Linehan WM, Kasid A. Expression of transforming growth factor alpha in normal human adult kidney and enhanced expression of transforming growth factors alpha and beta 1 in renal cell carcinoma. *Cancer Res* 1989; **49**: 6972–5.

71 Ivanov SV, Kuzmin I, We MH *et al.* Down-regulation of transmembrane carbonic anhydrases in renal cell carcinoma cell lines by wild-type von Hippel–Lindau transgenes. *Proc Natl Acad Sci USA* 1998; **95**: 12596–601.

72 Ohh M, Yauch RL, Lonergan KM *et al.* The von Hippel–Lindau tumor suppressor protein is required for proper assembly of an extracellular fibronectin matrix. *Mol Cell* 1998; **1**: 959–68.

73 Ruoslahti E. Integrins. *J Clin Invest* 1991; **87**: 1–5.

74 Hynes R. Integrins: versatility, modulation, and signaling in cell adhesion. *Cell* 1992; **69**: 11–25.

75 Rouslathi E. Fibronectin and its integrin receptors in cancer. *Adv Cancer Res* 1999; **76**: 1–20.

76 Yoshida MA, Ohyashiki K, Ochi H *et al.* Cytogenetic studies of tumor tissue from patients with nonfamilial renal cell carcinoma. *Cancer Res* 1986; **46**: 2139–47.

77 Yoshida MA, Ohyashiki K, Ochi H *et al.* Rearrangement of chromosome 3 in renal cell carcinoma. *Cancer Genet Cytogenet* 1986; **19**: 351–4.

78 Nordenson I, Ljungberg B, Roos G. Chromosomes in renal carcinoma with reference to intratumor heterogeneity. *Cancer Genet Cytogenet* 1988; **32**: 35–41.

79 Kovacs G, Erlandsson R, Boldog F *et al.* Consistent chromosome 3p deletion and loss of heterozygosity in renal cell carcinoma. *Proc Natl Acad Sci USA* 1988; **85**: 1571–5.

80 Kovacs G, Frisch S. Clonal chromosome abnormalities in tumor cells from patients with sporadic renal cell carcinomas. *Cancer Res* 1989; **49**: 651–9.

81 Anglard P, Brauch TH, Weiss GH *et al.* Molecular analysis of genetic changes in the origin and development of renal cell carcinoma. *Cancer Res* 1991; **51**: 1071–7.

82 Shuin T, Kondo K, Torigoe S *et al.* Frequent somatic mutations and loss of heterozygosity of the von Hippel–Lindau tumor suppressor gene in primary human renal cell carcinomas. *Cancer Res* 1994; **54**: 2852–5.

83 Reiter RE, Anglard P, Liu S, Gnarra JR, Linehan WM. Chromosome 17p deletions and p53 mutations in renal cell carcinoma. *Cancer Res* 1993; **53**: 3092–7.

84 Foster K, Crossey PA, Cairns P *et al.* Molecular genetic investigation of sporadic renal cell carcinoma: analysis of allele loss on chromosomes 3p, 5q, 11p, 17 and 22. *Br J Cancer* 1994; **69**: 230–4.

85 Presti JC Jr, Reuter VE, Cordon-Cardo C, Mazumdar N, Fair WR, Jhanwir SC. Allelic deletions in renal tumors: histopathological correlations. *Cancer Res* 1993; **53**: 5780–3.

86 Cohen AJ, Li FP, Berg S *et al.* Hereditary renal-cell carcinoma associated with a chromosomal translocation. *N Engl J Med* 1979; **301**: 592–5.

87 Kovacs G, Brusa P, de Riese W. Tissue-specific expression of a constitutional 3;6 translocation: development of multiple bilateral renal-cell carcinomas. *Int J Cancer* 1989; **43**: 422–7.

88 Koolen MI, van der Meyden AP, Bodmer D *et al.* A familial case of renal cell carcinoma and a t(2;3) chromosome translocation. *Kidney Int* 1998; **53**: 273–5.

89 Li FP, Decker HJH, Zbar B *et al.* Clinical and genetic studies of renal cell carcinomas in a family with a constitutional chromosome 3;8 translocation. *Ann Intern Med* 1993; **118**: 106–11.

90 Schmidt L, Li F, Brown RS *et al.* Mechanism of tumorigenesis of renal carcinomas associated with the constitutional chromosome 3;8 translocation. *Cancer J* 1995; **1**: 191–5.

91 Knudson AG. VHL gene mutation and clear-cell renal carcinomas. *Cancer J* 1995; **1**: 180–1.

92 Glassberg KI. Renal dysplasia and cystic disease of the kidney. In: Walsh P, Retik AB, Vaughan ED Jr, Wein AJ, eds. *Campbell's Urology*. Philadelphia: W.B. Saunders, 1996: 1778–81.

93 Osborne JP, Fryer A, Webb D. Epidemiology of tuberous sclerosis. *Ann NY Acad Sci* 1991; **615**: 125–7.

94 Kuntz M. Population studies. In: Gomez MR, ed. *Tuberous Sclerosis*. New York: Raven Press, 1988: 214.

95 Sampson JR, Patel A, Mee AD. Multifocal renal cell carcinoma in sibs from a chromosome 9 linked (TSC1) tuberous sclerosis family. *J Med Genet* 1995; **32**: 848–50.

96 Sampson JR. The kidney in tuberous sclerosis: manifestations and molecular genetic mechanisms. *Nephrol Dial Transplant* 1996; **11**: 34–7.

97 Kandt RS, Haines JL, Smith M *et al.* Linkage of an important gene locus for tuberous sclerosis to a chromosome 16 marker for polycystic kidney disease. *Nat Genet* 1992; **2**: 37–41.

98 European Consortium on Tuberous Sclerosis. Identification and characterization for the tuberous sclerosis gene on chromosome 16. *Cell* 1993; **75**: 1305–15.

99 Consortium TT. Identification of the TSC1 gene on chromosome 9q34. *Science* 1997; **277**: 805–8.

100 Kwiatkowska J, Jozwiak S, Hall F *et al.* Comprehensive mutational analysis of the TSC1 gene: observations on frequency of mutation, associated features, and nonpenetrance. *Ann Hum Genet* 1998; **62**: 277–85.

101 Young J, Povey S. The genetic basis of tuberous sclerosis. *Mol Med* 1998; **4**: 313–19.

102 Henske EP, Scheithauer BW, Short MP *et al.* Allelic loss is frequent in tuberous sclerosis kidney lesions but rare in brain lesions. *Am J Hum Genet* 1996; **59**: 400–6.

103 Carbonara C, Longa L, Grosso E *et al.* 9q34 loss of heterozygosity in a tuberous sclerosis astrocytoma suggests a growth suppressor-like activity also for the TSC1 gene. *Hum Mol Genet* 1994; **3**: 1829–32.

104 Jin F, Wienecke R, Xiao GH, Maize JC Jr, DeClue JE, Yeung RS. Suppression of tumorigenicity by the wild-type tuberous sclerosis 2 (Tsc2) gene and its C-terminal region. *Proc Natl Acad Sci USA* 1996; **93**: 9154–9.

105 Luttrell LM, Daaka Y, Lefkowitz RJ. Regulation of tyrosine kinase cascades by G-protein-coupled receptors. *Curr Opin Cell Biol* 1999; **11**: 177–83.

106 van Slegtenhorst M, Nellist M, Nagelkerken B *et al.* Interaction between hamartin and tuberin, the TSC1 and TSC2 gene products. *Hum Mol Genet* 1998; **7**: 1053–7.

107 Kovacs G. Papillary renal cell carcinoma: a morphologic and cytogenetic study of 11 cases. *Am J Path* 1989; **134**: 27–34.

108 Mancilla-Jimenez R, Stanley RJ, Blath RA. Papillary renal cell carcinoma: a clinical, radiologic and pathologic study of 34 cases. *Cancer* 1996; **38**: 2469.

109 Robson CJ, Churchill BM, Anderson W. The results of radical nephrectomy for renal cell tumours. *World J Urol* 1969; **101**: 297–301.

110 Zambrano NR, Lubensky IA, Merino MJ, Linehan WM, Walther MM. Histopathology and molecular genetics of renal tumors: toward unification of a classification system. *J Urol* 1999; **162**: 1246–58.

111 Bardelli A, Pugliese L, Comoglio PM. 'Invasive growth' signaling by the Met/HGF receptor: the hereditary renal carcinoma connection. *Biochim Biophys Acta* 1997; **1333**: M41–M51.

112 Kovacs G, Szucs S, Deriese W, Baumgartel H. Specific chromosomal aberration in human renal cell carcinoma. *Int J Cancer* 1987; **40**: 171–8.

113 Kovacs G, Fuzesi L, Emanuel A, Kung HF. Cytogenetics of papillary renal cell tumours. *Genes Chromosomes Cancer* 1991; **3**: 249–55.

114 Thrash-Bingham CA, Salazar H, Freed JJ, Greenberg RE, Tartof KD. Genomic alterations and instabilities in renal cell carcinomas and their relationship to tumor pathology. *Cancer Res* 1995; **55**: 6189–95.

115 Tonk V, Wilson KS, Timmons CF, Schneider NR, Tomlison GE. Renal cell carcinoma with translocation (X;1): further evidence for cytogenetically defined subtype. *Cancer Genet Cytogenet* 1995; **81**: 72–5.

116 Kardas I, Denis A, Babinska M *et al.* Translocation (X;1)(p11.2;q21) in a papillary renal cell carcinoma in a 14-year-old girl. *Cancer Genet Cytogenet* 1998; **101**: 159–61.

117 Sidhar SK, Clark J, Gill S *et al.* The t(X;1)(p11.2;q21.2) translocation in papillary renal cell carcinoma fuses a novel gene PRCC to the TFE3 transcription factor gene. *Hum Mol Genet* 1996; **5**: 1333–8.

118 Wetermen MA, Wilbrink M, Janssen I *et al.* Molecular cloning of the papillary renal cell carcinoma associated translocation (X;1)(p11q21) breakpoint. *Cytogenet Cell Genet* 1996; **75**: 2–6.

119 Hughson MD, Johnson LD, Silva FG, Kovacs G. Nonpapillary and papillary renal cell carcinoma: a cytogenetic and phenotypic study. *Mod Path* 1993; **6**: 449–56.

120 Henn W, Zwergel T, Wullich B, Thönnes M, Zang KD, Seitz G. Bilateral multicentric papillary renal tumors with heteroclonal origin based on tissue-specific karyotype instability. *Cancer* 1993; **72**: 1315–18.

121 Kovacs G, Tory K, Kovacs A. Development of papillary renal cell tumours is associated with a loss of Y-chromosome-specific DNA sequences. *J Path* 1994; **173**: 39–44.

122 Duh FM, Scherer SW, Tsui LC, Lerman MI, Zbar B, Schmidt L. Gene structure of the human MET proto-oncogene. *Oncogene* 1997; **15**: 1583–6.

123 Zbar B, Tory K, Merino M *et al.* Hereditary papillary renal cell carcinoma. *J Urol* 1994; **151**: 151–6.

124 Zbar B, Glenn G, Lubensky I *et al.* Hereditary papillary renal cell carcinoma: clinical studies in 10 families. *J Urol* 1995; **153**: 907–12.

125 Zbar B, Lerman M. Inherited carcinomas of the kidney. In: *Anonymous Advances in Cancer Research.* 1998: 163–201.

126 Schmidt L, Junker K, Weirich G *et al.* Two North American families with hereditary papillary renal carcinoma and identical novel mutations in the MET protooncogene. *Cancer Res* 1998; **58**: 1719–22.

127 Schmidt L, Duh F-M, Chen F *et al.* Germline and somatic mutations in the tyrosine kinase domain of the MET proto-oncogene in papillary renal carcinomas. *Nat Genet* 1997; **16**: 68–73.

128 Zhuang Z, Park WS, Pack S *et al.* Trisomy 7-harbouring nonrandom duplication of the mutant MET allele in hereditary papillary renal carcinomas. *Nat Genet* 1998; **20**: 66–9.

129 Fischer J, Palmedo G, von Knobloch R *et al.* Duplication and overexpression of the mutant allele of the MET proto-oncogene in multiple hereditary papillary renal tumours. *Oncogene* 1998; **17**: 733–9.

130 Bottaro DP, Rubin JS, Faletto DL *et al*. Identification of the hepatocyte growth factor receptor as the c-met proto-oncogene product. *Science* 1991; **251**: 802–4.

131 Giordano S, Zhen Z, Medico E, Gaudino G, Galimi F, Comoglio PM. Transfer of mitogenic and invasive response to scatter factor/hepatocyte growth factor by transfection of human MET protooncogene. *Proc Natl Acad Sci USA* 1993; **90**: 649–53.

132 Naldini L, Vigna E, Ferracini R *et al*. The tyrosine kinase encoded by the MET proto-oncogene is activated by autophosphorylation. *Mol Cell Biol* 1991; **4**: 1793–803.

133 Ponzetto C, Bardelli A, Zhen Z *et al*. A multifunctional docking site mediated signaling and transformation by the hepatocyte growth factor/scatter factor receptor family. *Cell* 1994; **77**: 261–71.

134 Menke A, McInnes L, Hastie ND, Schedl A. The Wilms' tumor suppressor WT1: approaches to gene function. *Kidney Int* 1998; **53**: 1512–18.

135 Bove KE. Wilms' tumor and related abnormalities in the fetus and newborn. *Semin Perinatol* 1999; **23**: 310–18.

136 Knudson AG, Strong LC. Mutation and cancer: a model for Wilms' tumor of the kidney. *J Natl Cancer Inst* 1976; **48**: 313–24.

137 Knudson AG, Hethcote HW, Brown BW. Mutation and childhood cancer: a probabilistic model for incidence of retinoblastoma. *Proc Nat Acad Sci USA* 1975; **72**: 5116–20.

138 Call KM, Glaser T, Ito CY *et al*. Isolation and characterization of a zinc finger polypeptide gene at the human chromosome 11 Wilms' tumor locus. *Cell* 1990; **60**: 509–20.

139 Gessler M, Konig A, Bruns GA. The genomic organization and expression of the WT1 gene. *Genomics* 1992; **12**: 807–13.

140 Haber DA, Sohn RL, Buckler AJ, Pelleteir J, Call KM, Housman DE. Alternative splicing and genomic structure of the Wilms tumor gene WT1. *Proc Natl Acad Sci USA* 1991; **88**: 9618–22.

141 Tadokoro K, Oki N, Fujhi H, Oshima A, Inque T, Yamada M. Genomic organisation of the human WT1 gene. *Jpn J Cancer Res* 1992; **83**: 1198–203.

142 Haber D, Englert C, Maheswaran S. Functional properties of WT1. *Med Pediatr Oncol* 1996; **27**: 453–5.

143 Englert C, Hou X, Maheswaran S *et al*. WT1 suppresses synthesis of the epidermal growth factor receptor and induces apoptosis. *EMBO J* 1995; **14**: 4662–75.

144 Kreidberg JA, Sariola H, Loring JM *et al*. WT-1 is required for early kidney development. *Cell* 1993; **74**: 679–91.

145 Grundy P, Telzerow P, Moksness JM, Breslow NE. Clinicopathologic correlates of loss of heterozygosity in Wilms' tumor patients: preliminary results. *Med Pediatr Oncol* 1996; **27**: 429–33.

146 Leiber MM, Tomera KM, Farrow GM. Renal oncocytoma. *J Urol* 1981; **125**: 481–5.

147 Brown JA, Takahashi S, Alcaraz A *et al*. Fluorescence in situ hybridization analysis of renal oncocytoma reveals frequent loss of chromosomes Y and 1. *J Urol* 1996; **156**: 31–5.

148 Herbers J, Schullerus D, Chudek J *et al*. Lack of genetic changes at specific genomic sites separated renal oncocytomas from renal cell carcinomas. *J Path* 1998; **184**: 58–62.

149 Psihramis KE, Dal Cin P, Dretler SP, Prout GR Jr, Sandberg AA. Further evidence that renal oncocytoma has malignant potential. *J Urol* 1988; **139**: 585–7.

150 Crotty TB, Lawrence KM, Moertel CA *et al*. Cytogenetic analysis of six renal oncocytomas and a chromophobe cell renal carcinoma: evidence that −Y, −1 may be a characteristic anomaly in renal oncocytomas. *Cancer Genet Cytogenet* 1992; **61**: 61–6.

151 Meloni AM, Sandberg AA, White RD. −Y,−1 as recurrent anomaly in oncocytoma. *Cancer Genet Cytogenet* 1992; **61**: 108–9.

152 Van den Berg E, Dijkhuizen T, Störkel S *et al*. Chromosomal changes in renal oncocytomas: evidence that t(5;11)(q35;q13) may characterize a second subgroup of oncocytomas. *Cancer Genet Cytogenet* 1995; **79**: 164–8.

153 Thrash-Bingham CA, Salazar H, Greenberg RE, Tartof KD. Loss of heterozygosity studies indicate that chromosome arm 1p harbors a tumor suppressor gene for renal oncocytomas. *Genes Chromosomes Cancer* 1996; **16**: 64–7.

154 Presti JC Jr, Rao PH, Chen Q *et al*. Histopathological, cytogenetic and molecular characterization of renal cortical tumors. *Cancer Res* 1991; **51**: 1544–52.

155 Sinke RJ, Dijkhuizen T, Janssen B *et al*. Fine mapping of human renal oncocytoma-associated translocation (5;11)(q35;q13) breakpoint. *Cancer Genet Cytogenet* 1997; **96**: 95–101.

156 Walter TA, Pennington RD, Decker H-J, Sandberg AA. Translocation t(9;11)(p23;q12): a primary chromosomal change in renal oncocytoma. *J Urol* 1989; **142**: 117–19.

157 Füzesi L, Gunawan B, Braun S, Boeckman W. Renal oncocytoma with a translocation t(9;11)(p23;q13). *J Urol* 1994; **152**: 471–2.

158 Neuhaus C, Dijkhuizen T, van den Berg E *et al*. Involvement of the chromosomal region 11q13 in renal oncocytoma: a case report and literature review. *Cancer Genet Cytogenet* 1997; **94**: 95–8.

159 Psihramis KE, Althausen AF, Yoshida MA, Prout G Jr, Sandberg AA. Chromosome anomalies suggestive of a malignant transformation in bilateral renal oncocytoma. *J Urol* 1986; **92**: 892–5.

160 Tallini G, Ladanyi M, Rosai J, Jhanwar SC. Analysis of nuclear and mitochondrial DNA alterations in thyroid and renal oncocytic tumors. *Cytogenet Cell Genet* 1994; **66**: 253–9.

161 Schwerdtle RF, Winterpacht A, Störkel S *et al*. Loss of heterozygosity studies and deletion mapping identify putative chromosome 14q tumor suppressor loci in renal oncocytomas. *Cancer Res* 1997; **57**: 5009–12.

162 Störkel S. Classification of renal cell carcinoma: correlation of morphology and cytogenetics. In: Vogelzang NJ, Scardino PT, Shipley WU, Coffey DS, eds. *Comprehensive Textbook of Genitourinary Oncology*. Baltimore: Williams & Wilkins, 1996: 179–86.

163 Grignon DJ, Eble JN. Papillary and metanephric adenomas of the kidney. *Semin Diagn Path* 1998; **15**: 41–53.

164 Kovacs G. Molecular cytogenetics of renal cell tumors. *Adv Cancer Res* 1993; **62**: 89–124.

165 Kovacs G, Fuzesi L, Emanuel A, Kung HF. Cytogenetics of papillary renal cell tumors. *Genes Chromosomes Cancer* 1991; **3**: 249–55.

166 Brown JA, Sebo TJ, Segura JW. Metaphase analysis of metanephric adenoma reveals chromosome Y loss with chromosome 7 and 17 gain. *Urology* 1996; **48**: 473–5.

167 Jones EC, Pins M, Dickerson GR, Young R. Metanephric adenoma of the kidney: a clinicopathologic, immunohistochemical, flow cytometric, cytogenetic and electron microscopic study of seven cases. *Am J Surg Path* 1995; **19**: 615–26.

168 Gatalica Z, Grujic S, Kovatich A, Petersen RO. Metanephric adenoma: histology, immunophenotype, cytogenetics, ultrastructure. *Mod Path* 1996; **9**: 329–33.

169 Renshaw AA, Maurici D, Fletcher JA. Cytologic and fluorescence in situ hybridization (FISH) examination of metanephric adenoma. *Diagn Cytopath* 1997; **16**: 107–11.

170 Fuhrman SA, Lasky LC, Limas C. Prognostic significance of morphologic parameters in renal cell carcinoma. *Am J Surg Pathol* 1982; **6**: 655–63.

171 Thrasher JB, Paulson DF. Prognostic factors in renal cancer. *Urol Clin North Am* 1993; **20**: 247–62.

172 Medeiros LJ, Gelb AB, Weiss LM. Renal cell carcinoma: prognostic significance of morphologic parameters in 121 cases. *Cancer* 1988; **61**: 1639–51.

173   Helpap B. Grading and prognostic significance of urologic carcinomas. *J Urol* 1992; **48**: 245–57.

174   Flint A, Grossman HB, Liebert M, Lloyd RV, Bromberg J. DNA and PCNA content of renal cell carcinoma and prognosis. *Am J Clin Pathol* 1995; **103**: 14–19.

175   Grignon DG, Abdel-Malak M, Mertens W. Prognostic significance of cellular proliferation in renal cell carcinoma: a comparison of synthesis-phase fraction and proliferating cell nuclear antigen index. *Mod Pathol* 1995; **8**: 18.

176   Gelb AB, Sudilowsky D, Wu CD, Weiss LM, Meideros LJ. Appraisal of intratumoral microvessel density, MIB-1 score, DNA content and p53 protein expression as prognostic indicators in patients with locally confined renal cell carcinoma. *Cancer* 1997; **80**: 1768–75.

177   Hofmockel G, Tsatalpas P, Muller H *et al.* Significance of conventional and new prognostic factors for locally confined renal cell carcinoma. *Cancer* 1995; **76**: 296–306.

178   Moch H, Sauter G, Buchholz N *et al.* Epidermal growth factor receptor expression is associated with rapid tumor cell proliferation in renal cell carcinoma. *Hum Pathol* 1997; **28**: 1255–9.

179   Screaton GR, Bell MV, Jackson DG, Cornelis FB, Gerth U, Bell JI. Genomic structure of DNA encoding the lymphocyte homing receptor CD44 reveals at least 12 alternatively spliced exons. *Proc Natl Acad Sci* 1992; **89**: 12160–4.

180   Gunthert U, Hofmann M, Rudy W *et al.* A new variant of glycoprotein CD44 confers metastatic potential to rat carcinoma cells. *Cell* 1991; **65**: 13–24.

181   Gilcrease MZ, Guzman-Paz M, Niehans G, Cherwitz D, McCarthy JB, Albores-Saavedra J. Correlation of CD44S expression in renal clear cell carcinomas with subsequent tumor progression or recurrence. *Cancer* 1999; **86**: 2320–6.

182   Paradis V, Ferlicot S, Ghannam E *et al.* CD44 is an independent prognostic factor in conventional renal cell carcinomas. *J Urol* 1999; **161**: 1984–7.

Further reading

Bardelli A, Ponzetto C, Comoglio PM. Identification of functional domains in the hepatocyte growth factor and its receptor by molecular engineering. *J Biotechnol* 1994; **37**: 109–22.

Bentz M, Bergerheim US, Li C *et al.* Chromosome imbalances in papillary renal cell carcinoma and first cytogenetic data of familial cases analysed by comparative genomic hybridization. *Cytogenet Cell Genet* 1996; **75**: 17–21.

Berg WJ, Divgi CR, Nanus DM, Motzer RJ. Novel approaches for advanced renal cell carcinoma. *Semin Oncol* 2000; **27**: 234–9.

Bernués M, Casadevall C, Miró R *et al.* Cytogenetic characterization of a familial papillary renal cell carcinoma. *Cancer Genet Cytogenet* 1995; **84**: 123–7.

Bladt F, Riethmacher D, Isenmann S, Aguzzi A, Birchmeier C. Essential role for the c-met receptor in the migration of myogenic precursor cells into the limb bud. *Nature* 1995; **376**: 768–71.

Boczko S, Fromowitz FB, Bard RH. Papillary adenocarcinoma of the kidney. *Urology* 1979; **14**: 491–5.

Dal Cin P, Van Poppel H, Sciot R *et al.* The t(1;12)(p36;q13) in a renal oncocytoma. *Genes Chromosomes Cancer* 1996; **17**: 136–9.

Englert C, Vidal M, Maheswaran S *et al.* Truncated WT1 mutants alter the subnuclear localization of the wild-type protein. *Proc Natl Acad Sci USA* 1995; **92**: 11960–4.

Fleming S. The impact of genetics on the classification of renal carcinoma. *Histopathology* 1993; **22**: 89–92.

Guinan PD, Vogelzang NJ, Fremgen AM *et al.* and members of the Cancer Incidence and End
Results Committee. Renal cell carcinoma: tumour size, stage and survival. *J Urol* 1995;
153: 901.

Hedborg F, Holmgren L, Sanddtedt B, Ohlsson R. The cell type-specific IGF2 expression during
human development correlates to the pattern of overgrowth and neoplasia in the
Beckwith–Weidemann syndrome. *Am J Pathol* 1994; **145**: 802–17.

Heider KH, Ratschek M, Zatloukal K, Adolf GR. Expression of CD44 isoforms in human renal
cell carcinomas. *Virchows Arch* 1996; **428**: 267–73.

Hoffman DMJ, Gitilitz BJ, Belldegrun A, Figlin RA. Adoptive cellular therapy. *Semin Oncol*
2000; **27**: 221–33.

Huebner K, Ohta M, Lubinski J, Berd D, Maguire HC Jr. Detection of specific genetic alterations
in cancer cells. *Semin Oncol* 1996; **23**: 22–30.

Jeffers M, Schmidt L, Nakaigawa N *et al.* Activating mutations for the met tyrosine kinase
receptor in human cancer. *Proc Natl Acad Sci USA* 1997; **94**: 11445–50.

Kovacs G, Hoene E. Multifocal renal cell carcinoma: a cytogenetic study. *Virchows Arch A
Pathol Anat Histopathol* 1987; **412**: 79–82.

Kovacs G, Ishikawa I. High incidence of papillary renal cell tumours in patients on chronic
haemodialysis. *Histopathology* 1993; **22**: 135–9.

Kovacs G, Szücs S, Eichner W, Maschek H, Wahnschaffe U, De Riese W. Renal oncocytoma: a
cytogenetic and morphologic study. *Cancer* 1987; **59**: 2071.

Kovacs G, Welter C, Wilkens L, Blin N, Deriese W. Renal oncocytoma: a phenotypic and
genotypic entity of renal parenchymal tumours. *Am J Path* 1989; **134**: 967–71.

Kovacs G. Molecular cytogenetics of renal cell tumours. *Adv Cancer Res* 1993; **62**:
89–124.

Kovacs G. Molecular differential pathology of renal cell tumours. *Histopathology* 1993;
22: 1–8.

Kovacs G. The value of molecular genetic analysis in the diagnosis and prognosis of renal cell
tumours. *World J Urol* 1994; **12**: 64–8.

LeRoith D, Beserga R, Helman L, Roberts CT Jr. Insulin-like growth factors and cancer. *Ann Int
Med* 1995; **122**: 54–9.

Mayer B, Jauch KW, Gunthert U *et al.* De novo expression of CD44 and survival in gastric
cancer. *Lancet* 1993; **342**: 1019–22.

Meloni AM, Bridge J, Sandberg AA. Reviews on chromosome studies in urological tumours. I.
Renal tumours. *J Urol* 1992; **148**: 253–65.

Meloni AM, Dobbs RM, Pontes JE, Sandberg AA. Translocation (X;1) in papillary renal cell
carcinoma: a new cytogenetic subtype. *Cancer Genet Cytogenet* 1993; **65**: 1–6.

Mydlo JH, Bard RH. Analysis of papillary renal adenocarcinoma. *Urology* 1987; **20**: 529–34.

Park M, Dean M, Kaul K, Braun MJ, Gonda MA, Vande WG. Sequence of MET protooncogene
cDNA has features characteristic of the tyrosine kinase family of growth-factor receptors.
Proc Natl Acad Sci USA 1987; **84**: 6379–83.

Reeve AE. Role of genetic imprinting in Wilms' tumour and overgrowth disorders. *Med Paediatr
Oncol* 1996; **27**: 470–5.

Shipley JM, Birdsall S, Clark J *et al.* Mapping the X chromosome breakpoint in two papillary
renal cell carcinoma cell lines with a t(X;1)(p11.2;q21.2) and the first report of a female case.
Cytogenet Cell Genet 1995; **71**: 280–4.

Stauder R, Eisterer W, Thaler J, Gunthert U. CD44 variant isoforms in non-Hodgkin's
lymphoma: a new independent prognostic factor. *Blood* 1995; **85**: 2885–99.

Tanabe KK, Ellis LM, Saya H. Expression of CD44R1 adhesion molecule in colon carcinomas
and metastases. *Lancet* 1993; **341**: 725–6.

Terpe HJ, Störkel S, Zimmer V *et al.* Expression of CD44 isoforms in renal cell tumours: positive
correlation to tumour differentiation. *Am J Pathol* 1996; **148**: 453–63.

Thrasher JB. Molecular markers in renal cell carcinoma: not quite ready for 'Prime Time'. *Cancer* 1999; **86**: 2195–7.

Weidner KM, Sachs M, Birchmeier W. The Met receptor tyrosine kinase transduces motility, proliferation and morphogenic signals of scatter factor/hepatocyte growth factor in epithelial cells. *J Cell Biol* 1993; **121**: 141–54.

Weterman MA, Wilbrink M, Geurts van Kessel A. Fusion of the transcription factor TFE3 gene to a novel gene, PRCC, in t(X;1)(p11;q21)-positive papillary renal cell carcinomas. *Proc Natl Acad Sci USA* 1996; **93**: 15294–8.

Zbar B, Lerman M. Inherited carcinomas of the kidney. *Adv Cancer Res* 1998; **75**: 164–201.

2: Cytokines and Angiogenesis Inhibitor Treatments

S. Chowdhury & M. Gore

Introduction

Although renal cell carcinoma accounts for only approximately 2% of all malignancies, its incidence is increasing [1,2]. A significant proportion of patients with localized disease can be cured by nephrectomy; however, at presentation approximately 50% of patients will have locally advanced or metastatic disease [3]. Up to one-third of patients who initially present with localized disease will subsequently relapse after nephrectomy, usually with metastatic disease [3]. The outlook for patients with metastatic disease remains poor, with a 5-year survival of less than 10% [2].

Until relatively recently medroxyprogesterone acetate (MPA) had been the standard therapy for metastatic renal cell carcinoma. In a review of 173 patients treated in 10 trials, Harris [4] showed a response rate to MPA of 10%. MPA still has a role in the management of certain patients with metastatic disease because it can increase appetite and weight, with little if any toxicity.

Renal cell carcinoma is an inherently chemo-resistant tumour, possibly because of over-expression of the multidrug resistance gene, MDR-1. There have been many trials of single agent and combination chemotherapy regimens; however, response rates are low and characteristically of short duration [4,5] and only 5-fluorouracil and vinblastine have demonstrated modest activity [4,5]. Thus, there is no role for chemotherapy alone in the treatment of renal cell carcinoma, but there have been improvements in survival as a result of the development of cytokine therapy.

Prognostic factors

Metastatic renal cell carcinoma encompasses a heterogeneous group of patients and it is important to identify prognostic factors which predict survival before applying toxic therapy. Assessment of these factors can assist in decisions regarding patient management as well as in categorizing patients in clinical studies, thus aiding trial interpretation. The initial analysis of these factors was carried out by Elson and colleagues [6]. This retrospective study looked at 610 patients treated in the Eastern Cooperative Oncology Group (ECOG) phase II studies for advanced renal cell carcinoma between 1975 and 1984.

Risk group	No. of risk factors	n	Median survival (months)
1	0–1	113	12.8
2	2	141	7.7
3	3	151	5.3
4	4	123	3.4
5	5	82	2.1

Table 2.1 Prognostic groups and their impact on survival (Elson *et al.* [6])

Table 2.2 Prognostic groups and their impact on survival (Motzer *et al.* [10])

Risk group	No. of risk factors	% of patients	Median survival (months)
Favourable	0	25	20
Intermediate	1–2	53	10
Poor	3 or more	22	4

Risk factors that enabled the authors to stratify patients into appropriate risk groups were identified. These included performance status (performence status 1, 2 and 3 counting as 1, 2 and 3 risk factors respectively), recent diagnosis (<1 year), number of metastatic sites, weight loss and the use of prior cytotoxic chemotherapy (Table 2.1).

Other studies analysing prognostic factors in patients with metastatic renal cell carcinoma have defined different parameters, but performance status and a measure of disease extent consistently appear to be important indicators of survival [7–9]. A recent retrospective study by Motzer and colleagues looked at the relationship between pretreatment clinical features and survival in 670 patients with advanced renal cell carcinoma treated in the Memorial Sloan-Kettering Cancer Centre clinical trials between 1975 and 1996 [10]. Five pretreatment features were associated with a shorter survival in the multivariate analysis: low Karnofsky performance status, high serum lactate dehydrogenase, low haemoglobin, an elevated serum calcium and the absence of prior nephrectomy.

Using these factors the authors stratified patients into three separate risk groups (see Table 2.2). While these and the previously mentioned prognostic factors are useful in aiding management decisions, they are not prescriptive and each patient should be assessed individually.

Tumour immunology and cytokines

The immune system has evolved to detect and destroy molecules or pathogens that are recognized as 'non-self' but not to react to host tissues. Manipulation of the immune system for cancer treatment attempts either to make the tumour appear more 'foreign' when compared with normal tissues or to magnify host immune responses to tumours. Cytokines are soluble proteins produced by mononuclear cells of the immune system that act as messengers between cells. They have a wide range of biological effects, particularly on cells of the immune system and haemopoietic lineage.

The variable natural history of metastatic renal cell carcinoma, and occasional observed spontaneous regression, suggest a role for the immune system in control of tumour progression and provide a rationale for the use of biological therapy. In addition, metastases may regress after nephrectomy, and improvement in host immune response post nephrectomy has been observed [11]. Further evidence of an immune response is provided by the fact that tumour infiltrating lymphocytes can be detected in renal cell carcinoma tissue [12]. In addition, the presence of specific cytotoxic T lymphocytes (CTLs) within this population suggests the presence of antigens for their development, and analysis of CTLs has revealed four separate antigens defined in renal cell carcinoma [13]. Cytokine therapy has become important in biological therapy for advanced renal cell carcinoma. The activity of cytokines is shown in separate survival analyses by Fossa *et al.* (Table 2.3) [9], Jones *et al.* (Table 2.4) [8] and Motzer *et al.* [10]. In the analysis by Motzer and colleagues, cytokine therapy was shown to have a statistically significant survival advantage when compared with patients treated with chemotherapy, with a median survival of 12.9 months as compared with 6.3 months. The benefit of cytokine therapy appeared to be greatest in those with more favourable prognostic disease. The median survival times for favourable risk, intermediate risk and poor risk patients were 26, 12 and 6 months respectively.

Interferons

Interferons were the first cytokines to be identified and are a family of proteins produced by cells in response to viral infection or stimulation with double-stranded RNA, antigens or mitogens [14]. They have a wide range of actions including immunomodulatory activity, antiviral activity, antiproliferative effects on normal and malignant cells, inhibition of angiogenesis and enhancement of expression of a variety of cell surface antigens. Their direct antiproliferative activity is thought to play a major part in their antitumour effects, but other actions may prove important. No universal mechanism has been identified to explain how interferons inhibit the growth of tumours except that they prolong the G0/G1 phase of the cell cycle.

The majority of clinical research has centred on the use of interferon-alpha (IFN-α) as it appears to have the greatest activity in renal cell cancer. Most studies have reported response rates of 15–20% with IFN-α and median response durations of 6–10 months [14]. A dosing range of 2–10 million IU/m^2 given intramuscularly or subcutaneously has been most commonly used, although an optimum treatment regimen or duration has not been defined. Despite numerous clinical trials, it was not known until recently whether therapy with IFN-α improved survival. A Medical Research Council study [15] addressed this issue by comparing subcutaneous IFN-α (10 mU s.c. 3 times/week for 12 weeks; n = 174) with oral MPA (300 mg daily for 12 weeks; n = 176). The trial was stopped in November 1997 when data were available for 335 patients. There was a 28% reduction in the risk of death in the IFN-α group (hazard ratio 0.72; 95% CI: 0.55–0.94; P = 0.017). IFN-α gave an improvement in 1-year survival of 12% (MPA 31%, IFN-α 43%) and an improvement in median survival of 2.5 months (MPA 6 months, IFN-α 8.5 months). The authors noted the small benefit of IFN-α and its potential toxicity. However, IFN-α should become the standard control arm in future trials for advanced renal cell carcinoma.

Unlike with chemotherapy, the time taken to respond to interferons may be prolonged and varies widely. Most patients who are going to respond will have done so by 3–4 months and it is unusual for patients who progress on interferons to subsequently respond. However, there are reports of responses starting to occur at 6 and 9 months. There is also the question of treatment duration in patients with either stabilization of disease or a partial or complete remission. Our current practice is to continue treatment indefinitely for those patients with stable disease or in remission, provided they are able to tolerate the side-effects and treatment is stopped as soon as progressive disease occurs. Toxicity associated with interferon therapy includes flu-like symptoms, rashes, gastrointestinal complaints, liver dysfunction, neurological complaints and fatigue, which are highly dose and schedule dependent.

The benefit of IFN-α appears to be greatest in patients in the good or moderate prognostic categories of disease [9]. Table 2.3 shows the impact of IFN-α on survival in renal cancer, and is derived from a case–control study involving 231 patients. Controls were obtained from a US database (Eastern Cooperative Oncology Group, ECOG) of patients treated in non-biological therapy trials.

Table 2.3 The impact of interferon-alpha on survival in renal cancer (Fossa *et al.* [9])

Prognostic group	Median survival ECOG (months)	Median survival IFN-α (months)	P
Good	11.4	23.3	<0.001
Moderate	8.1	11.3	0.1014
Poor	5.0	6.9	NS

A trial of gamma interferon vs. placebo in metastatic renal cell carcinoma [16] showed similar response rates in both groups (4.4% interferon vs. 6.6% placebo; $P = 0.54$). The median time to progression was 1.9 months in both arms of the study ($P = 0.49$) and there was no significant difference in median survival (12.2 months with interferon vs. 15.7 months with placebo; $P = 0.52$). These results show that, in the dosages tested, not all cytokines have activity in metastatic renal cell carcinoma.

Interleukin 2

Interleukin 2 (IL-2) is the other cytokine that has shown significant activity against renal cell carcinoma. IL-2 is produced primarily by T cells. It has no intrinsic antitumour activity, but has a wide range of actions and plays a central role in immune regulation. Its primary action is to stimulate growth of activated T cells that bear the IL-2 receptor, but it also potentiates the activity of cytotoxic T cells and production of other cytokines. The initial work on IL-2 was carried out by Rosenberg and colleagues at the National Cancer Institute, using high-dose i.v. bolus IL-2. The initial publication in 1985 has been followed by a number of publications summarizing response rates and toxicity. A report of 255 patients with renal cell carcinoma treated in seven separate phase II trials using high-dose bolus single agent IL-2 [17] has recently been updated showing an overall response rate of 15% (7% complete response (CR) and 8% partial response (PR)) [18]. Responses were noted in all sites of disease including bone, intact primary tumours and visceral metastases and in patients with large tumour burdens. The major response duration for all complete responses has yet to be reached, but is at least 80 months (range 7–131 months). The median duration of response for partial responders is 20 months and the median survival for all 255 patients is 16.3 months, with 10–20% of patients estimated to be alive 5–10 years after treatment.

A major limitation to the use of high-dose bolus IL-2 is its significant toxicity. The toxicity manifests itself as a vascular leak syndrome with fluid retention, oedema and ultimately multi-organ dysfunction. The most common major toxicities seen are hypotension and oliguria, which require vasopressor support in >50% of the 255 patients [17]. This toxicity limits treatment to patients who are relatively fit and the use of IL-2 to specialist centres. Other important toxicities affect the cardiovascular, neurological, haematological and gastrointestinal systems.

There have been attempts over the last 15 years to reduce toxicity by modifying the treatment dosage regimen. The high-dose i.v. bolus IL-2 regimen was compared with a lower dose i.v. bolus to see if toxicity could be reduced while maintaining efficacy [19]. In this study 125 patients with metastatic renal cell carcinoma were randomized, but the received dose intensity difference was less than 10 because patients were able to tolerate more doses in the lower dose arm. Response rates between the two study arms were comparable and were 15% in the lower dose arm (7% CR and 8% PR) and 20% in the high-dose arm (3% CR and 17% PR). As expected, toxicity was considerably reduced in the lower dose arm. Thus it appears that low-dose i.v. bolus IL-2 is an acceptable alternative to the standard high-dose i.v. bolus IL-2.

IL-2 can also be administered by continuous intravenous infusion (CVI), and this method of delivery takes into account the short half-life of IL-2 ($T_{1/2}$ 12.9 min). Response rates vary considerably between studies, but in an overview of published trials using CVI IL-2 a response rate of 13.6% in 789 patients was seen (2.7% CR, 10.9% PR) [20]. The complete response rate and median response duration appear similar to high-dose bolus infusions, but toxicity using CVI IL-2 appears lower than that seen with the high-dose bolus strategy.

IL-2 can also be injected subcutaneously (s.c.), and this has been exploited to allow it to be given in the outpatient setting. A summary of phase II trials of single agent s.c. IL-2 shows a response rate of 17.9% in 190 patients (3.2% CR, 14.7% PR) [20]. Although the response rate appears comparable to intravenous administration, the database is small and durability of responses and hence effect on survival is yet to be established. The optimal dose, schedule and route of administration for IL-2 in patients with renal cell carcinoma has yet to be defined. Response rates appear similar with all three methods of administration, although data on response duration and overall survival are awaited before definitive comparisons can be made.

The impact of single agent IL-2 on survival has not yet been demonstrated in a randomized phase III trial. However, Jones and colleagues [8] compared the survival of 327 patients receiving CVI IL-2 with a set of matched controls from the ECOG database. Treatment with IL-2 was associated with a prolongation of survival in patients with good or moderate prognostic disease (see Table 2.4).

IL-2 was given in the early trials with lymphocyte activated killer (LAK)

Table 2.4 The impact of interleukin 2 on survival in renal cancer (Jones *et al.* [8])

Prognostic group	Median survival ECOG (months)	Median survival IL-2 (months)	P
Good	12.6	20.4	0.0001
Moderate	7.2	11.4	0.0013
Poor	5.6	6.3	NS

cells. We now know that the results with IL-2 and LAK cells are similar to those seen with IL-2 alone [20]. In a prospective randomized trial of high-dose i.v. bolus IL-2 alone or with LAK cells conducted by Rosenberg and colleagues [21], no significant difference in overall survival was seen between the two groups. It is now no longer practice for IL-2 to be given with LAK cells.

Another strategy used to potentially enhance the activity of IL-2 is to give it in combination with tumour infiltrating lymphocytes (TILs). TILs are found in high numbers in renal cell carcinoma and can be expanded *ex vivo* in the presence of IL-2. Murine and clinical models have suggested synergy between TILs and IL-2 to activate the cellular immune response and cause tumour regression. In a pilot study by Figlin and colleagues [22] involving 55 patients treated with nephrectomy followed by TILs plus low-dose IL-2, 19 patients (34.6%) responded and 5 (9%) achieved a complete response. In the subgroup of 23 patients who received CD8+ TILs, the overall response rate was 43.5%. In the light of this encouraging single institution study, a randomized multicentre study was conducted to compare CD8+ TILs plus low-dose IL-2 vs. low-dose IL-2 alone [23]. All patients underwent nephrectomy from which tissue was obtained to generate CD8+ TILs. In the intention-to-treat analysis there was no significant difference in response rate (9.4% vs. 11.4%) and 1-year survival rate (55% vs. 47%) in the TIL/IL-2 and IL-2 groups, respectively. However, it is difficult to draw meaningful conclusions from this study as only 48% of patients who were randomized to the TIL/IL-2 arm actually received TIL therapy. The major cause for this was cell processing failures, with insufficient yield of viable cells, although in the pilot study 96% of intended patients were treated with CD8+ TILs (23 of 24). In patients who have initially responded to IL-2 there remains the possibility of retreatment with IL-2 at relapse. However, it seems that retreatment rarely produces a second response and thus alternative approaches should be considered in these patients [24].

Interleukin 2 and interferon-alpha

Synergistic antitumour effects are seen in murine tumour models combining IL-2 and IFN-α and provide a rationale for their use in the clinical setting. The exact mechanisms of synergy are unknown, but it is possible that administration of IFN-α may increase immunogenicity of tumour cells via an enhancement of their histocompatibility and tumour associated antigens, thus increasing their lysis by CTLs, the number of which is increased by IL-2.

Clinical trials investigating IFN-α and IL-2 combination therapy have used differing routes of administration, treatment schedules, cytokine doses, patient selection and response criteria, making comparisons difficult. However, an overview of phase I and II trials showed a response rate of 20% in over 1400 patients with metastatic renal cell carcinoma [20], with approximately

25% of responders achieving a complete response. A French multicentre randomized trial investigated the efficacy of single agent vs. combination IL-2 and IFN-α [25]. A total of 425 patients were randomized to receive either IL-2 alone (18 mU/m^2/day CVI on days 1–5 and days 12–15; as two induction cycles followed by four maintenance cycles), IFN-α alone (18 mU s.c. 3 times/week for 10 weeks), or a combination of IL-2 and IFN-α (same dose IL-2, but only 6 mU IFN-α 3 times/week, during the two induction and subsequent maintenance periods). Intention-to-treat analysis showed a significantly improved response rate after 10 weeks (IL-2: 6.5%; IFN-α: 7.5%; IL-2 and IFN-α: 20%; P <0.01) and 1-year event-free survival (IL-2: 15%; IFN-α: 12%; IL-2 and IFN-α: 20%; P = 0.01) for patients receiving combination therapy. However, there was no significant difference in overall survival between the three groups (IL-2: 12 months; IFN-α: 13 months; IL-2 and IFN-α: 17 months; P = 0.55).

This study identified a subgroup of patients who had little chance of benefiting from treatment. These patients had more than one metastatic site, liver involvement, an interval between diagnosis of the primary tumour and development of metastases of less than 1 year or a performance status of >1.

This study also assessed the benefit of crossover therapy after failure of IL-2 or IFN-α [26]. A total of 113 patients with progressive disease after first-line treatment received either IFN-α (n = 48) or IL-2 (n = 65) as second-line treatment; however, only four patients achieved a PR (1 with IFN-α, 3 with IL-2). Three of these patients had stable disease or had responded to first-line treatment. Only one patient with confirmed disease progression after IL-2 subsequently responded to IFN-α. Thus in patients who progress rapidly during first-line treatment additional benefit from further cytokine treatment is unlikely.

Other cytokines

Several other interleukins have been tested in phase I and II trials in renal cell carcinoma, but antitumour activity has been low, with response rates of less than 5%. Interleukin 12 (IL-12), which promotes cell-mediated immunity through its regulatory effects on T and NK cells, is one of the more promising new agents. In a randomized phase II trial of IL-12 vs. IFN-α in advanced renal cell carcinoma, 30 patients were treated with IL-12 and 2 (7%) achieved a partial response, while no responses were seen in the IFN-α arm [27].

Animal models have noted a synergy between IL-2 and IL-12 and this interaction has been shown in a study which assessed *in vivo* stimulation of IL-12 secretion by subcutaneous low-dose IL-2 in metastatic renal cell carcinoma [28]. Evaluating IL-12 variations in relation to clinical response, a marked significant increase in IL-12 values occurred in patients with disease response or stabilization of disease, whereas patients with progressive disease showed a significant decline in IL-12 levels during IL-2 administration. Thus IL-2 may stimulate release of IL-12 and this is possibly associated with a favourable prognosis. Further studies of IL-12 as part of combination therapy with IL-2 are needed to see if this synergy can be exploited.

Biochemotherapy

The lack of cross-resistance, non-overlapping toxicity and potential synergy between chemotherapy and biological therapy has led to several trials combining cytokines and chemotherapeutic agents (so-called biochemotherapy) in metastatic renal cell carcinoma. A recent phase III study involving 160 patients compared IFN-α plus vinblastine (VLB) with vinblastine alone [29]. This study showed a significant benefit for biochemotherapy in terms of both median survival (IFN-α + VLB: 67.6 weeks; VLB: 37.8 weeks; $P = 0.0049$) and response rate (IFN-α + VLB: 16.5%; VLB: 2.5%; $P = 0.0025$). The increase in survival is both clinically and statistically significant, and long-term survivors who remained in remission after 4–5 years were noted.

This study did not address the role of vinblastine in the combination and it could be argued that the benefit seen is due solely to IFN-α. A phase III study by Fossa and colleagues [30] compared IFN-α with or without vinblastine. It found no statistically significant differences in activity or survival between the two regimens. Combination treatment was associated with a higher response rate (24% vs. 11%) and a trend to longer median survival (55 vs. 47 weeks). The role of vinblastine in combination with cytokines requires further investigation, but this agent is likely to contribute only modestly to antitumour activity.

The most extensively studied chemotherapeutic agent used in combination with cytokines in the treatment of renal cell carcinoma is 5-fluorouracil (5-FU). The administration of IFN-α with 5-FU modulates the effects of 5-FU, resulting in synergy due to the blocking of thymidine incorporation into DNA. Increased efficacy was shown in *in vitro* models, but this was not reflected in the results of a phase II trial in which there were no objective clinical responses when IFN-α + 5-FU was given to patients and where median survival was only 5 months [31].

The highest response rates in metastatic renal cell carcinoma are obtained using a combination of IFN-α, IL-2 and 5-FU (bolus). This was first described by Atzpodien and colleagues [32] and is an outpatient-based regimen of subcutaneous IFN-α, IL-2 and bolus intravenous 5-FU. Atzpodien and colleagues' initial study demonstrated a response rate of 48.6% (4 CR, 13 PR out of 35 patients) These workers went on to confirm the activity of this regimen in a randomized trial comparing IFN-α, IL-2 and 5-FU with oral tamoxifen

Reference	n	Response rate (%)	Median survival
32	46	19	Not reported
56	34	38	Not reported
57	55	16	12 months
33	41*	39	42 months
58	55	31	23 months
25	61*	8	Not reported
34	111	2	12 months
59	62	19	33% at 2 years
37	55	31	10.7 months
60	16	25	93 weeks

Table 2.5 Treatment of renal cell carcinoma with IFN-α + IL-2 + 5-FU

*Randomized data.

[33]. There was a response rate of 39% in the IFN-α, IL-2 and 5-FU arm, whereas no responses occurred in patients treated with tamoxifen. Furthermore, overall and progression-free survival were both significantly improved in the biochemotherapy arm (overall survival: IFN-α, IL-2 and 5-FU median not reached after 42 months vs. 14 months for tamoxifen, $P < 0.04$; progression-free survival: 13 vs. 4 months, $P < 0.01$).

This combination has been tested by several other groups, and response rates vary widely (see Table 2.5). This may be a result of differences in patient characteristics between study groups or of different scheduling of the drugs, as exemplified by a study by Ravaud and colleagues [34], which gave a response rate of only 1.8%.

The optimal method of scheduling and delivery of these agents has yet to be established. Our own group has explored an alternative way of delivering 5-FU within this combination. 5-FU is principally active in the S-phase of the cell cycle and may be more effective when given as a protracted venous infusion (PVI). PVI 5-FU-containing regimens have given high response rates in neoadjuvant treatment of breast cancer [35] and relapsed ovarian cancer [36]. A recent study from our own group using IFN-α, IL-2 and 5-FU (PVI) showed an overall response rate of 31% in 55 patients (CR: 3 patients; PR: 14 patients) [37]. The European Organization for Research and Treatment of Cancer (EORTC) and Cancer Research Campaign (CRC) have mounted a trial of this approach in the adjuvant setting. Despite high response rates seen with the IFN-α, IL-2 and 5-FU combination, the majority of patients relapse. The concept of continuing immune stimulation in responders is an attractive one, and our own group and Atzpodien's are investigating the feasibility of this approach.

Angiogenesis inhibitors

Angiogenesis is the growth of new microvessels. The growth of tumours beyond 1–2 mm^3 depends on angiogenesis, which is necessary for the supply of nutrients and also provides the route for metastasis. In adults the vascular endothelium is a quiescent tissue with a low cell division rate and thus pathological angiogenesis must occur to allow tumour development. A number of pro-angiogenic factors have been identified which include basic fibroblast growth factor and vascular endothelial growth factor, as well as antiangiogenic factors such as angiostatin and endostatin. The balance between these factors is important in tumour dormancy and control of micrometastases, where the apoptotic rate remains high until angiogenesis occurs. This change is termed the 'angiogenic switch', a complex process resulting in a shift in the balance between stimulators and inhibitors of angiogenesis, during which inhibitors are downregulated [38].

Neovascularization provides not only a perfusion stimulus for tumour growth but also a paracrine effect, which results from endothelium-derived growth factors and cytokines that stimulate growth and migration of tumour cells. This paracrine effect is thought to result from increased endothelial cell survival and growth. This two-cell-compartment model of tumour growth may influence the design of future clinical trials.

The close relationship between angiogenesis and tumour growth and metastasis makes it an attractive target for cancer therapy. Also, the amplification factor seen in the relationship between tumour and vascular endothelial cells means that suppression of one endothelial cell could inhibit the growth of approximately 100 tumour cells [39]. Initial experience with angiogenesis inhibitors in animal models and from early clinical trials in advanced cancer has led to general guidelines about their use [38].

Long-term therapy is necessary and anti-angiogenic therapy should not be interrupted, because of the ability of microvessels to regrow quickly. Resistance does not appear to be a problem with long-term use. The theoretical basis for this is that endothelial cells, unlike tumour cells, are not considered to be mutating and thus are unlikely to generate resistant clones. It is recommended that a combination of anti-angiogenic agents with different mechanisms of action should be given, as this approach appears to be more effective [40]. Such combinations in animal models have been curative, whereas single agents alone are merely inhibitory [41].

Angiogenesis inhibitors used in clinical trials to treat renal cell carcinoma

TNP-470

TNP-470 is a fumigillin analogue and was one of the first angiogenesis inhibitors to undergo clinical testing. Fumigillin was originally isolated from *Aspergillus fumigatus* contaminating endothelial cell cultures [42] and is a potent inhibitor of endothelial growth *in vitro* and *in vivo*. A number of analogues of fumigillin were synthesized and TNP-470 was selected as the least toxic compound with the greatest anti-angiogenic effect [42].

A recent phase II trial of TNP-470 was carried out in 33 patients with metastatic renal cell carcinoma [43]. There was only 1 partial response of short duration (response rate 3%) but 6 patients (18%) had stabilization of disease for 6 months or longer. At a median follow-up of 14 months, median survival was 56 weeks. Therapy was reasonably tolerated, although neuro-cortical toxicities were common (67% of patients) and led to the withdrawal of five patients from treatment. Fatigue and asthenia were also common, being seen in 60% of patients. This patient group had been heavily pretreated, and it is unclear whether this resulted in accrual of patients with indolent disease (median interval from diagnosis of metastatic disease to study initiation was 14 months). It is not apparent whether prolonged overall and progression-free survival in several patients was due to TNP-470 or merely a reflection of the natural history of their disease. Nevertheless, further studies using TNP-470 are warranted and combinations with other angiogenesis inhibitors, cyto-toxic drugs and cytokines are indicated [41,42].

An attractive option would be the combination of TNP-470 with IFN-α, which is known to have both anti-angiogenic and direct antitumour activity. Future studies should also address ways of increasing exposure to TNP-470, which animal studies suggest is necessary to maximize its anti-angiogenic properties. In the study mentioned above, exposure was likely to have been suboptimal as the half-lifes of TNP-470 and its active metabolite are only 2 and 6 minutes, respectively. It may also be that the greatest benefit in using TNP-470 to delay progression in renal cell carcinoma is seen in the adjuvant or minimal disease setting.

THALIDOMIDE

Thalidomide has been discovered to have powerful anti-angiogenic activity [44]. Its mechanism of action is complex and includes breakdown of mRNA of a number of molecules such as fibroblast growth factor (FGF) and tumour necrosis factor-alpha (TNF-α). In a recent phase II study from our own group low-dose thalidomide (100 mg orally every night) was tested in 66 patients with metastatic cancer, including several with renal cell carcinoma [45]. There were three partial responses and 13 stabilizations of previously progressive disease (3 for >3 months) in the 18 patients with renal cell carcinoma that were treated. Treatment was well tolerated and no WHO grade 3 or 4 toxicities were seen. The main toxicity was lethargy (38 patients grade 1, eight patients grade 2), but, conversely, several patients experienced improvement in sleep and appetite. Initial results from an on-going study from our own group using thalidomide at 600 mg orally every night show two partial responses and 10 stabilizations of disease for >12 weeks (7 for >24 weeks) in the 17 patients with renal cell carcinoma that have been assessed to date.

The exact mechanism of action of thalidomide is unknown and requires further investigation. A possible mechanism in renal cell carcinoma is inhibition of TNF-α, which is known to be secreted by renal cell carcinomas. This cytokine enhances neo-angiogenesis and stimulation of renal carcinoma cells by IL-6, and contributes to many systemic features of advanced malignancy, for example cachexia and malaise. Future studies of thalidomide should address this possibility by measuring pretreatment and serial levels of TNF-α. Two new classes of thalidomide have been developed [46]: one class of compounds are potent phosphodiesterase 4 inhibitors, which also inhibit TNF-α but have little effect on T-cell activation. The other class of compounds, similar to thalidomide, are not phosphodiesterase 4 inhibitors but inhibit TNF-α and stimulate T-cell proliferation and IL-2 and IFN-γ production. Introduction of these compounds into clinical practice may help elucidate the mechanisms by which thalidomide exerts its activity.

The ability of thalidomide to inhibit TNF-α production could be exploited by combining it with IFN-α, IL-2 and 5-FU. The side-effects with this combination are likely to be a result of IL-2-induced TNF-α production. TNF-α has little if any activity when used in renal cell carcinoma [47], and may even stimulate growth of renal carcinoma cells. Thus combining thalidomide with biochemotherapy may provide a way of decreasing side-effects while increasing efficacy.

New agents

Several other anti-angiogenic agents have shown potential activity in phase I/II trials. Jones and colleagues [48] used a combination of low molecular weight heparin, captopril and marimastat, all of which have anti-angiogenic activity *in vitro* and in animal models. In this study, 17 patients were treated, six of whom had renal cell carcinoma. One patient obtained a partial response and 1 had stabilization of disease. In five of the first six patients treated, plasma vascular endothelial growth factor levels were noted to have decreased. This regimen was well tolerated and had activity in renal cell carcinoma, and the biochemical data showed a reduction in angiogenic factors post-treatment.

SU5416 is a potent angiogenesis inhibitor, and the first drug in humans to directly block vascular endothelial growth factor (VEGF)-mediated Flk-1 (endothelial cell receptor) signalling. In a phase I trial of 63 patients, stabilization of disease for more than 6 months was seen in several tumour types, including renal cell carcinoma [49]. Thus, SU5416 is a promising new agent acting via a novel mechanism of action, and phase II studies are planned.

Vitaxin is a monoclonal antibody targeting endothelial integrin $\alpha\upsilon\beta3$. In animals, no expression of integrin $\alpha\upsilon\beta3$ is seen in established blood vessels from normal tissue, whereas high expression is seen in tumour associated blood vessels. In a phase I study, 15 patients with a variety of malignancies, two of which were renal carcinomas, were treated. There was one partial response and six patients had stable disease (tumour type not reported) [50]. Thus, integrin $\alpha\upsilon\beta3$ appears to be a clinically relevant anti-angiogenic target, and phase II studies are planned.

Matrix metalloproteinases (MMPs) have important roles in tumour metastasis and angiogenesis. Degradation of the basement membrane is needed for angiogenesis by invasion and migration of endothelial cells into tumour stroma. Specific inhibitors of these enzymes have been developed and include marimastat, CGS27023a, AG3340 and BAY 12-9566. Myalgia and arthralgia are the main side-effects seen with some of these agents. In a phase I study of BAY 12-9566 in 29 patients with a variety of malignancies, stabilization of disease was seen in seven patients (tumour type not reported) [51]. Again this compound is being further assessed in on-going phase II and III studies.

There is currently considerable interest in anti-angiogenesis as a treatment strategy in cancer patients. There are several anti-angiogenic agents in development and many have entered clinical trials. Two of the most interesting compounds are angiostatin and endostatin, both of which were isolated by Folkman and colleagues. Angiostatin is a proteolytic degradation product of plasminogen [52] and is a specific inhibitor of endothelial proliferation. It is the first angiogenesis inhibitor that can cause regression of human cancer xenografts in mice. A microscopic dormant state in which virtually all neovascularization has been blocked is achieved by prolonged blockade of angiogenesis [53].

Endostatin, a proteolytic degradation product of collagen type XVIII [54], has also been shown to cause tumour regression in murine carcinoma models. Tumours recurred when treatment was stopped but regressed again when endostatin therapy was recommenced. Interestingly, when therapy was withdrawn for a second time no tumour recurrence was observed [55].

Conclusion

Patients with metastatic renal cell carcinoma have a poor prognosis and thus there remains the continued need for clinical research into new treatments. Cytokine therapy has been shown to improve overall survival in metastatic renal cell carcinoma, as demonstrated by three randomized controlled studies [15,29,33]. Our knowledge of the molecular biology of renal cell carcinoma is ever increasing, allowing new therapeutic options such as anti-angiogenesis agents, tumour vaccines, monoclonal antibodies, antisense oligonucleotides and gene therapy to be developed.

References

1   Ries LAG, Kosary CL, Hankey BF *et al*. *SEER Cancer Statistics Review, 1973–1994*. NIH Publications 97-2789. Bethesda: National Cancer Institute, 1997.

2   Motzer RJ, Bander NH, Nanus DM. Renal-cell carcinoma. *N Engl J Med* 1996; **335**: 865–75.

3   Ritchie AWS, Oliver PTD. Tumours of the kidney (other than nephroblastoma). In: Peckham M, Pinedo H, Veronesi U, eds. *Oxford Textbook of Oncology*. Oxford: Oxford University Press, 1995: 1480–98.

4   Harris DT. Hormonal therapy and chemotherapy of renal cell carcinoma. *Semin Oncol* 1983; **10**: 422–30.

5   Yagoda A, Abi-Bached B, Petrylak D. Chemotherapy for advanced renal cell carcinoma 1983–1993. *Semin Oncol* 1995; **22**: 42–60.

6   Elson P, Witte R, Trump DL. Prognostic factors for survival in patients with recurrent or metastatic renal cell carcinoma. *Cancer Res* 1988; **48**: 7310–13.

7   Palmer PA, Vinke J, Philip T *et al*. Prognostic factors for survival in patients with advanced renal cell carcinoma treated with recombinant interleukin-2. *Ann Oncol* 1992; **3**: 475–80.

8   Jones M, Selby P, Franks C *et al*. The impact of interleukin-2 on survival in renal cell cancer: a multivariate analysis. *Cancer Biother* 1993; **8**: 275–88.

9   Fossa SD, Kramer A, Droz JP. Prognostic factors and survival in patients with metastatic renal cell carcinoma treated with chemotherapy or interferon-alpha. *Eur J Cancer* 1994; **30A** (Suppl.): 1310–14.

10 Motzer RJ, Mazumdar M, Bacik J *et al*. Survival and prognostic stratification of 670 patients with advanced renal cell carcinoma. *J Clin Oncol* 1999; **17**: 2530–40.

11 Dadian G, Riches PG, Henderson DC *et al*. Immunological parameters in peripheral blood of patients with renal cell carcinoma before and after nephrectomy. *Br J Urol* 1994; **74**: 15–22.

12 Finke JH, Tubbs R, Connelly B *et al*. Tumour-infiltrating lymphocytes in patients with renal cell carcinoma. *Ann N Y Acad Sci* 1988; **532**: 387–94.

13 Van den Eynde BJ, Gaugler B, Probst-Kepper M *et al*. A new antigen recognised by cytolytic T lymphocytes on a human kidney tumor results from reverse strand transcription. *J Exp Med* 1999; **190**: 1793–800.

14 Lineham WM, Shipley WU, Parkinson DR. Cancer of the kidney and ureter. In: Devita VT, Hellman S, Rosenberg SA, eds. *Cancer: Principles and Practice of Oncology*, 5th edn. New York: Lippincott-Raven, 1997: 1271–300.

15 Medical Research Council Renal Cancer Collaborators. Interferon-alpha and survival in

metastatic renal carcinoma: early results of a randomised controlled trial. *Lancet* 1999;
353: 14–17.

16   Gleave ME, Elhilali M, Fradet Y *et al*. Interferon gamma-1b compared with placebo in
metastatic renal-cell carcinoma. *N Engl J Med* 1998; **338**: 1265–71.

17   Fyfe G, Fisher RI, Rosenberg SA *et al*. Results of 255 patients with metastatic renal cell
carcinoma who received high-dose recombinant interleukin therapy. *J Clin Oncol* 1995;
13: 688–96.

18   Fisher RI, Rosenberg SA, Fyfe G *et al*. Long-term survival update for high-dose
recombinant interleukin-2 in patients with renal cell carcinoma. *Cancer J Sci Am* 2000; **6**
(Suppl. 1): 55–7.

19   Yang JC, Topalian SL, Parkinson D *et al*. Randomised comparison of high-dose and low-
dose intravenous interleukin-2 for the therapy of metastatic renal cell carcinoma: an
interim report. *J Clin Oncol* 1994; **12**: 1572–6.

20   Bukowski RM. Natural history and therapy of metastatic renal cell carcinoma: the role of
interleukin-2. *Cancer* 1997; **80**: 1198–220.

21   Rosenberg SA, Lotze MT, Yang JC *et al*. Prospective randomised trial of high-dose
interleukin-2 alone or in conjunction with lymphokine-activated killer cells for the
treatment of patients with advanced cancer. *J Natl Cancer Inst* 1993; **85**: 622–32.

22   Figlin RA, Pierce WC, Kaboo R *et al*. Treatment of metastatic renal cell carcinoma with
nephrectomy, interleukin-2 and cytokine primed or CD8+ selected tumour infiltrating
lymphocytes from primary tumour. *J Urol* 1997; **158**: 740–5.

23   Figlin RA, Thompson JA, Bukowski RM *et al*. Multicentre, randomised phase III trial of
CD8+ tumour-infiltrating lymphocytes in combination with recombinant interleukin-2 in
metastatic renal cell carcinoma. *J Clin Oncol* 1999; **17**: 2521–9.

24   Sherry RM, Rosenberg SA, Yang JC. Relapse after response to interleukin-2-based
immunotherapy: patterns of progression and response to treatment. *J Immunother* 1991;
10: 371–5.

25   Negrier S, Escudier B, Lasset C *et al*. Recombinant human interleukin-2, recombinant
interferon-alpha or both in metastatic renal cell carcinoma. *N Engl J Med* 1998; **338**:
1272–8.

26   Escudier B, Chevreau C, Lasset C *et al*. Cytokines in metastatic renal cell carcinoma: Is it
useful to switch to interleukin-2 or interferon after failure of a first treatment? *J Clin Oncol*
1999; **17**: 2039–43.

27   Berg WJ, Bukowski R, Thompson JA *et al*. A randomised phase II trial of recombinant
human interleukin-12 versus interferon alpha-2a in advanced renal cell carcinoma. *Proc
Am Soc Clin Oncol* 1998; **17**: 1226.

28   Lissoni P, Fumagalli L, Rovelli F *et al*. In vivo stimulation of IL-12 secretion by
subcutaneous low-dose IL-2 in metastatic cancer patients. *Br J Cancer* 1998; **77**: 1957–
60.

29   Pyrhonen S, Salminen E, Ruutu M *et al*. Prospective randomised trial of interferon alpha-2a
plus vinblastine versus vinblastine alone in patients with advanced renal cell cancer. *J Clin
Oncol* 1999; **17**: 2859–67.

30   Fossa SD, Martinelli G, Otto U *et al*. Recombinant interferon alpha-2a with or without
vinblastine in metastatic renal cell carcinoma: results of a European multicentre phase III
study. *Ann Oncol* 1992; **3**: 301–5.

31   Murphy BR, Rynard SM, Einhorn LH *et al*. A phase II trial of interferon alpha-2a plus
fluorouracil in advanced RCC. *Invest New Drugs* 1992; **10**: 225–30.

32   Atzpodien J, Kirchner H, Lopez Hanninen E *et al*. Interleukin-2 in combination with
interferon-A and 5-fluorouracil for metastatic renal cell cancer. *Eur J Cancer* 1993; **29A**
(Suppl. 5): 6–8.

33 Atzpodien J, Kirchner H, Franzke A *et al*. Results of a randomised clinical trial comparing sc interleukin-2, sc interferon-alpha 2a and IV bolus 5-fluorouracil against oral tamoxifen in progressive metastatic renal cell carcinoma patients. *Proc Am Soc Clin Oncol* 1997; **16**: 1164.

34 Ravaud A, Audhuy B, Gomez F *et al*. Subcutaneous interleukin-2, interferon alpha-2a and continuous infusion of fluorouracil in metastatic renal cell carcinoma: a multicentre phase II trial. *J Clin Oncol* 1998; **16**: 2728–32.

35 Smith IE, Walsh G, Jones A *et al*. High complete remission rates with primary neoadjuvant infusional chemotherapy for large early breast cancer. *J Clin Oncol* 1995; **13**: 424–9.

36 Ahmed FY, Mainwaring PN, Macfarlane V *et al*. Infusional chemotherapy (cisplatin, epirubicin, 5-FU: ECF) for patients with epithelial ovarian carcinoma. *9th NCI-EORTC Symposium on New Drug Therapy*, Amsterdam, 1996.

37 Allen MJ, Vaughan M, Webb A *et al*. Protracted venous infusion of 5-fluorouracil in combination with subcutaneous interleukin-2 and alpha interferon in patients with metastatic renal cell cancer: a phase II study. *Br J Cancer* 2000; **83**: 980–5.

38 Folkman J. Antiangiogenic therapy. In: Devita VT, Hellman S, Rosenberg SA, eds. *Cancer: Principles and Practice of Oncology*, 5th edn. New York: Lippincott-Raven, 1997: 3075–85.

39 Modzelewski RA, Davies P, Watkins SC *et al*. Isolation and identification of fresh tumour-derived endothelial cells from a murine RIF-1 fibrosarcoma. *Cancer Res* 1994; **54**: 336.

40 Kato T, Sato K, Kakinuma H *et al*. Enhanced suppression of tumour growth by combination of angiogenesis inhibitor O-(chloroacetyl-carbamoyl) fumagillol (TNP-470) and cytotoxic agents in mice. *Cancer Res* 1994; **54**: 5143–7.

41 Teicher BA, Holden SA, Ara G *et al*. Potentiation of cytotoxic cancer therapies by TNP-470 alone and with other anti-angiogenic agents. *Int J Cancer* 1994; **57**: 920–5.

42 Ingber D, Fujita T, Kishimoto S *et al*. Synthetic analogues of fumagillin that inhibit angiogenesis and suppress tumour growth. *Nature* 1990; **348**: 555–7.

43 Stadler WM, Kuzel T, Shapiro C *et al*. Multi-institutional study of the angiogenesis inhibitor TNP-470 in metastatic renal carcinoma. *J Clin Oncol* 1999; **17**: 2541–5.

44 D'Amato RJ, Loughman MS, Flynn E *et al*. Thalidomide is an inhibitor of angiogenesis. *Proc Natl Acad Sci USA* 1994; **91**: 4082–5.

45 Eisen T, Boshoff C, Mak I *et al*. Continuous low dose thalidomide: a phase II study in advanced melanoma, renal cell, ovarian and breast cancer. *Br J Cancer* 2000; **82**: 812–17.

46 Corral LG, Haslett PA, Muller GW *et al*. Differential cytokine modulation and T cell activation by two distinct classes of thalidomide analogues that are potent inhibitors of TNF-α. *J Immunol* 1999; **163**: 380–6.

47 Boshoff C, Jones AL. Tumour necrosis factor. In: Gore ME, Riches P, eds. *Immunotherapy in Cancer*. London: John Wiley, 1996: 77–103.

48 Jones PH, Elliot M, Dobbs N *et al*. Phase I/II study of combination antiangiogenesis therapy with marimastat, captopril and fragmin. *Proc Am Soc Clin Oncol* 1999; **18**: 1723.

49 Rosen L, Mulay M, Mayers A *et al*. Phase I dose-escalating trial of SU5416, a novel angiogenesis inhibitor in patients with advanced malignancies. *Proc Am Soc Clin Oncol* 1999; **18**: 618.

50 Gutheil JC, Campbell TN, Pierce PR *et al*. Phase I study of vitaxin, an anti-angiogenic humanised monoclonal antibody to vascular integrin αvβ3. *Proc Am Soc Clin Oncol* 1998; **17**: 832.

51 Goel R, Hirte H, Major P *et al*. Clinical pharmacology of the metalloproteinase (MMP) and angiogenesis inhibitor Bayer 12-9566 in cancer patients. *Proc Am Soc Clin Oncol* 1999; **18**: 616.

52   O'Reilly MS, Holmgren L, Shing Y *et al.* Angiostatin: a novel angiogenesis inhibitor that mediates the suppression of metastases by a Lewis lung carcinoma. *Cell* 1994; **21**, 79: 315–28.

53   O'Reilly MS, Holmgren L, Chen C *et al.* Angiostatin induces and sustains dormancy of human primary tumours in mice. *Nat Med* 1996; **2**: 689–92.

54   O'Reilly MS, Boehm T, Shing Y *et al.* Endostatin: an endogenous inhibitor of angiogenesis and tumour growth. *Cell* 1997; **24**, 88: 277–85.

55   Boehm T, Folkman J, Browder T *et al.* Antiangiogenic therapy of experimental cancer does not induce acquired drug resistance. *Nature* 1997; **390**: 404–7.

56   Hofmockel G, Langer W, Theiss M *et al.* Immunotherapy for metastatic renal cell carcinoma using a regimen of interleukin-2, interferon-alpha and 5-fluorouracil. *J Urol* 1996; **156**: 40.

57   Joffe JK, Banks RE, Forbes MA *et al.* A phase II study of interferon-alpha, interleukin-2 and 5-fluorouracil in advanced renal carcinoma: clinical data and laboratory evidence of protease activation. *Br J Urol* 1996; **77**: 638–49.

58   Ellerhorst JA, Sella A, Amato RJ *et al.* Phase II trail of 5-fluorouracil, interferon-alpha and continuous infusional interleukin-2 for patients with metastatic renal cell carcinoma. *Cancer* 1997; **80**: 2128–32.

59   Tourani JM, Pfister C, Berdah JF *et al.* Outpatient treatment with subcutaneous interleukin-2 and interferon-alpha administration in combination with fluorouracil in patients with metastatic renal cell carcinoma: results of a sequential nonrandomised phase II study. Subcutaneous administration propeukin program cooperative group. *J Clin Oncol* 1998; **16**: 2505–13.

60   Elias L, Lew D, Figlin RA *et al.* Infusional interleukin-2 and 5-fluorouracil with subcutaneous interferon-alpha for the treatment of patients with advanced renal cell carcinoma: a southwest oncology group phase II study. *Cancer* 2000; **89**: 597–603.

3: Surgical Management of Metastatic Renal Cancer

D. F. Badenoch

Introduction

In 1958 Flocks and Kadesky [1] developed the first system for staging renal cell carcinoma. This was later modified by Robson, Churchill and Anderson, and Robson *et al.*'s [2] system has been used in clinical practice by urologists ever since. The TNM staging system was first applied to renal cell carcinoma in 1974, and most recently has been revised by the UICC in 1997 [3,4] (Table 3.1).

Using these staging classifications, it has been shown in many studies that prognosis is related to clinical stage at presentation. Preoperative staging in renal cell carcinoma aims to delineate operability and exclude the presence of metastases before radical nephrectomy is undertaken. Excision of a primary renal cell carcinoma in the presence of metastases may be undertaken in limited circumstances. Nephrectomy is appropriate if the primary is causing uncontrollable symptoms, where there is a solitary metastasis and if there is synchronous or metachronous disease or metastases in the contralateral kidney.

Nephrectomy in the presence of metastatic disease remains a contentious issue among urologists. Nonetheless, there are still those who advocate a nephrectomy to be carried out in the management of metastatic renal cell carcinoma. As has been well reviewed by Montie [5], the procedure of radical nephrectomy is an invasive and potentially dangerous one and those surgeons who advocate it in the presence of metastases should have some evidence that it will improve the patient's life expectancy or at least the quality of life.

The rationale for nephrectomy in the presence of metastases

The role of nephrectomy in the induction of spontaneous regression of metastases

The first report of spontaneous regression of metastases following nephrectomy was by Bumpus in 1928 [6]. The incidence of such regression of metastases after nephrectomy is variably reported, but is probably in the region of

Table 3.1 The 1997 UICC TNM classification of renal cell carcinoma

pT1	Tumour ≤7.0 cm in greatest dimension limited to the kidney
pT2	Tumour >7.0 cm in greatest dimension limited to the kidney
pT3	Tumour extends into major veins, or invades adrenal or perinephric tissues but not beyond Gerota's fascia:
	pT3a: Tumour invades adrenal gland or perinephric tissues not beyond Gerota's fascia
	pT3b: Tumour grossly extends into renal veins or vena cava
	pT3c: Tumour grossly extends into vena cava above the diaphragm
pT4	Tumour invades beyond Gerota's fascia
pN0	No regional lymph node metastases
pN1	Metastasis in one regional lymph node
pN2	Metastasis in more than one regional lymph node
pN3	Metastasis in a lymph node >5.0 cm in greatest dimension
pM0	No distant metastasis
pM1	Distant metastasis

1% of cases. Few of these instances have histological confirmation of metastases, and it may be that in many cases the observation is merely of resolution of areas of consolidation secondary to infection [7–9]. It should be remembered that nephrectomy is not without risk and there is an operative mortality of approximately 3–5%. This is a major consideration in an evaluation of the benefits of nephrectomy in this particularly poor risk group of patients, and there is little objective evidence to support the strategy of performing nephrectomy in order to induce spontaneous regression of metastases.

The palliation of local symptoms

There has been support at times for removal of the primary tumour in the presence of metastatic disease in order to palliate symptoms caused by the primary tumour, the most common of these being disabling haematuria or local pain. The latter is rarely amenable to surgical intervention and the former is generally better managed by radiological embolization in order to abolish bleeding from the particular vessel or group of vessels that is causing the persistent haematuria [10,11].

Nephrectomy for psychological support

Although it is a natural urge for surgeons to perform surgery, and there are times when the patient and/or family may put pressure on the surgeon to perform radical nephrectomy in the presence of metastases, such an action cannot be satisfactorily supported in order to benefit the psychological requirements of the patient. More usually, this is done purely for the psychological benefit of the surgeon and should not be encouraged.

In order to improve response to chemotherapy, hormone therapy or immunotherapy

Although there has been some supportive evidence in animal tumour systems showing that removal of a large tumour burden can improve non-specific immunological function, the extrapolation to the human model is not proven. The idea of debulking surgery in this context has little objective support. There remain the rare anecdotal cases where immunotherapy has been shown to diminish the extent of the primary tumour. In this context, a nephrectomy might be entertained following effective immunotherapy with downstaging of the primary tumour [12–14].

Renal vein and inferior vena caval metastases

The pattern of spread of renal cell carcinoma in invading the renal veins and extending into the main renal vein as a tumour thrombus is well described and well recognized [15]. In addition a small number will go on to thrombus within the inferior vena cava itself. This is usually without direct invasion of the vessel wall. The relative frequency with which this occurs was not appreciated until quite recently. However, with modern preoperative evaluation by CT or MRI scans, the situation can be well recognized. When vena caval extension is recognized, this should be carefully followed with views of the chest in order to rule out extension to the supra-diaphragmatic vena cava or even into the right atrium [16,17].

Previously vena caval extensions were considered to describe a dire prognosis with little prospect for cure. However, where this alone is the totality of spread of the tumour, the patient can have the embolus removed and the outlook is by no means gloomy. Clayman *et al.* [18] in 1980 showed a significant chance of 1-year survival in those patients with vena caval extension successfully operated on. Even where the tumour extends into the right atrium, surgical excision can be considered in appropriate cases. Libertino *et al.*, in 1987 [19], reported a 10-year survival of 6-% in 32 patients without regional or metastatic disease but vena caval thrombosis, the majority of these being infra-diaphragmatic extensions.

The possibility of resection of caval thrombi has been significantly improved by collaboration between urologists and vascular and cardiac surgeons. Where the thrombus is situated above the diaphragm, then cardiac bypass with circulatory arrest must be available. There now exist several series where satisfactory results for this form of surgery have been obtained, with operative mortality rates which are from 5 to 10% [20–23]. Clearly this requires full and informed consent of the patient.

Occasionally there is invasion into the inferior vena cava wall, which requires resection of part of the vena cava. Generally the vena cava can be repaired adequately leaving a decent lumen for blood flow without the need for grafting, although the placement of a vascular graft on the vena cava is on occasion necessary [24].

The surgery of metastases

It occasionally arises that a solitary metastasis from renal cell carcinoma appears following the initial radical nephrectomy. This may be within a lung field or even in another area such as the bladder or contralateral adrenal gland. In such cases where the patient is otherwise fit and well, it is reasonable and sensible to think in terms of surgical excision of the metastatic lesion. Clearly if this is within the chest then a thoracic surgical colleague must be approached. Case reports of long-term survival in these circumstances exist, and provided that the patient is fully aware of the risk this is something that can be sensibly pursued [25–27].

Surgery for metastasis or metachronous tumour in the contralateral kidney

The development of a tumour in the contralateral kidney having previously undergone nephrectomy arises in up to 7% of patients with renal cell cancer. In these circumstances, where feasible, conservative surgery retaining as much viable kidney as possible must be considered provided that no further metastases exist. Full preoperative work to assess the exact extent of the tumour—which nowadays will involve spiral CT scans and/or MRI scans in order to look at the vascular anatomy more closely—is required, and then partial nephrectomy or even enucleation of the tumour can be performed [28–30]. It is always helpful to consider regional hypothermia in this procedure. It has been elegantly shown by Wickham *et al.* [31] that this enables prolonged renal artery clamping to take place so that excision of the tumour with or without partial nephrectomy can be carried out in a controlled fashion. Provided that the amount of kidney tissue left is adequate, this may allow the patient to forgo the need for subsequent dialysis. Full review of the patient by nephrology colleagues is required as part of the preoperative evaluation.

Conclusion

Although overall the prospect in renal cell carcinoma once metastases have developed is poor, evidence accrued over the last 20 years indicates that an aggressive surgical policy to renal vein and inferior vena caval metastatic spread is reasonable provided there are no other metastases and that the patient is fit. This requires extremely careful preparation and collaboration with disciplines of vascular and cardiac surgery. Likewise, if conservative surgery to the contralateral kidney is performed, regional hypothermia and collaboration with nephrologists is necessary. The operation of radical nephrectomy in the presence of metastases in order to induce spontaneous regression cannot be supported and there appears to be little logic in palliative radical nephrectomy in the face of metastases given the balance of risks involved.

References

1   Flocks RH, Kadesky MC. Malignant neoplasms of the kidney: an analysis of 353 patients followed 5 years or more. *J Urol* 1958; **79**: 196–201.
2   Robson CJ, Churchill BM, Anderson W. The results of radical nephrectomy for renal cell carcinoma. *J Urol* 1969; **101**: 297–301.
3   Harmer M. *TNM Classification of Malignant Tumours*, 2nd edn. Geneva: International Union Against Cancer, 1974.
4   Fleming ID, Cooper JS, Henson DE *et al. Cancer Staging Manual*, 5th edn. Philadelphia: Lippincott-Raven, 1997: 231–2.
5   Montie JE. Chapter 23a. In: Carlton EE, ed. *Controversies in Urology*. Yearbook Medical Publishers, 1989.
6   Bumpus HC Jr. The apparent disappearance of pulmonary metastasis in a case of hypernephroma following nephrectomy. *J Urol* 1928; **20**: 185.
7   Badenoch DF, Ross HB, Badenoch MP. Renal carcinoma presenting as a goitre. *Br J Urol* 1987; **59**: 361–2.
8   Montie JE, Stewart BH, Straffon RA, Banowsky LH, Hewitt CB, Montague DK. The role of adjunctive nephrectomy in patients with metastatic renal cell carcinoma. *J Urol* 1977; **117**: 272–5.
9   de Kernion JB, Ramming KP, Smith RB. Natural history of metastatic renal cell carcinoma. *J Urol* 1978; **120**: 148–52.
10 Wallace S, Chuang VP, Swanson D. Embolization of renal carcinoma: experience with 100 patients. *Radiology* 1981; **138**: 563.
11 Gottesman JE, Crawford ED, Grossman HB. Infarction—nephrectomy for metastatic renal carcinoma. *Cancer* 1985; **25**: 248.
12 McNicholls DW, Segura JW, Deweerd JH. Renal cell carcinoma: long term survival and late recurrences. *J Urol* 1981; **126**: 17.
13 Oliver RTD, Miller RM, Mehta A, Barnett MJ. A phase II study of surveillance in patients with metastatic renal cell carcinoma and assessment of response of such patients to therapy on progression. *J Mol Biother* 1988; **1**: 14–20.
14 Marcus SG, Choyke PL, Reitr R. Regression of metastatic renal cell carcinoma after cytoreductive nephrectomy. *J Urol* 1993; **150**: 154–66.
15 Skinner DJ, Colvin RB, Vemillion CD, Pfister RC, Leadbetter WF. Diagnosis and management of renal carcinoma: clinical and pathologist study of 309 cases. *Cancer* 1971; **28**: 1165.
16 Kearney GP, Waters WB, Klein LA, Richie JP, Gittes RF. Results of inferior vena cava resection for renal cell carcinoma. *J Urol* 1977; **118**: 474.
17 Giuliani L, Martorana G, Giberti C, Bonamini A, Gittes RF. Results of inferior vena cava resection for renal cell carcinoma. *Eur Urol* 1987; **13**: 22.
18 Clayman RV, Gonzalez R, Fraley EE. Renal cell carcinoma invading the inferior vena cava: clinical review and anatomical approach. *J Urol* 1980; **123**: 157.

19 Libertino JA, Zinman L, Watkins E Jr. Long-term results of resection of renal cell cancer with extension into inferior vena cava. *J Urol* 1987; **137**: 21.

20 Marshall FF, Reitz BA, Diamond DA. New technique for management of renal cell carcinoma involving right atrium: hypothermia and cardiac arrest. *J Urol* 1984; **131**: 103.

21 Vaislic CD, Puel P, Grondin P *et al*. Cancer of the kidney invading the vena cava and heart: results of 11 years of treatment. *J Thorac Cardiovas Surg* 1986; **91**: 604.

22 Novick OC, Cosgrove DM. Surgical approach for removal of renal cell carcinoma extending into the vena cava and the right atrium. *J Urol* 1980; **123**: 947.

23 Montie JE, Jackson CL, Cosgrove DM, Streem SB, Novick AC, Pontes JE. Resection of large inferior vena cava thrombi from renal cell carcinoma with the use of circulatory arrest. *J Urol* 1988; **139**: 25.

24 Shefft P, Novick AC, Straffon RA, Stewart BH. Survey for renal carcinoma extending into the inferior vena cava. *J Urol* 1978; **120**: 28.

25 Middleston RG. Surgery for metastatic renal cell carcinoma. *J Urol* 1967; **97**: 973.

26 Sosa RE, Muecke EC, Vaughan ED, McCarron JP. Renal cell carcinoma extending into the inferior vena cava: the prognostic significance of the level of vena cava involvement. *J Urol* 1984; **132**: 1097.

27 O'Dea MJ, Zincke H, Utz DC, Bernatz PE. Treatment of renal cell carcinoma with solitary metastases. *J Urol* 1978; **120**: 540.

28 Carini M, Selli C, Barbanit G, Lapini A, Turini D, Costantini A. Conservative surgical treatment of renal cell carcinoma: clinical experience and re-appraisal of indications. *J Urol* 1988; **140**: 725.

29 Marberger M, Pugh RCB, Auvert H *et al*. Conservative surgery of renal cell carcinoma: the EIRSS experience. 1981; **53**: 528.

30 Rosenthal CL, Kraft R, Zing EJ. Organ preserving surgery in renal cell carcinoma: tumour enucleation versus partial kidney resection. *Eur Urol* 1984; **10**: 222.

31 Wickham JEA, Coe N, Ward JP. One hundred cases of nephrolithotomy under hypothermia. *J Urol* 1974; **112**: 702.

Kidney Cancer: Commentary

J. Waxman

Although renal cell carcinoma is one of the less common malignancies, it is one of the tumours for which there has been the most changes in management in the last decade. These changes lead the way for many other malignancies.

The development of cytokine therapy for renal cell carcinoma has provided a significant benefit for patients. Durable remissions have been obtained through immunotherapy and I have seen examples of this in my own clinical practice with patients in remission 12 years from their presentation with metastatic disease.

Treatment with cytokines was initially extremely toxic; however, treatment regimens have been refined and are now less toxic. This allows the patient to be treated at home rather than in hospital. Alongside these immunological developments we have seen developments in the surgical treatment of this condition. Currently surgery is more frequently being offered to patients with limited numbers of metastases allowing cure to be contemplated. These changes have led to the identification of moleculer markers of kidney cancer that assist the pathologist in his work and define prognosis.

There have also been changes in our understanding of the molecular processes of renal cell carcinoma and in particular in the role of tumour suppressor genes.

We hope that over the next decade we will see further progress in immunotherapy such that a greater proportion of patients with metastatic kidney cancer can be cured.

Part 2
Bladder Cancer

4: The Molecular Biology of Bladder Cancer

P. E. Keegan, D. E. Neal & J. Lunec

Introduction

While great progress has been made in understanding the molecular biology of bladder cancer, attempts to use this information to influence favourably treatment options and patient outcomes are still unproven. The clinical application of basic research has centred on the development of prognostic markers to select aggressive treatment for patients with high risk tumours. The assumption is that the clinical behaviour of a bladder tumour can be predicted by its particular expression of tumour-suppressor genes, oncogenes and other molecular prognostic markers. Many potential targets for novel diagnostic and therapeutic approaches have also been identified. The rapid development of this field has led to a confusing picture, with different molecular markers being reported simultaneously as candidates for further study. Attempts to exploit this information for future patient benefit may require new approaches in the conduct of prognostic marker studies and perhaps the use of alternative statistical techniques, such as neural network analysis.

Basic science

In tumours the accumulation of genetic alterations, usually at the somatic level, leads to the loss of normal control of cell growth and differentiation. Often these genes are involved in the control of cell proliferation, either by activation of proto-oncogenes or by inactivation of tumour-suppressor genes (TSGs). Secondary changes lead to altered interactions of the cancer cell with its microenvironment through peptide growth factors, receptors, adhesion molecules and regulators of angiogenesis.

Cytogenic studies

Chromosomal deletions are common in cancer and for a given epithelial cancer seem to be non-random. Previously, cytogenetic analysis was used to identify loss of genetic material at specific sites. More recently, techniques including polymerase chain reaction (PCR)-based assays have uncovered more discrete abnormalities.

Loss of heterozygosity studies

TSG function is thought to be lost as a result of chromosome deletions containing one allele, accompanied by a defect in the remaining allele arising, for example, by point mutation. This concept is exploited by loss of heterozygosity (LOH) analyses that identify sites in the genome near possible TSGs. Where heterozygosity for a polymorphic DNA marker sequence, detected in normal tissue, is lost in analysis of matched tumour tissue, this indicates the marker is present in a deleted region. A panel of such markers that map to different regions of a chromosome can be used to define the extent of a deleted region. By comparing deletions for a number of tumours, a minimal region of common deletion is identified. Once a region has been found to be deleted commonly in bladder cancers, it can be searched for expressed sequences, which can then be assessed as candidate TSGs. This process has been helped greatly by advances in mapping the human genome. Table 4.1 shows TSGs and predicted TSG loci implicated in transitional cell carcinoma.

Comparative genomic hybridization and fluorescence *in situ* hybridization studies

Other molecular genetic techniques have been used to identify regions where genes are overexpressed in bladder cancer. Fluorescence *in situ* hybridization

Table 4.1 Gene loci implicated in transitional cell carcinoma and associated tumour-suppressor genes (adapted from [86])

Genetic location	Frequency of deletion/mutation	Tumour-suppressor gene/product
3p	48%	
4p	22%	
4q	24%	
8q	23%	
9p21	20–45%	CDKN2A(p16) and p14ARF
9q22	10–30%	PTEN
	LOH in 50%	PTCH
	Mutated in 4%	
9q34	LOH in 50%	TSC1
9q32–33	LOH in 50%	DBCCR1
11p	40%	
11q	15%	
13q14	30%	Rb
14q	10–40%	
17p13	10–70%	p53
18q		DCC/SMAD

Table 4.2 Oncogenes and potential oncogene loci genetically altered in transitional cell carcinoma (adapted from [86])

Gene	Observation
HRAS	Mutated in 6–44%
ERBB2	Amplified in 10–14%
CCND1	Amplified in 10–20%
(MYC) or other 8q gene	8q gain
	MYC overexpression
1q22–24	Amplification
3p24	Amplification
6p22	Amplification
8q21–22	Amplification
10p13–14	Amplification
10q22–23	Amplification
12q15	Amplification
20q	Amplification

(FISH) involves labelling of normal metaphase spreads simultaneously with different coloured fluorescent probes, derived from both normal and tumour tissue. A decrease or increase in the fluorescent signal from the tumour probe relative to the normal probe alters the colour balance, and indicates regions of possible gene deletion or amplification, respectively. Comparative genomic hybridization is an extension of this technique to involve the entire cellular chromosomal complement. These and other approaches have led to identification of some of the oncogenes and potential oncogene loci altered in bladder cancer presented in Table 4.2.

Cell cycle control and tumour-suppressor genes

Before discussing in detail studies of individual TSGs important in bladder cancer, it will be useful to document some of the molecular pathways by which these key molecules are thought to interact and function.

The cell growth and division cycle consists of a DNA synthesis phase (S phase), mitotic phase (M phase—during which chromosome condensation and segregation into dividing daughter cells takes place), and two intervening gap phases (G1 and G2). During G1, cells may either advance towards another division or withdraw from the cycle into a resting state (G0). In contrast to the S, G2 and M phases, progression through G1 is normally dependent on positive and negative extracellular signalling. For cancer cells to remain in the cell cycle they must overcome the normal regulatory mechanisms that restrict uncontrolled transit through the G1 phase [1].

Some key molecular pathways for cell cycle control are illustrated in Fig. 4.1. The function of the retinoblastoma (p105) phosphoprotein and its family

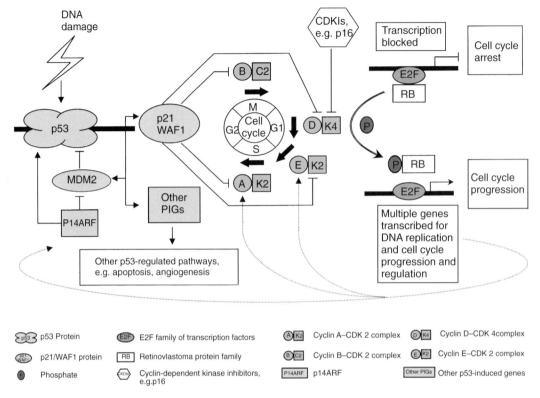

Figure 4.1 p53-mediated cell cycle arrest results from the stimulation of p21/WAF1 transcription, which in turn inhibits cyclin–CDK activity. This results in hypophosphorylated retinoblastoma protein accumulation which subsequently blocks E2F-dependent transcription, causing cell cycle arrest. Interactions with MDM2, p14ARF and cyclin-dependent kinase inhibitors (CDKIs) are also shown. The illustrated molecular pathways are fundamental for cell cycle arrest and are likely to be perturbed at some level in all cancers.

members (p107 and p130) is central to cell cycle regulation. These proteins control the cell cycle by interacting with the E2F family (E2F1–5) of transcription factors. These promote transcription of the genes necessary for DNA replication and cell cycle progression. During the G0/G1 phase of the cell cycle the retinoblastoma protein is hypophosphorylated, in which state it can bind E2F1 and repress its function. When retinoblastoma protein becomes phosphorylated on progression into the S phase, it no longer binds E2F and stops repressing E2F function, allowing the cell cycle to progress. A family of proteins called cyclins, in association with cyclin-dependent kinases (CDKs), phosphorylates retinoblastoma, and thereby promotes cell cycle progression. The complex of cyclin D to CDK4 is initially responsible for phosphorylation of retinoblastoma during G1. The cyclin E–CDK2 complex accelerates the process. Other cyclin–CDK complexes act to maintain retinoblastoma proteins in the phosphorylated state at other points in the cycle until cells complete mitosis and re-enter the G1 phase [2].

One of the best-characterized pathways for negative growth regulation operating through the above pathway involves the stimulation of transcription of the WAF1/CIP/SDI/p21 gene by activated p53. This encodes the p21/WAF1 protein, which is an inhibitor of cyclin–CDK activity (cyclin-dependent kinase inhibitor—CDKI). Hypophosphorylated retinoblastoma protein then accumulates, blocking E2F-dependent transcription and causing cell cycle arrest. This is not the only mechanism of negative growth regulation by p53, which also can have a direct inhibitory effect on the DNA synthesis machinery. Other specific CDK inhibitors, for example p16 (often mutated in bladder cancer), negatively regulate cell cycle progression in a p53-independent manner. More recently the p19ARF tumour-suppressor gene has been shown to both activate p53 and inhibit MDM2 function. MDM2 normally has the key role of keeping p53-mediated functions in check by binding to p53—both enhancing its degradation and blocking transcription of p53-induced genes (PIGs). The molecular pathways illustrated in Fig. 4.1 are fundamental to the process of the control of the cell cycle and are likely to be perturbed at some level in all cancers [3].

Apoptosis

Programmed cell death (apoptosis) eliminates cells during normal embryonic development and also during the normal turnover of cells in healthy adult tissues. When cells develop damage to DNA, they may undergo apoptosis—by means of p53-dependent or -independent pathways. In this way, cells at risk of cancerous development are effectively eliminated [4], and failure to undergo apoptosis can be considered a mechanism of carcinogenesis. Radiotherapy and DNA damaging agents used in chemotherapy may induce apoptosis in tumour tissue. Studies of apoptotic pathways (see Fig. 4.2) may therefore help identify prognostic factors that predict treatment response. In this context controversy exists as to whether p53 mutations in bladder cancer lead to enhanced or reduced chemosensitivity [5].

Recently multiple genes that encode proteins which regulate levels of reactive oxygen species within cells have been reported to be induced by p53, before the onset of apoptosis [6]. This has led to a proposed model of p53-induced apoptosis through transcriptional induction of p53-related genes, the formation of reactive oxygen species and the oxidative degradation of cellular components culminating in cell death. The validity of this model in different circumstances remains to be established. Cell cycle arrest and the induction of apoptosis are the main downstream effects of p53 activation.

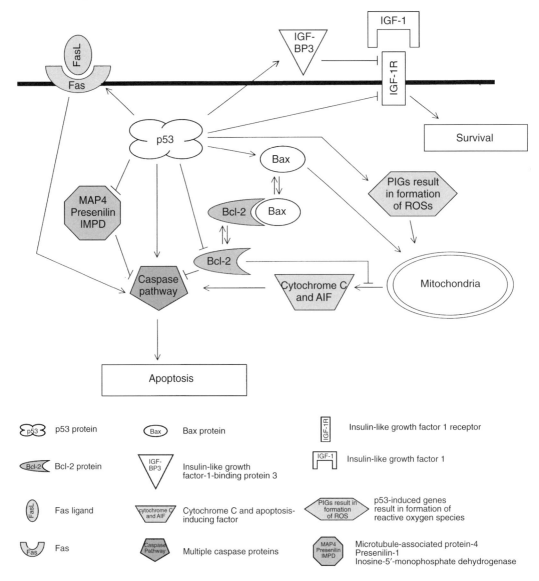

Figure 4.2 Pathways for p53-mediated apoptosis (adapted from Sionov & Haupt [85] with the permission of Nature Publishing Group). p53 promotes expression of pro-apoptotic genes (including PIGs, Bax, IGF-BP3 and Fas) and represses expression of survival-promoting genes (including IGF-1R, Bcl-2, MAP4, Presenilin, IMPD). p53 activates caspase pathways directly stimulating apoptosis as well as via pathways involving cell surface receptors (e.g. Fas) and mitochondria (e.g. release of apoptosis inducing factor (AIF) and cytochrome C). The ratio of Bax to Bcl-2 (and their family members) is also important in determining whether apoptosis takes place.

p53

The protein encoded by the p53 tumour-suppressor gene, located on chromosome 17p13.1, is a 393 amino acid, 53-kDa nuclear phosphoprotein critical for cellular response to genotoxic insult [7]. It is well accepted that inactivation of p53 function is a key event in tumorigenesis. The gene is lost or mutated in over 50% of human tumours [8], the most common specific gene defect yet discovered in cancer. Furthermore it is likely that many tumours with non-mutated, wild type p53 will have alterations either in the pathways which regulate p53 function or in the downstream pathways concerned with effecting a p53-mediated response. This suggests therefore that p53 function is aberrant in a greater number of human tumours than originally estimated [4].

Most translational research into bladder cancer has involved the application of immunohistochemical techniques. The levels of p53 in normal cells are usually below the threshold for detection by immunohistochemical methods [9]. Mutations in p53 may increase the stability of the protein, resulting in a prolonged half-life and detectable accumulation. Cordon-Cardo and colleagues [10] compared p53 genetic sequencing with p53 immunohistochemistry (IHC) in bladder cancer, and estimated the accuracy of detection of p53 mutations by IHC at 90.3%. Many studies have cited this work when defining positive p53 IHC as being greater than a threshold of 20% positive nuclear staining. However, this paper did not report which individual threshold of p53 positivity best predicted mutations, and actually studied nine threshold values. Others have reported that positive p53 IHC occurs frequently in bladder cancer, even in the absence of mutations [11]. Interestingly this study suggested that positive p53 IHC (50% nuclear staining threshold) predicted worse survival in tumours without p53 mutations. Abnormally upregulated wild type p53 detected by IHC may therefore have prognostic value. The dual detection of both mutated and abnormally expressed non-mutated p53 might even enhance the prognostic value of p53 IHC in bladder cancer [12].

Positive staining in the absence of mutation can occur when levels of non-mutated wild type p53 are abnormally expressed [13], such as following cellular stress due, for example, to ultraviolet light damage or hypoxia. The stability of p53 is also altered by binding to intracellular proteins such as MDM2 or the expression of certain oncogenes. False negatives, in which there is no detectable protein product from a p53 mutation, are thought to occur relatively rarely compared with stabilization by point mis-sense mutations [14].

Following reports that abnormalities of the p53 gene occurred commonly in bladder cancer [15,16] and that increased p53 IHC was associated with high stage and grade, there have been over 40 published studies on p53 IHC and its relationship to clinical outcome in bladder cancer. In order for p53 to be a valuable marker for routine clinical use, IHC must provide prognostic information that is independent of conventional prognostic factors. This may be assessed using multivariate analysis. Many such studies have concluded that p53 IHC can provide independent prognostic information whilst others have failed to demonstrate a relationship independent of traditional prognostic factors such as stage, grade, frequency of recurrence, presence of carcinoma *in situ* and multifocality. Where p53 IHC has not been found independent of grade as a molecular prognostic factor it could still be of some value if it can be more objectively determined. It is well documented that the discordance between pathologists in assessing grade can be as high as 50% [17]. Other studies have even failed to find any prognostic value for p53 IHC regardless of whether it is independent. Some of the studies on p53 IHC and its prognostic value are presented in Table 4.3.

INTERPRETING P53 EXPRESSION

Difficulties arise in comparing these studies which result from a number of variables. Differences in tissue fixing, antigen retrieval, antibody source and definition of p53 positivity all lead to significant differences in results [18].

Recently the statistical pitfalls associated with the inappropriate use of cut-points in prognostic marker studies have been highlighted [19–22]. The importance of p53 IHC in predicting clinical outcome has certainly been overstated in some studies as a result of this problem. Power calculations should also be stated when studies report a negative finding in order to put negative conclusions in perspective [23].

Some studies have concentrated on specific stages of bladder cancer while others have included all stages. Important differences also exist in the treatment modalities received by patients. Some studies have assessed the prognostic value of p53 IHC in clearly defined groups of patients all receiving the same treatment (see Table 4.3). Others have studied more heterogeneous groups of patients whose various treatments were less clearly defined.

Where patients with a single clearly defined stage of disease, who have all been treated similarly, have been studied some interesting results have been reported. In carcinoma *in situ* (CIS) p53 IHC has been reported to be an independent prognostic marker for progression [24]. Positive p53 IHC post therapy (4 weeks following 6 weekly instillations) was a prognostic indicator for progression in 60 patients with CIS treated with intravesical BCG therapy, but it was not independent of having had a clinical BCG response [25]. In Ta disease p53 IHC was found to have independent prognostic value for progression in 54 patients [26] and for progression and recurrence in 59 patients [27].

Table 4.3 Studies of p53 IHC and its prognostic value in bladder cancer

Reference	Year	Study size	Type of tumours	p53 antibody used	% positive staining cut-off levels used	Comments	Independent prognostic information in multivariate analysis	Possible bias from explicit choice of optimal threshold
37	1996	109	T2–T4	Monoclonal Do-1	20	Prognostic indicator for survival of T3b disease (preop DXT)	Yes in subgroup analysis (Independent of tumour size and pathological downstaging)	
27	1997	59	TaG1	Monoclonal Do-7	0, 5	0% threshold and not 5% threshold p53 IHC was independent predictor of progression and recurrence	Yes (Independent of tumour size, focality and recurrence)	Yes
87	1996	98	Ta, Tis, T1	Monoclonal 1801	20	In patients failing to respond to BCG post-BCG p53 IHC predicts progression	Yes (Independent of pre-BCG stage, pre-BCG p53 status and BCG response)	
33	1995	90	T2–T4	Monoclonal 1801	20	Neoadjuvant MVAC followed by cystectomy	Yes (Independent of performance status, grade, stage, size, multifocality, ureteral obstruction and palpable mass)	
34	1995	44	T2–T4	Monoclonal 1801	20, 40, 60, 80	Independent predictor of survival at 40% cut-off	Yes (Independent of grade, stage, lymph node status, chemotherapy and PCNA positivity)	Yes
38	1994	243	Ta–T4	Monoclonal 1801	10	Cystectomy patients	Yes (Independent of grade, stage and lymph node status)	

Continued p. 68

Table 4.3 *Continued*

Reference	Year	Study size	Type of tumours	p53 antibody used	% positive staining cut-off levels used	Comments	Independent prognostic information in multivariate analysis	Possible bias from explicit choice of optimal threshold
28	1995	69	T1	Monoclonal 1801	20, 40, 60, 80		Yes (Independent of grade, age, sex and proliferative activity)	
30	1997	32	T1	Monoclonal Do-7	20	Predicted which T1 responded/failed to respond to BCG in selected patients	Yes (Independent of Bcl-2, capthesin-D, Ki67, c-erbB-2, c-myc) ?too many variables for small sample	
26	1993	54	Ta	Monoclonal 1801	20		Yes (Independent of age, sex, grade and BCG therapy)	
24	1994	33	CIS	Monoclonal 1801	20		Yes (Independent of age, sex, associated Ta tumour and BCG therapy)	
29	1993	21	pT1	Polyclonal rabbit CM1	0, 10, 30, 50, 70, 90	>10% p53 predicted progression	Not done (small study)	Yes
5	1997	88	?	Monoclonal 1801	10	Adjuvant chemotherapy resulted in reduced recurrence in p53 positive but not p53 negative tumours	Not applicable	
40	1996	265	Ta–T1	Polyclonal rabbit BC11	0	p53, Rb and HER-2/neu	No	Yes

88	1994	234	Ta–T4	Polyclonal rabbit CM1	20	p53, EGFR and c-erbB-2 (EGFR was independent prognostic marker)	No
41	1993	212	Ta–T4	Polyclonal rabbit CM1	20	p53 predicted survival in whole group but was not independent in MVA	No
36	1995	154	T2–T4	Monoclonal 1801	30	Response to DXT	No
39	1996	106	Ta–T4	Polyclonal sheep	Own scoring system	—	No
43	1995	97	Ta–T4	Monoclonal 1801	10	—	No
42	1998	83	Ta–T4	Monoclonal Do-7	10	Mixed stage and treatments. No independent value for p53 in this study	No
25	1997	60	CIS	?	20	p53 post-BCG prognostic indicator for progression but non-independent to BCG response	No
47	1997	59	Ta–T1	Monoclonal 1801	20	p53 not independent prognostic marker but p53 and Rb together were	No
44	1997	51	Ta–T4	Monoclonal Do-7	20	DNA ploidy and p53	No
35	1996	41	T2–T4	Monoclonals Do-1, Do-7	5, 20, 50	p53 and Bcl-2 in cystectomy patients	No
32	1994	28	pT1	Monoclonals 1801, Do-7	10, 25, 50, 75	—	No
31	1998	25	T1	?	0, 5, 10, 20, 35, 40, 45, 55, 65	Despite MPV type approach no prediction of BCG response	Yes

This later study based its threshold for p53 positivity on patient outcome, thereby possibly introducing bias.

In 69 patients T1 bladder cancer p53 IHC was shown to predict progression independent of grade, age, sex and proliferative activity as determined by proliferating cell nuclear antigen (PCNA) positivity [28]. This result confirmed that of a previous study of 21 T1 patients where positive p53 IHC also predicted progression [29]. Multivariate analysis was avoided in this study due to small sample size, but bias due to an explicit choice of an optimal cut-point may have also been introduced. The response of T1 tumours to BCG has also been studied. In 32 patients p53 IHC in pretreatment samples predicted for BCG response [30]. By contrast, p53 IHC failed to predict BCG response in a further group of 25 patients [31]. In another study of 28 tumours, p53 was not found to be a prognostic marker in T1 disease. The considerable variation in p53 expression reported in different studies confirms the variability of inter- and intra-tumour staining with different immunohistochemical methods [32].

p53 positivity independently predicted poor survival in 90 patients with invasive disease, treated with neoadjuvant MVAC prior to radical surgery [33]. In muscle invasive disease, positive p53 IHC has also been reported to independently predict survival in 44 patients undergoing radical cystectomy [34]. There is a problem with interpretation in this study because of the explicit choice of the best threshold to predicate for outcome. In a similar study of 41 patients no prognostic value was found, even as a non-independent marker of survival in univariate analysis [35]. A study of 154 patients with invasive tumours who received radical radiotherapy failed to find any predictive value of p53 IHC for local recurrence or survival [36]. Similarly in 109 patients with muscle invasive disease also treated with radiotherapy, p53 IHC was not of prognostic value for the whole group [37]. This paper, however, performed subgroup analysis and found that in 30 selected patients with T3b disease, positive p53 IHC appeared to have prognostic value independent of grade, tumour size, pretreatment haemoglobin level and radiotherapy pathological response for predicting survival.

In a study of 243 patients who had radical surgery for both superficial and muscle invasive disease, positive p53 IHC was a predictor of recurrence and overall survival independent of grade, stage and lymph node status [38]. For organ confined disease it was the only independent predictor of survival. These authors suggested that p53 status could help identify patients who might benefit from radical surgery and adjuvant therapy. In 88 patients with transitional cell carcinoma treated by radical cystectomy and randomized to receive adjuvant chemotherapy or observation, retrospective p53 IHC analysis appeared to show only patients with abnormal p53 status had a recurrence and survival benefit from chemotherapy [5].

There have been numerous studies which have failed to establish a role for p53 IHC as an independent prognostic factor in bladder cancer. In three large studies with polyclonal antibodies, p53 IHC failed to independently predict clinical outcome. Underwood *et al.* [39] applied a staining index that combined percentage staining and intensity to 106 superficial and invasive tumours with a sheep polyclonal antibody to p53, and did not find a predictive value. Using a polyclonal rabbit antibody, Tetu *et al.* [40] found positive p53 IHC predicted time to recurrence in univariate analysis in 264 superficial tumours (Ta = 208, T1 = 56). Multivariate analysis, however, failed to identify p53 expression as an independent predictor of recurrence. Similarly, using a polyclonal rabbit antibody in 212 tumours (Ta = 39, T1 = 57, T2–4 = 116) positive p53 IHC was shown to predict poor outcome but did not have independent prognostic valve [41]. The differences in findings with polyclonal as compared with monoclonal antibodies might relate to possible increased cross-reactivity or increased sensitivity, resulting in greater detection of non-mutant p53 expression, perhaps resulting in a decreased prognostic value [12]. Alternatively the value of p53 IHC as an independent prognostic marker with monoclonal antibodies may have been overestimated. This is certainly the case for at least some of the published studies where the threshold of percentage nuclear staining used to define positivity was based on the point which produced the smallest *P*-value in survival analysis [22].

Many more studies of patients with various stages of disease and types of treatment have also failed to report a prognostic value for p53 IHC in bladder cancer independent of established factors [42–44]. It is possible, however, that by simultaneously studying heterogeneous groups of patients with mixed stage, grade and treatments received, prognostic value for p53 IHC in defined subgroups of patients could be obscured.

While the clinical use of p53 IHC remains controversial it is arguably the most studied molecular prognostic test in bladder cancer. This has led in the United States to a National Institutes of Health funded, prospective multi-institutional randomized trial to evaluate the role of chemotherapy for organ confined bladder cancer based on p53 analysis as determined by immunohistochemistry. At present p53 is the only example of a molecular prognostic marker influencing bladder cancer treatment, with assignment of patients, based on p53 IHC results, to either three cycles of adjuvant chemotherapy or observation as part of this study.

PCR-based direct DNA sequencing studies have confirmed p53 mutations to be more common in invasive tumours, but in contrast to p53 IHC studies have not demonstrated, perhaps because of small study size, a prognostic value independent of traditional factors. Recently a functional assay in yeast has been used to measure p53 mutations that result in loss of p53 function. In this study p53 mutations, as detected by this elegant technique, predicted the response of 24 T1G3 and 2 CIS tumours to BCG instillation therapy [45]. This study did not compare these results with either direct sequencing or p53 IHC. This method cannot be applied to most routinely processed paraffin embedded samples. As complex molecular biological techniques are un- likely to be introduced into standard clinical practice in the near future, IHC remains the most likely method for assessment in clinical practice of molecular prognostic information.

Retinoblastoma

The retinoblastoma (Rb) gene product binds to the E2F transcription factor and blocks transcription of genes critical for cell cycle progression. Rb is inactivated by phosphorylation, thereby releasing this negative control. Mutations or deletions of this gene can contribute to the loss of cell cycle regulation seen in cancer. The large size of this gene has precluded extensive sequencing studies. The development of more efficient and readily accessible automated DNA sequencing systems may remove this barrier.

Several studies have assessed the role of Rb IHC as a prognostic marker in bladder cancer. Wright *et al.* [46] found positive p53 IHC and negative Rb IHC to be associated with muscle invasion and high grade, in addition to an increased tumour cell growth fraction as assessed by Ki67 IHC. In a further study of 74 cases, lack of positive Rb IHC correlated with grade but did not predict time to recurrence [40]. Cordon-Cardo *et al.* [47] studied 59 superficial tumours (Ta = 28, T1 = 31) with both p53 and Rb IHC. A com- bination of p53 positive IHC and Rb negative IHC was an independent predictor of disease progression in this study, as shown in 45 T1 tumours treated by transurethral resection, and 185 invasive tumours treated by radical cystectomy. In these studies multivariate analysis was not done and normal Rb staining was compared with abnormal expression defined as either negative or strong staining, based on the observation that these patients did equally badly [48,49]. A recent study has suggested that abnormally strong Rb IHC in bladder cancer is associated with loss of p16 function (see below) [50].

In 97 patients treated with radiotherapy Pollack *et al.* [51] found nega- tive Rb IHC independently predicted pathological response, but did not predict patient outcome. Despite this finding, in 24 patients with stage T3b disease loss of Rb expression predicted a poor outcome, although this was not independent of p53 IHC in multivariate analysis. By contrast, in a similar study by Jahnson *et al.* [36] no prognostic value was observed for negative Rb IHC as a prognostic indicator for muscle invasive disease treated by radiotherapy.

Further studies are required to establish a clear role for Rb IHC as independent from established prognostic factors and from p53 IHC in bladder cancer. Its use in combination with p53 IHC, however, appears promising, and is supported by theoretical models which suggest that inactivation of both Rb and p53 pathways may be required for transformation and immortalization of urothelial cells. As the phosphorylation status of Rb is a key factor in determining cell cycle progression this also warrants assessment for its prognostic value in bladder cancer.

p14ARF and p16

Deletions involving 9p and/or 9q occur in 60% of bladder tumours [52]. Recently, studies have focused on the INK4 locus at chromosome 9p21 which encodes p16 and p15, both cyclin-dependent kinase inhibitors, and p14ARF, which is analogous with p19ARF in mice, and which binds MDM2 thereby activating p53 function. Interestingly, part of the genetic sequence that encodes p16 (INK4A) is shared by p14ARF but due to translation in an *alternative reading frame* (hence ARF) the protein products are unrelated.

In a study of 85 Ta and 21 T1 bladder tumours, INK4A deletions, which affect both p16 and p14ARF, predicted recurrence in univariate analysis. The number of tumours at presentation, however, was the only significant prognostic marker for recurrence in a multivariate analysis that included INK4A deletions, stage, grade and tumour size [53]. The p16 gene can be inactivated by methylation of its promoter region in addition to inactivation by mutation. This study also performed p16 IHC and showed that neither normal urothelium nor tumours with p14ARF/p16 deletions or a methylated p16 promoter had detectable p16 expression. While this might limit the use of p16 IHC, abnormally strong Rb IHC in bladder cancer is associated with loss of p16 function [50]. This further strengthens the observation that tumours both with negative and abnormally high Rb IHC do badly. Less is known about the potential prognostic role of p14ARF in bladder cancer. A recent study of 19 bladder tumour cell lines showed inactivation of both the p14ARF/p53 and the CDKN2A(p16)/Rb pathways in all but one line [54]. Clearly the role of p14ARF and its prognostic significance requires evaluation in bladder cancer.

p21/WAF1

p21/WAF1 is a cyclin-dependent kinase inhibitor important for p53-mediated cell cycle arrest. Mutations of WAF1 are not found commonly in bladder cancer, or in any other tumour for that matter, and WAF1 knock-out mice are not cancer prone [55,56]. This has led to the conclusion that WAF1 does not mediate the tumour-suppressor properties of p53. In a series of 173 patients with primary bladder cancer, p21/WAF1 immunoreactivity was inversely correlated with tumour stage, grade, p53 protein accumulation and Ki67 expression, but was not found to have a prognostic value in superficial disease. WAF1 positivity in muscle invasive disease, however, was shown to be significantly correlated with improved survival [57]. In 242 patients treated with cystectomy for bladder cancer, positive p21 IHC predicted better out-come, and was independent of grade, stage and p53 IHC in multivariate analysis. Higher rates of recurrence and decreased survival were seen in the p53 positive, WAF1 negative tumours [58]. By contrast, in 186 patients with Ta–T4 disease p21 IHC was not related to stage, grade or prognosis even in univariate analysis [59].

Loss of function of tumour-suppressor genes is central to the development and progression of bladder cancer. Furthermore, assessment by IHC has shown potential for their use as molecular prognostic markers. Other studies have focused on the abnormal expression of proto-oncogenes, peptide growth factors and receptors, adhesion molecules, proliferation markers and regulators of angiogenesis. The growing list of potential molecular prognostic markers described in bladder cancer is presented in Table 4.4.

MDM2, EGFR, proliferation antigens and angiogenesis

The MDM2 oncogene was first described as an amplified gene on double minute chromosomes present in a transformed mouse cell line (3T3DM) hence its name *Murine Double Minute* gene 2 [60]. The MDM2 protein binds to p53 and blocks transcription of p53-induced genes and also promotes p53 degradation. The transcription of the MDM2 gene is positively regulated by p53, thus MDM2 acts as an autoregulatory feedback inhibitor of p53 func-tion. Its critical importance as a regulator of p53 has been elegantly demon-strated by knock-out mice experiments [61,62]. While mice lacking MDM2 genes are non-viable, mice which lack both MDM2 and p53 genes are viable. Consequently MDM2 is thought to protect the normal cell from p53 over-activity [63].

Lianes *et al.* [64] reported greater than 20% nuclear staining with MDM2 IHC in 30% of 87 bladder tumours and found an association with low grade and stage. MDM2 overexpression was also associated with positive p53 IHC in 16 tumours in this study. By contrast, positive p53 IHC and positive MDM2 IHC were not co-correlated in 25 tumours studied by Barbareschi *et al.* [65], who suggested that combining MDM2 and p53 evaluation might be of prog-

Table 4.4 Potential molecular prognostic markers described in bladder cancer. For review see Stein *et al.* [89]

Tumour-suppressor genes and cell cycle inhibitors
  p53
  p21/WAF1
  Rb
  p16
  p14ARF
Oncogenes
  MDM2
  Cyclin-dependent kinases
  Ras
  c-myc
  c-jun
Components of apoptosis pathways
  Apoptosis counts
  Bcl-2
  Bax
Epidermal growth factor receptor family
  Epidermal growth factor receptor
  c-erbB-2
Metalloproteinases
Angiogenesis and angiogenesis inhibitors
  Microvessel density count
  Vascular endothelial growth factor
  Thrombospondin-1
Cell adhesion molecules
  Large families of adhesion molecules include:
  Cadherins
  Selectins
  Integrins
  Immunoglobulin-like cellular adhesion molecules
Blood group antigens
Proliferation markers
  Mitotic count
  Silver stained nucleolar organizer regions
  Ki67
  Proliferating cell nuclear antigen
Determinants of response to chemotherapy and radiotherapy
  Multidrug resistance genes
  DNA repair genes
  Drug-metabolizing enzyme polymorphisms

nostic relevance. The prognostic value of simultaneous p53 and MDM2 IHC in 61 patients with superficial bladder cancer has been reported. Schmitz-Drager *et al.* [66] confirmed p53 IHC (>5% intense nuclear staining with monoclonal antibody Do-1) to independently predict progression, but MDM2 IHC (>5% intense nuclear staining with monoclonal antibody Ab-1, clone IF2) alone had no prognostic value. However, combined p53 and MDM2 IHC proved a highly significant predictor of progression independent of smoking, multifocal disease and p53 accumulation in multivariate analysis. This study also showed no correlation between positive p53 IHC and positive MDM2 IHC. It also showed 49% of T1 lesions overexpressed MDM2 compared with 22% of muscle invasive tumours.

Combined p53 and MDM2 IHC has also been shown to correlate strongly with basement membrane degradation in 29 superficial tumours (Ta = 23, T1 = 6) [67]. In a study of 106 tumours (Ta–T4), combined p53 and MDM2 IHC predicted survival in univariate analysis, but stage, type of therapy and Ki67 were the only independent markers for survival in multivariate analysis in this study [68]. More recently, in 84 tumours treated by cystectomy the combined p53 and MDM2 IHC category and stage were independent of grade, cell proliferation and apoptotic markers for predicting progression and survival in multivariate analysis [69].

Multiple isoforms of MDM2 protein have been described. Novel forms of alternatively spliced MDM2 transcripts have also been reported and found more commonly in muscle invasive bladder cancer [70]. Which isoforms of MDM2 expressed in bladder cancer are recognized by the various MDM2 antibodies used for MDM2 IHC is unknown. Clearly, this may have important implications when selecting which antibody should be used for MDM2 IHC.

Epidermal growth factor receptor (EGFR)

EGFR is a cell surface receptor. Ligand binding can result in both homodimerization and heterodimerization, with c-erbB-2 and c-erbB-3, with subsequent activation of tyrosine kinase activity. The resulting phosphorylation of secondary messenger proteins through the Ras–Map kinase pathway then promotes changes including DNA synthesis and cell proliferation. Following reports that EGFR was overexpressed in invasive tumours [71] EGFR IHC was shown to be a predictor of survival in 101 patients independent of other factors including size, stage and grade (Ta–T4) [72]. Subsequently, when this series was extended to 212 patients EGFR IHC had value independent from stage, grade and other risk factors for predicting stage progression in addition to survival [73]. In 110 Ta and T1 tumours EGFR IHC predicted progression independently of T category [74]. However, it was not found to have prognostic value for survival in the entire cohort of 234 (Ta–T4) patients independent from the other prognostic factors studied. S-phase fraction (SPF), a marker of proliferation, was an independent marker for survival in the whole cohort in this study.

EGFR IHC did not have value in superficial tumours for predicting survival and recurrence free survival, as shown by univariate analyses. Despite this, a prognostic value for EGFR IHC was reported, independent of other prognostic factors, following multivariate analysis in the same group using these same end-points. In 173 invasive bladder tumours (T1–T4) treated with cystectomy, EGFR IHC was not found to have a prognostic value independent of stage [75]. This was also the finding in 85 patients with invasive disease [76]. Studies in defined groups of patients with the same stage of disease and treatment received may help establish if EGFR IHC has a future role as a prognostic marker. Its use appears more promising in superficial disease.

Proliferation antigens

Many studies have assessed the role of proliferation antigens as prognostic markers in bladder cancer. Methods used include mitotic count, silver stained nucleolar organizer regions (AgNOR), Ki67 IHC and PCNA IHC. In general an increase in proliferation has been found to be associated with increasing stage and grade. Several studies have suggested proliferation markers are useful for predicting prognosis in bladder cancer [77,78]. The role of MIB-1 IHC, which is a proliferation marker similar to Ki67, as a prognostic marker independent of p53 IHC, stage, grade, size and growth has also been demonstrated in bladder cancer [79]. The prognostic value of this marker in both univariate and multivariate analysis may have been overestimated in some studies of other malignancies. This problem results from the selection and use of a threshold value in the proliferation marker that gives the smallest *P*-value in survival analysis [22].

Angiogenesis and angiogenesis inhibitors

Angiogenesis, quantified by measuring mean blood vessel density (MVD), has been claimed to be of prognostic value in superficial [80] and muscle invasive bladder cancer [81], although these claims have been the subject of debate [22]. mRNA levels of vascular endothelial growth factor (VEGF), a potent stimulator of angiogenesis, have been reported to be of prognostic value in bladder cancer [82]. However, a prognostic role for VEGF IHC independent of established prognostic factors has not yet been reported. Thrombospondin (TSP) is induced by p53 and is a potent inhibitor of angiogenesis. It may therefore have tumour-suppressor activity by inhibiting the potential of a tumour to develop a blood supply. The bladders of 163 patients who underwent radical cystectomy for invasive disease were examined for TSP expression by IHC [83]. Patients with low TSP expression were found to have increased recurrence rates and decreased survival. TSP status was independent of stage, lymph node involvement and grade as a predictor of recurrence and survival, but was not independent of positive p53 IHC status.

Combinations of prognostic markers

The simultaneous measurement of a number of molecular prognostic markers is likely to be necessary to provide clinically useful prognostic information. Questions then arise as to which prognostic markers should be combined to predict the behaviour of an individual bladder tumour. The value of new molecular markers over conventional markers is often assessed by multivariate analysis. Arguably, then, molecular markers for use in combinations should have value independent not only of conventional factors but also of each other. To study combinations of prognostic markers, current practice is often to define a threshold for each marker which is positive or negative, and then compare outcome between the patient groups. This can result either in severe bias or in loss of power, depending on how thresholds are chosen [22].

Recently artificial neural network (ANN) analysis has been used to predict patient outcome in bladder cancer with combined conventional prognostic markers and EGFR, c-erbB-2 and p53 status as assessed by IHC [84]. Techniques such as ANN analysis provide a possible way of combining multiple potential prognostic markers with conventional prognostic information to predict an individual patient's prognosis. Furthermore, where a prognostic factor has been measured as a continuous variable statistical problems introduced by its categorization could be avoided. In this recent study, however, molecular information was entered as categorical variables (i.e. positive or negative expression).

Conclusion

Molecular biology studies have provided not only a host of potential molecular prognostic factors but also a sound theoretical basis why such factors may predict prognosis in bladder cancer. Many potential targets for novel diagnostic and therapeutic approaches have been identified in the process of their discovery. The challenge remains of translating this information into treatment which favourably influences patient outcome. Just as a significant sophistication has developed in the conduct of clinical trials, prognostic factor studies are now receiving greater critical attention. It is likely that with high quality studies, in clearly defined patient groups, immunohistochemical analysis of combinations of molecular markers will provide clinically useful prognostic information.

References

1   Sherr CJ. Cancer cell cycles. *Science* 1996; **274**: 1672–7.

2   Velculescu VE, El-Deiry WS. Biological and clinical importance of the p53 tumor suppressor gene. *Clin Chem* 1996; **42**: 858–68.

3   Helin K, Peters G. Tumor suppressors: from genes to function and possible therapies. *Trends Genet* 1998; **14**: 8–9.

4   Gottlieb TM, Oren M. p53 in growth control and neoplasia. *Biochim Biophys Acta* 1996; **1287**: 77–102.

5   Cote RJ, Esrig D, Groshen S, Jones PA, Skinner DG. p53 and treatment of bladder cancer. *Nature* 1997; **385**: 123–5.

6   Polyak K, Xia Y, Zweier JL, Kinzler KW, Vogelstein B. A model for p53-induced apoptosis. *Nature* 1997; **389**: 300–5.

7   Cox LS, Lane DP. Tumour suppressors, kinases and clamps: how p53 regulates the cell cycle in response to DNA damage. *Bioessays* 1995; **17**: 501–8.

8   Hollstein M, Sidransky D, Vogelstein B, Harris CC. p53 mutations in human cancers. *Science* 1991; **253**: 49–53.

9   Finlay CA, Hinds PW, Tan TH, Eliyahu D, Oren M, Levine AJ. Activating mutations for transformation by p53 produce a gene product that forms an hsc70–p53 complex with an altered half-life. *Mol Cell Biol* 1988; **8**: 531–9.

10 Cordon-Cardo C, Dalbagni G, Saez GT *et al.* p53 mutations in human bladder cancer: genotypic versus phenotypic patterns. *Int J Cancer* 1994; **56**: 347–53.

11 Abdel-Fattah R, Challen C, Griffiths TRL, Robinson MC, Lunec J. Alterations of TP53 in microdissected transitional cell carcinoma of the human urinary bladder: high frequency of TP53 accumulation in the absence of detected mutations is associated with poor prognosis. *Br J Cancer* 1998; **17**: 2230–8.

12 Keegan PE, Lunec J, Neal DE. p53 and p53-regulated genes in bladder cancer. *Br J Urol* 1998; **82**: 710–20.

13 Hall PA, Lane DP. p53 in tumour pathology: can we trust immunohistochemistry? — Revisited! *J Pathol* 1994; **172**: 1–4.

14 Baas IO, Mulder JW, Offerhaus GJ, Vogelstein B, Hamilton SR. An evaluation of six antibodies for immunohistochemistry of mutant p53 gene product in archival colorectal neoplasms. *J Pathol* 1994; **172**: 5–12.

15 Sidransky D, Von Eschenbach A, Tsai YC *et al.* Identification of p53 gene mutations in bladder cancers and urine samples. *Science* 1991; **252**: 706–9.

16 Fujimoto K, Yamada Y, Okajima E *et al.* Frequent association of p53 gene mutation in invasive bladder cancer. *Cancer Res* 1992; **52**: 1393–8.

17 Ooms EC, Anderson WA, Alons CL, Boon ME, Veldhuizen RW. Analysis of the performance of pathologists in the grading of bladder tumours. *Hum Pathol* 1983; **14**: 140–3.

18 Messing EM, Catalona W. Urothelial tumours of the urinary tract. In: Walsh PC, Retik AB, Vaughan ED, Wein AJ, eds. *Campbell's Urology*, 7th edn. Philadelphia: WB Saunders, 1997: 2327–410.

19 Hilsenbeck SG, Clark GM, McGuire WL. Why do so many prognostic factors fail to pan out? *Breast Cancer Res Treatment* 1992; **22**: 197–206.

20 Altman DG, Lausen B, Sauerbrei W, Schumacher M. Dangers of using 'optimal' cutpoints in the evaluation of prognostic factors. *J Natl Cancer Inst* 1994; **86**: 829–35.

21 Hilsenbeck SG, Clark GM. Practical p-value adjustment for optimally selected cutpoints. *Statistics Med* 1996; **15**: 103–12.

22 Keegan PE, Matthews JNS, Lunec J, Neal DE. Review: Statistical problems with 'optimal' cut-points in studies of new prognostic factors in urology. *BJU Int* 2000; **85**: 392–7.

23 Theodorescu D. Editorial comment. *J Urol* 1998; **159**: 791.

24 Sarkis AS, Dalbagni G, Cordon-Cardo C *et al*. Association of P53 nuclear overexpression and tumor progression in carcinoma in situ of the bladder. *J Urol* 1994; **152**: 388–92.

25 Ovesen H, Horn T, Steven K. Long-term efficacy of intravesical bacillus calmette-guerin for carcinoma in situ: relationship of progression to histological response and p53 nuclear accumulation. *J Urol* 1997; **157**: 1655–9.

26 Sarkis AS, Zhang ZF, Cordon-Cardo C *et al*. p53 nuclear overexpression and disease progression in Ta bladder carcinoma. *Int J Oncol* 1993; **3**: 355–60.

27 Casetta G, Gontero P, Russo R, Pacchioni D, Tizzani A. p53 expression compared with other prognostic factors in Oms grade-I stage-Ta transitional cell carcinoma of the bladder. *Eur Urol* 1997; **32**: 229–36.

28 Serth J, Kuczyk MA, Bokemeyer C *et al*. p53 immunohistochemistry as an independent prognostic factor for superficial transitional cell carcinoma of the bladder. *Br J Cancer* 1995; **71**: 201–5.

29 Thomas DJ, Robinson MC, Charlton R, Wilkinson S, Shenton BK, Neal DE. P53 expression, ploidy and progression in pT1 transitional cell carcinoma of the bladder. *Br J Urol* 1994; **73**: 533–7.

30 Lee E, Park I, Lee C. Prognostic markers of intravesical Bacillus Calmette-Guerin therapy for multiple, high-grade, stage T1 bladder cancers. *Int J Urol* 1997; **4**: 552–6.

31 Lebret T, Becette V, Baragelatta M *et al*. Correlation between p53 over expression and response to Bacillus Calmette-Guerin therapy in a high risk select population of patients with T1G3 bladder cancer. *J Urol* 1998; **159**: 788–91.

32 Gardiner RA, Walsh MD, Allen V *et al*. Immunohistological expression of p53 in primary pT1 transitional cell bladder cancer in relation to tumour progression. *Br J Urol* 1994; **73**: 526–32.

33 Sarkis AS, Bajorin DF, Reuter VE *et al*. Prognostic value of p53 nuclear overexpression in patients with invasive bladder cancer treated with neoadjuvant MVAC. *J Clin Oncol* 1995; **13**: 1384–90.

34 Kuczyk MA, Bokemeyer C, Serth J *et al*. p53 overexpression as a prognostic factor for advanced stage bladder cancer. *Eur J Cancer* 1995; **31A**: 2243–7.

35 Glick SH, Howell LP, White RW. Relationship of p53 and bcl-2 to prognosis in muscle-invasive transitional cell carcinoma of the bladder. *J Urol* 1996; **155**: 1754–7.

36 Jahnson S, Risberg B, Karlsson MG, Westman G, Bergstrom R, Pedersen J. p53 and Rb immunostaining in locally advanced bladder cancer: relation to prognostic variables and predictive value for the local response to radical radiotherapy. *Eur Urol* 1995; **28**: 135–42.

37 Wu CS, Pollack A, Czerniak B *et al*. Prognostic value of p53 in muscle-invasive bladder cancer treated with preoperative radiotherapy. *Urology* 1996; **47**: 305–10.

38 Esrig D, Elmajian D, Groshen S *et al*. Accumulation of nuclear p53 and tumor progression in bladder cancer. *N Engl J Med* 1994; **331**: 1259–64.

39 Underwood MA, Reeves J, Smith G *et al*. Overexpression of p53 protein and its significance for recurrent progressive bladder tumours. *Br J Urol* 1996; **77**: 659–66.

40 Tetu B, Fradet Y, Allard P, Veilleux C, Roberge N, Bernard P. Prevalence and clinical significance of HER/2neu, p53 and Rb expression in primary superficial bladder cancer. *J Urol* 1996; **155**: 1784–8.

41 Lipponen PK. Over-expression of p53 nuclear oncoprotein in transitional-cell bladder cancer and its prognostic value. *Int J Cancer* 1993; **53**: 365–70.

42 Pfister C, Buzelin F, Casse C, Bochereau G, Buzelin JM, Bouchot O. Comparative analysis of Mib1 and p53 expression in human bladder tumours and their correlation with cancer progression. *Eur Urol* 1998; **33**: 278–84.

43 Nakopoulou L, Constantinides C, Papandropoulos J *et al*. Evaluation of overexpression of p53 tumor suppressor protein in superficial and invasive transitional cell bladder cancer: comparison with DNA ploidy. *Urology* 1995; **46**: 334–40.

44 Raitanen MP, Tammela TL, Kallioinen M, Isola J. P53 accumulation, deoxyribonucleic acid ploidy and progression of bladder cancer. *J Urol* 1997; **157**: 1250–3.

45 Pfister C, Flaman JE, Dunet F, Grise P, Frebourg T. p53 mutations in bladder tumors inactivate the transactivation of the p21 and Bax genes, and have a predictive value for the clinical outcome after Bacillus Calmette-Guerin therapy. *J Urol* 1999; **162**: 69–73.

46 Wright C, Thomas D, Mellon K, Neal DE, Horne CH. Expression of retinoblastoma gene product and p53 protein in bladder carcinoma: correlation with Ki67 index. *Br J Urol* 1995; **75**: 173–9.

47 Cordon-Cardo C, Zhang ZF, Dalbagni G *et al.* Cooperative effects of p53 and pRB alterations in primary superficial bladder tumors. *Cancer Res* 1997; **57**: 1217–21.

48 Grossman HB, Leibert M, Antelo M *et al.* p53 and RB expression predict progression in T1 bladder cancer. *Clin Cancer Res* 1998; **4**: 829–34.

49 Cote RJ, Dunn MD, Chatterjee SJ *et al.* Elevated and absent pRb expression is associated with bladder cancer progression and has cooperative effects with p53. *Cancer Res* 1998; **58**: 1090–4.

50 Benedict WF, Lerner SP, Zhou J, Shen X, Tokunaga H, Czerniak B. Level of retinoblastoma protein expression correlates with p16 (MTS-1/INK4A/CDKN2) status in bladder cancer. *Oncogene* 1999; **18**: 1197–203.

51 Pollack A, Czerniak B, Zagars GK *et al.* Retinoblastoma protein expression and radiation response in muscle-invasive bladder cancer. *Int J Radiat Oncol Biol Phys* 1997; **39**: 687–95.

52 Cairns P, Shaw ME, Knowles MA. Initiation of bladder cancer may involve deletion of a tumour-suppressor gene on chromosome 9. *Oncogene* 1993; **8**: 1083–5.

53 Orlow I, LaRue H, Osman I *et al.* Deletions of the INK4A gene in superficial bladder tumours: association with recurrence. *Am J Pathol* 1999; **155**: 105–13.

54 Markl IDC, Jones PA. Presence and location of TP53 mutation determines pattern of CDKN2A/ARF pathway inactivation in bladder cancer. *Cancer Res* 1998; **58**: 5348–53.

55 Lacombe L, Orlow I, Silver D *et al.* Analysis of p21WAF1/CIP1 in primary bladder tumors. *Oncol Res* 1996; **8**: 409–14.

56 Malkowicz SB, Tomaszewski JE, Linnenbach AJ, Cangiano TA, Maruta Y, McGarvey TW. Novel p21WAF1/CIP1 mutations in superficial and invasive transitional cell carcinomas. *Oncogene* 1996; **13**: 1831–7.

57 Braithwaite KL, Mellon JK, Neal DE, Lunec J. WAF1 expression in transitional cell carcinoma (TCC) of the bladder: inverse relationship to p53 accumulation and association with good prognosis. Abstract no. 3534. American Association for Cancer Research, 1997.

58 Stein JP, Ginsberg DA, Grossfeld GD *et al.* Effect of p21WAF1/CIP1 expression on tumour progression in bladder cancer. *J Natl Cancer Inst* 1998; **90**: 1072–9.

59 Lipponen P, Aaltomaa S, Eskelinen M, Ala-Opas M, Kosma VM. Expression of p21 (waf1/cip1) protein in transitional cell bladder tumours and its prognostic value. *Eur Urol* 1998; **34**: 237–43.

60 Fakharzadeh SS, Trusko SP, George DL. Tumorigenic potential associated with enhanced expression of a gene that is amplified in a mouse tumor cell line. *EMBO J* 1991; **10**: 1565–9.

61 Jones SN, Roe AE, Donehower LA, Bradley A. Rescue of embryonic lethality in Mdm2-deficient mice by absence of p53. *Nature* 1995; **378**: 206–8.

62 Montes de Oca Luna R, Wagner DS, Lozano G. Rescue of early embryonic lethality in mdm2-deficient mice by deletion of p53. *Nature* 1995; **378**: 203–6.

63 Piette J, Neel H, Marechal V. Mdm2: keeping p53 under control. *Oncogene* 1997; **15**: 1001–10.

64 Lianes P, Orlow I, Zhang ZF *et al.* Altered patterns of MDM2 and TP53 expression in human bladder cancer. *J Natl Cancer Inst* 1994; **86**: 1325–30.

65 Barbareschi M, Girlando S, Fellin G, Graffer U, Luciani L, Dalla Palma P. Expression of mdm-2 and p53 protein in transitional cell carcinoma. *Urol Res* 1995; **22**: 349–52.

66 Schmitz-Drager BJ, Kushima M, Goebell P *et al*. p53 and Mdm2 in the development and progression of bladder cancer. *Eur Urol* 1997; **32**: 487–93.

67 Ozdemir E, Kakehi Y, Okuno H, Habuchi T, Okada Y, Yoshida O. Strong correlation of basement membrane degradation with p53 inactivation and/or MDM2 overexpression in superficial urothelial carcinomas. *J Urol* 1997; **158**: 206–11.

68 Korkolopoulou P, Christodoulou P, Kapralos P *et al*. The role of p53, MDM2 and c-erb B-2 oncoproteins, epidermal growth factor receptor and proliferation markers in the prognosis of urinary bladder cancer. *Pathol Res Pract* 1997; **193**: 767–75.

69 Shiina H, Igawa M, Shigeno K *et al*. Clinical significance of mdm2 and p53 expression in bladder cancer: a comparison with cell proliferation and apoptosis. *Oncology* 1999; **56**: 239–47.

70 Sigalas I, Calvert AH, Anderson JJ, Neal DE, Lunec J. Alternatively spliced mdm2 transcripts with loss of p53 binding domain sequences: transforming ability and frequent detection in human cancer. *Nat Med* 1996; **2**: 912–17.

71 Neal DE, Marsh C, Bennett MK *et al*. Epidermal-growth-factor receptors in human bladder cancer: comparison of invasive and superficial tumours. *Lancet* 1985; **1** (8425): 366–8.

72 Neal DE, Sharples L, Smith K, Fennelly J, Hall RR, Harris AL. The epidermal growth factor receptor and the prognosis of bladder cancer. *Cancer* 1990; **65**: 1619–25.

73 Mellon K, Wright C, Kelly P, Horne CH, Neal DE. Long-term outcome related to epidermal growth factor receptor status in bladder cancer. *J Urol* 1995; **153**: 919–25.

74 Lipponen P, Eskelinen M. Expression of epidermal growth factor receptor in bladder cancer as related to established prognostic factors, oncoprotein (c-erbB-2, p53) expression and long-term prognosis. *Br J Cancer* 1994; **69**: 1120–5.

75 Sriplakich S, Jahnson S, Karlosson MG. Epidermal growth factor receptor expression: predictive value for outcome after cystectomy for bladder cancer? *BJU Int* 1999; **83**: 498–503.

76 Nguyen PL, Swanson PE, Jaszcz W *et al*. Expression of epidermal growth factor receptor in invasive transitional cell carcinoma of the urinary bladder: a multivariate survival analysis. *Am J Clin Pathol* 1994; **101**: 166–76.

77 Mulder H, Van Hootegem JCSP, Sylvester R *et al*. Prognostic factors in bladder carcinoma: histologic parameters and expression of a cell cycle-related nuclear antigen (Ki-67). *J Path* 1992; **166**: 37–43.

78 Bush C, Price P, Norton J *et al*. Proliferation in human bladder carcinoma measured by Ki-67 antibody labelling: its potential clinical importance. *Br J Cancer* 1991; **64**: 357–60.

79 Popov Z, Hoznek A, Colombel M *et al*. The prognostic value of p53 nuclear overexpression and MIB-1 as a proliferative marker in transitional cell carcinoma of the bladder. *Cancer* 1997; **80**: 1472–81.

80 Philip EA, Stephenson TJ, Reed MWR. Prognostic significance of angiogenesis in transitional cell carcinoma of the human urinary bladder. *Br J Urol* 1996; **77**: 352–7.

81 Dickinson AJ, Fox SB, Persad RA, Hollyer J, Sibley GN, Harris AL. Quantification of angiogenesis as an independent predictor of prognosis in invasive bladder carcinomas. *Br J Urol* 1994; **74**: 762–6.

82 Crew JP, O'Brien T, Bradburn M *et al*. Vascular endothelial growth factor is a predictor of relapse and stage progression in superficial bladder cancer. *Cancer Res* 1997; **57**: 5281–5.

83 Grossfeld GD, Ginsberg DA, Stein JP *et al*. Thrombospondin-1 expression in bladder cancer: association with p53 alterations, tumor angiogenesis, and tumor progression. *J Natl Cancer Inst* 1997; **89**: 219–27.

84 Qureshi KN, Naguib RG, Hamdy FC, Neal DE, Kilian Mellon J. Neural network analysis of clinicopathological and molecular markers in bladder cancer. *J Urol* 2000; **163**: 630–3.

85 Sionov RV, Haupt Y. The cellular response to p53: the decision between life and death. *Oncogene* 1999; **18**: 6145–57.

86 Knowles MA. The genetics of transitional cell carcinoma: progress and potential clinical application. *BJU Int* 1999; **84**: 412–27.

87 Lacombe L, Dalbagni G, Zhang ZF *et al.* Overexpression of p53 protein in a high-risk population of patients with superficial bladder cancer before and after bacillus Calmette-Guerin therapy: correlation to clinical outcome. *J Clin Oncol* 1996; **14**: 2646–52.

88 Lipponen PK, Aaltomaa S. Apoptosis in bladder cancer as related to standard prognostic factors and prognosis. *J Pathol* 1994; **173**: 333–9.

89 Stein JP, Grossfeld GD, Ginsberg DA *et al.* Prognostic markers in bladder cancer: a contemporary review of the literature. *J Urol* 1998; **160**: 645–59.

5: Surgery for Advanced Bladder Cancer

D. W. W. Newling

Introduction

Bladder cancer is the second most common urological malignancy, with around 53 000 new cases per year in the US, causing approximately 12 000 deaths. Seventy-five per cent of bladder cancers present as superficial tumours, and, of these, 70% require no more than transurethral resection of the tumours with or without intravesical immunotherapy or chemotherapy. The remaining 25% present with more advanced disease, and of these, the 20% of those presenting initially with superficial tumours who subsequently develop invasive features, the surgical options were until recently somewhat limited [1].

Until the beginning of the 1970s, radical cystectomy and incontinent diversion still carried a mortality of around 20%. With the advent of continent reservoirs, neo-bladders, improvements in transurethral techniques and the increasing awareness of the value of partial cystectomy for circumscribed lesions in the dome and posterior wall, the surgical options and the possibilities for the patients with invasive cancer have improved dramatically. Improvements in radiotherapeutic techniques and the arrival of active chemotherapeutic agents have also added another dimension to the management of patients with advanced bladder tumours. These patients can now benefit from planned combination therapy of their tumours instead of always relying on monotherapeutic cystectomy [2]. It is not the purpose of this chapter to describe details of all the operative procedures. The important oncological and surgical principles will be given the most attention, along with an update of the various results of the procedures carried out.

Transurethral resection

This principal treatment modality for superficial tumours also has two important roles to play in the management of invasive disease. The first and foremost is in the accurate staging of that disease process, and the second is the possible use of transurethral resection combined with other treatment modalities in the treatment of solitary small T1 and T2 tumours.

The staging

For the accurate staging of a bladder tumour it is important that the examination is carried out under anaesthesia so that a thorough bi-manual assessment of the tumour can be made. The bi-manual must be performed before the transurethral resection and again afterwards. Only then may the difference between a T2 and a T3 tumour be identified. It should be remembered that transurethral resection is only one part of the process of staging bladder tumours, and an intravenous pyelogram with possibly retrograde studies, CT scans and MRIs may also have important roles to play. After transurethral resection the oedema in the bladder wall and possibly some leakage of the bladder content can give rise to misleading appearances on the CT scan. It is therefore advisable that the CT scan be carried out before the transurethral resection.

The first procedure in transurethral resection of bladder tumours is a careful urethrocystoscopy, which should preferably be carried out with rigid instruments, although flexible cystoscopy plays an important role in the follow-up of superficial tumours. Having ascertained that the urethra is of a reasonable calibre to allow the passage of the resectoscope and that there is no suspicious tissue therein, the initial inspection of the bladder should be carried out with a 70° telescope, with the use of a 120° telescope in the presence of a large medium lobe which makes viewing of the interurethric and trigonal region difficult. Once the tumours are identified the plan of resection should be made. This takes into account such factors as the size of the tumours and their location; for instance, the resection of a tumour in the trigonal region may generate so much gas that smaller tumours in the vault cannot be seen. The location of the ureteric orifices must be confirmed and, if necessary, a ureteric catheter can be passed.

For staging it is important that the exophytic tumour is submitted in a separate pot, to a deeper biopsy. The deeper biopsy can often best be performed with a cold cup forcep, thus avoiding charring of the underlying tissue which may make pathological infiltration difficult. Immediately after the procedure a map should be drawn of the bladder with a description of all the tumours present, and the pathologist must be made aware of the location of all the lesions. At the end of the procedure the bladder should again be inspected with the 70° telescope. The use of videos will enable findings to be checked at a later date, by the original operator or by a colleague. In order to improve the accuracy of transurethral resection for staging, many urologists elect to carry out a second cystoscopy and re-biopsy of invasive tumours, particularly poorly differentiated ones, after 4–6 weeks. Although this may slightly delay necessary subsequent therapy, it does allow the clinician and the patient to confirm whether or not the potentially dangerous tumour has been completely eliminated [3].

Transurethral resection for invasive tumours with therapeutic intent

In the early 1980s, Soquet, a Belgian urologist, produced a series of cases of transurethral resection or partial cystectomy for invasive bladder tumours where the patients received methotrexate postoperative therapy for 6 months. Hall, in the UK, and Herr, in the US, had suggested, independently and at approximately the same time, that the use of controlled perforation to resect small, invasive tumours of the bladder with a low pressure resectoscope might be justified. The early results with systemic chemotherapy, particularly using cisplatin and methotrexate based treatments, made this an intriguing possibility for preserving bladders and avoiding immediate cystectomy. The technique is applicable only for tumours in the extraperitoneal part of the bladder. The resection needs to be carried out with a low pressure Inglesis-type resectoscope to prevent widespread dissemination of tumour tissue in the retroperitoneum. It is important that the gap in the bladder wall should be of the order of 0.5 cm in diameter, otherwise the outer layer of the bladder may act as a sort of flap valve permitting urine only into the retroperitoneum and not back into the bladder. After the resection the bladder must be drained through a catheter for a minimum of 5 days. Using this technique Hall *et al.* [4] showed that for a defined group of patients and a defined group of tumours this treatment yielded as good results, in his hands, as early cystectomy.

Partial cystectomy

Partial cystectomy of a single, muscle invasive bladder tumour is possible in most areas of the bladder. In the past there was a tendency, because of the high mortality of radical cystectomy, for people to attempt partial cystectomy on patients with more advanced tumours and most particularly patients with carcinoma *in situ* elsewhere in the bladder. This meant that the partial cystectomy fell into some disrepute. It remains, however, a useful operation in the elderly and frail, in patients with marked local symptoms but who have metastatic disease, and in patients who refuse cystectomy or have tumours invading from other organs or tumours in a diverticulum. It is of vital importance that the rest of the bladder is healthy and has not undergone pre-malignant changes over a wider field. Random biopsies therefore play an important role in the initial staging of the tumour. It must be possible to excise the tumour with at least 1 cm of normal bladder and not leave the patient with a bladder of such small capacity or low compliance that incontinence is going to be an inevitable outcome. The bladder capacity before the operation should be at least 300 cm^3

and if the operation is being considered for a female patient there must be no history of urge incontinence. Opinions are divided over the simultaneous administration of intravesical cytotoxics but it would seem reasonable to fill the bladder with a cytotoxic solution such as epirubicin or mitomycin before spillage of tumour-containing urine. Other workers consider that if the bladder is filled with water with its known cytotoxic effect, this is adequate and does not place the operator or other staff at any danger from exposure to cytotoxic agents [5]. For larger tumours partial cystoscopy might form part of a combined brachytherapeutic regime where iridium wires or gold seeds can be left behind in the bed of the tumour, or in the surrounding bladder when the tumour has been excised [6].

Radical cystectomy

In the early 1970s radical cystectomy was a formidable operation accompanied by a mortality of around 20%, by considerable long-term morbidity and by an incontinent abdominal stoma. In recent series, Koch & Smith [7] and Thomas *et al.* [8] have described a mortality of between 2 and 3%, with around 75% of patients in remission of their cancer 5 years from surgery. The majority of centres are now offering orthotopic bladder replacement or a continent abdominal stoma, and the complications are related mainly to the urinary tract reconstruction rather than to the operation of cystectomy itself.

Preoperative management

It is important that the patient comes to the operating theatre in a good general condition. Urinary tract infection must be treated, the patient must be in an optimal nutritional state and where necessary may have been transfused. In this respect, few people use autologous blood because it is important that the patient maintains a good circulatory blood and fluid volume during a long operation, and therefore to begin the operation in an anaemic state is not a good idea.

The use of combination therapies in the treatment of advanced, muscle invasive bladder cancer includes the use of neoadjuvant therapy and radiotherapy. In a recent large Medical Research Council (MRC)/European Organization for Research and Treatment of Cancer (EORTC) study of neoadjuvant chemotherapy using cisplatin, methotrexate and vinblastine, researchers were disappointed to find that three courses of the CMV therapy did not lead to an improvement in overall survival when accompanied by definitive radiotherapy or cystectomy [9]. A recently completed Southwest Oncology Group (SWOG) study suggests that if the chemotherapy is quadruple chemotherapy, using M-VAC, there may be an advantage in overall survival for those patients who go on to cystectomy (C. Sternberg, personal communication, 1999).

Radiotherapy is used in two different contexts when combined with cystectomy. It has been used in a variety of regimes, prior to a planned cystectomy or as definitive therapy to be followed by salvage cystectomy if necessary for recurrence. At a recent consensus meeting on the management of bladder cancer, the majority of contributors found few indications for giving preoperative radiotherapy prior to the performance of a cystectomy. Nevertheless there are still some centres which somewhat empirically give 1500–2000 rads in five daily treatments a week before cystectomy. This adds little in the way of discomfort for the patient but others consider that it is hazardous, particularly if the urinary tract reconstruction is going to involve orthotopic bladder substitution or a reservoir employing the large bowel, which may have been irradiated [10]. The performance of radical cystectomy differs between men and women and therefore the principles of the operations will be considered separately for the two sexes.

Radical cystectomy in men

The majority of patients undergoing radical cystectomy will be having a radical cysto-prostatectomy. Only a few, those with clear involvement of the urethra by tumour, will need to have the urethra removed as well. The operation is performed under a general anaesthetic with the patient in the supine position, the iliac crest over the break in the table which should give a hyperextension of approximately 40°. This enables a better view of the pelvis and a lengthening of the space between the umbilicus and the pubic symphisis. The site of a possible stoma should have already been marked in collaboration with a stoma nurse, and the long midline incision should pass on the opposite side of the navel to the side of a possible stoma sack. The operation is greatly helped by the use of a retractor fixed to the operating table, such as an Omnitract or a Buckwalther retractor. After incision in the midline, the space of the cave of Retzius is opened by blunt dissection before beginning a lymph node dissection. The majority of urologists finding pathological lymph nodes present will abort the operation and proceed to some other systemic therapy, perhaps considering a salvage cystectomy at a later date. The majority of urologists also favour a bilateral lymph node dissection, starting on the side of the tumour. All the lymphatics should be removed from an area bounded laterally by the genito-femoral nerve and medially by the bladder wall. Distally the dissection should reach the lymph node of Cloquet, where lymph vessels pass under the inguinal ligament. The involvement of the lymph nodes in transitional cell carcinoma is an important prognostic factor, with the 3-year survival rate falling dramatically. Patients with high grade and high stage

Table 5.1 The therapeutic value of lymph node dissection in patients following radical cystectomy, with pathological nodes incidences and survival (Waters *et al.* [11])

Author	Period	*n*	N+	%	Strata	>5-year survival (%)
Whitmore	1940–55	230	55	24	Overall	4
Laplante	1955–63	324	12		N4	0
					T4 N1–3	8
					T3 N1–3	13
Dretler	1955–67	302	54	18	Overall	17
Bredael	1964–73	174	26		Overall	4
Reid	1964–74	135	24	18	Overall	26
Smith, Whitmore	1966–77	662	134	20	N1	17
					N2	5
					N3	5
					N4	0
Skinner	1971–79	153	36	24	Overall	35
Zincke	1960–80	–	57	–	Overall	10
Roehrborn	1971–86	280	42	15	N1	23
					N2, N3	18
Takashi	1978–88	86	19	22	Overall	25
Lerner *et al.*	1971–89	591	132	22	<P3b	50
					>P3b	18
Vieweg	1980–88	627	140	22	<P3b	55
					>P3b	22
Bretheau, Ponthieu	1970–90	248	40	16	N1	22
					N2	8
Kuriki	1984–92	131	22	17	Overall	34.5

tumours have a greater incidence of positive lymph nodes and naturally a much poorer prognosis. In a recent review by Waters *et al.* [11], 5-year survival rates of up to 50% were reported with positive nodes in the presence of a T2 tumour but the figure was as low as 17% if the local tumour stage was T4 (see Table 5.1).

After the lymph node dissection, the next step is the mobilization of the sigmoid colon and caecum with upward displacement of the gastrointestinal tract, which can be packed away behind a large gauze. The ureters may then be mobilized and should be divided from the bladder as low as possible. Frozen section of the distal end of the ureter is important if the tumour has a high grade or if there is carcinoma *in situ* in the bladder. It is helpful to tie the ureters at the distal end in order that dilatation can occur during the rest of the cystectomy, making the intestinal anastomosis somewhat easier. There is considerable dispute over whether or not the internal iliac arteries should be ligated at this stage to limit blood loss. In all patients with widespread vascular disease there may be a risk of necrosis in the gluteal tissues even if the iliac vessels are ligated below the superior gluteal artery.

The following step is to mobilize the bladder with the prostate and seminal vesicles and the rectum (Fig. 5.1). With the urachus retracted forwards the peritoneum over the front of the rectum at the back of the bladder can be divided. It is important at this stage that the correct plane is found in front of at least one layer of the fascia of Deneuvielliers to be certain that the vesicles, prostate and ampulla of the vas can be mobilized adequately (Fig. 5.2). The prostate and vesicular structures can be freed by blunt dissection in this relatively bloodless field. By starting with the obliterated umbilical artery superiorly, the vascular pedicles can then be individually ligated or clipped to mobilize the bladder on both sides. The remainder of the dissection is very similar to a standard retropubic radical prostatectomy. The endo-pelvic fascia will be incised on both sides and the prostate mobilized. The dorsal vein of the penis should be mobilized from the front of the urethra and carefully ligated. The prostate, bladder and perivesical tissues can then be removed intact. If potency is important for the patient then both neurovascular bundles should be preserved by incising the prostatic fascia and by blunt dissection mobilizing the bundles off the prostate (Fig. 5.3). Particular care must be taken at the apex of the prostate where the bundles may again be damaged.

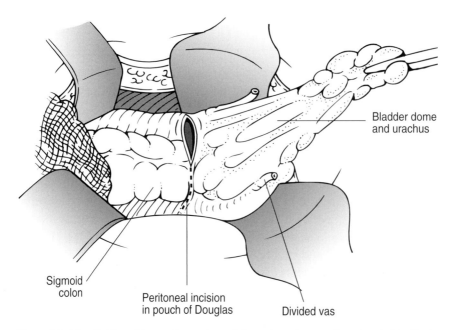

Figure 5.1 After division of the urachus at the umbilicus, the peritoneum lateral to the bladder is divided toward the obliterated umbilical artery. The peritoneal incision is then further extended into the retrovesical peritoneal pouch. Reproduced from *Altas Urol Clin North Am*, October, 1997, with the permission of W. B. Saunders.

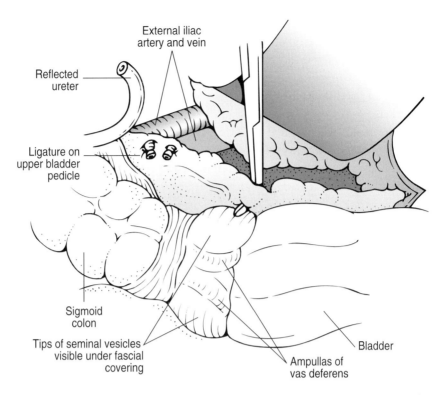

Figure 5.2 The upper part of the lateral bladder pedicle is divided to allow further exposure of the posterior bladder and rectum. The bladder pedicle is divided adjacent to the seminal vesicles. Reproduced from *Atlas Urol Clin North Am*, October, 1997, with the permission of W. B. Saunders.

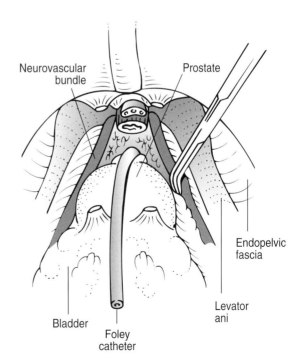

Figure 5.3 The plane between the rectum and prostate is developed and connects to the retrovesical plane. The lateral prostatic fascia is divided to free the neurovascular bundles. Reproduced from *Atlas Urol Clin North Am*, October, 1997, with the permission of W. B. Saunders.

URETHRECTOMY

If the urethra is to be removed in the same session then the patient must be placed in the half lithotomy position, thus enabling the second team to remove the urethra at the time that the urinary diversion is being prepared. Through a midline perineal incision the urethra can be mobilized from the pelvic diaphragm to the last centimetre of the glans of the penis itself, by a process of inversion. It is probably not necessary to remove the last centimetre of the urethra, which can lead to considerable bleeding from the erectile tissue of the glans.

Radical cystectomy in women

It is probably seldom that a radical cystectomy is carried out on its own. The procedure for advanced bladder cancer is usually an anterior exenteration and until recently this was followed by the formation of a continent reservoir or ileal conduit in the manner of Bricker. Recently it has been shown that it is possible to perform an exenteration and to make an orthotopic bladder without necessarily making the patient incontinent. The patient is placed in the hyperextended supine position with the iliac crest located just below the break in the operating table. The legs should be placed in a modified frogleg position if an orthotopic diversion is planned. The first stages of the operation are very similar in women to those in men. The bladder is initially mobilized from the urachus downwards, after pelvic lymph node dissection and ligation of the ureters. Again, the question of ligation of the internal iliac artery needs to be considered. Personally, I find in females that it is advisable to do so as it reduces considerably the bleeding from the uterine vessels. Female patients are generally younger than the male patients and do not run the same vascular risk as was outlined above.

After division of the lateral pedicles, the bladder and uterus specimen are retracted anteriorly, exposing the pouch of Douglas (Fig. 5.4). The peritoneal reflections lateral to the rectum must be incised and the uterus and cervix mobilized until the vagina comes clearly into view. The vagina should be incised just distal to the cervix to enable the exenteration to be carried out. The bladder should be freed of the anterior vaginal surface to enable a good cuff of vagina to remain (Fig. 5.5). The final part of the dissection involves the careful separation of as much urethral tissue as possible from the bladder neck in order to make the subsequent anastomosis simpler. In order to prevent prolapse and particularly an enterocoele, it is important that the top of the vagina, after closure, be attached to Cooper's ligament.

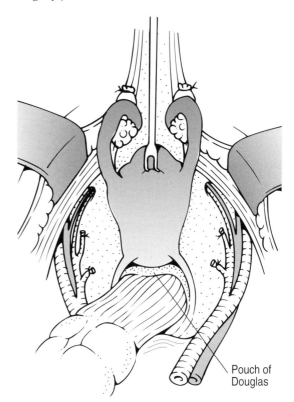

Figure 5.4 The bladder, uterus, overies and fallopian tubes are retracted. Reproduced from *Atlas Urol Clin North Am*, October, 1997, with the permission of W. B. Saunders.

Pouch of Douglas

Urinary diversion

The vast majority of patients undergoing cystectomy can now enjoy a continent urinary diversion, either to the skin or to their own urethra. There remain, however, some absolute contraindications to this. Renal function must be reasonable and a creatinine level >200 μmol/L is generally agreed as an absolute contraindication. Patients with compromised intestinal or liver function should not undergo a continent deviation. Weak, elderly patients can probably better manage an external appliance. Patients over 70 sometimes have problems with continence after an orthotopic reconstruction, and patients who have a lack of understanding of the importance of regular emptying of the continent reservoir or an orthotopic bladder may also run into difficulties [12].

Early complications of cystectomy and urinary diversion

Probably the most commonly seen complication of such a large procedure is

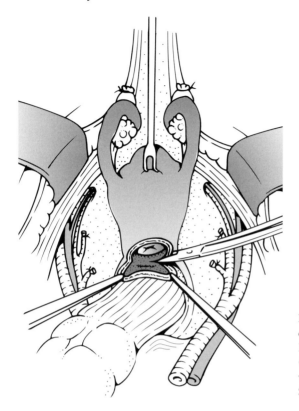

Figure 5.5 The vagina is
excised just distal to the cervix.
Reproduced from *Atlas Urol
Clin North Am*, October, 1997,
with the permission of W. B.
Saunders.

postoperative bleeding. It is important that at the end of the operation the
blood volume and blood pressure are high enough to be certain that any significant bleeding can be corrected before the abdomen is closed. However,
there are inevitably cases that need to return to theatre for haemostasis which
may be locally achieved or may necessitate late ligation of the internal iliac
arteries. Bleeding from mesenteric vessels following continent or incontinent
urinary diversion after radiotherapy is quite frequent and results from con-
traction of the fatty tissues of the mesentery around these vessels, liberating
the ligatures. It is important when carrying out a salvage cystectomy after
radiotherapy to ensure that the mesentery is long enough to reach the skin
when performing the inevitable ileal conduit. Acute complications from the
urinary diversion include ischaemia of an ileal conduit, torsion of an orthotopic bladder or continent cutaneous diversion. Urinary leakage or persistent
lymphatic leakage can lead to prolonged ileus, necessitating prolonged naso-
gastric drainage and intravenous therapy. Many surgeons feel that it is expedient when carrying out cystectomy with continent or incontinent diversion to

carry out a gastrostomy or jejunostomy to avoid the use of prolonged naso-gastric drainage with the accompanying respiratory problems. One of the greatest worries of surgeons after cystectomy and diversion is the loss of drains or splints and it is therefore imperative that during the operation all tubes are securely sutured and the drainage is visible at all times. If during the course of the cystectomy the internal iliac artery was ligated there is a risk, particularly in elderly patients, of gluteal necrosis and the gluteal region must be inspected every day for this complication.

Late complications

URETERIC OBSTRUCTION

Regardless of the diversion employed, i.e. continent or incontinent, there is a risk of uretero-enteric stenosis. In the first instance the upper urinary tract should be evaluated some 3 or 4 weeks after the procedure then again after 6 months. If there is no evidence of upper tract impairment or obstruction then subsequent intravenous pyelograms and renograms could probably be carried out on an annual basis. Dilatation of the upper tract, if perceived to be due to stenosis of the uretero-ileal anastomosis, may be treated by the positioning of a Wall stent or some other sort of splint either via a nephrostomy or endo-scopically from the reservoir or conduit itself. Consistent dilatation which does not respond to these endoscopic procedures will probably require a re-anastomosis over double J or other stents, which should be left for approxi-mately 6 weeks.

TUMOUR RECURRENCE

If the urethra has been employed as the urine outlet then cytology should be performed half yearly for the first 5 years to ensure there is no evidence of tumour recurrence, and if necessary 'cystoscopy' of the orthotopic bladder should be performed. In patients with high risk tumours, regardless of the di-version used, regular chest radiographs and if necessary CT scans should be performed in the first 3 years every 6 months and annually for the first 10 years to exclude metastases. Urethral recurrence after orthotopic bladder replace-ment occurs in around 6% of patients. When this occurs it is a relatively simple procedure to convert the neo-bladder into a continent reservoir by a narrowed length of ileum or a Kock valve, and the urethra can then excised [13].

METABOLIC PROBLEMS

Apart from the metabolic problems as a result of ureteric obstruction, and the subsequent development of renal failure, there are few difficulties with the use of an ileal conduit. If the conduit is selected at least 15 cm from the ileocaecal valve there is little risk of bile salt loss. With the use of long segments of ileum, ileocaecum or colon for a continent reservoir, there is the long-term risk of the development of hyperchloraemic and possibly hypokalaemic acidosis. Vitamin B_{12} deficiency following the use of 70–120 cm of ileum does not usually develop within the first 3 years. It is probably expedient in all patients who have a continent reservoir or an orthotopic bladder to monitor the electrolytes every 3 months for the first year and every 6 months for the following 5 years. If a large segment of ileum has been used then serum B_{12} should be measured annually after 3 years. In all patients who have large segments of ileum excluded, there is a risk of osteoporosis. The most important facet of avoidance of this complication is the correction of acidosis occurring in the medium to long term [14].

Conclusion

The outlook for patients with advanced bladder cancer has greatly improved during the last 15 years. This improvement has come largely through more accurate staging, and therefore early intervention to cure the cancer, and the advances in techniques of urinary diversion, which enable patients to enjoy a good quality of life after cystectomy.

As with all major surgery in the last 20 years, major improvements in patient preparation, anaesthesia and the handling of the metabolic consequences of these interventions have been, and still are, of immense importance. Thus many patients with muscle invasive bladder cancer can be offered early cystectomy and continent urinary diversion with nerve sparing techniques. This means that many more patients, who formerly faced a grim future, are now prepared to accept the risks of cystectomy and urinary diversion in order to guarantee prolonged survival with a reasonable quality of life.

References

1   Stein JP, Skinner DG. Radical cystectomy in women. *Atlas Urol Clin North Am* 1997; 5, 2: 37–64.
2   Anderson L, Esposti PL, Fosså SD. Induction chemotherapy in association with pre-operative radiotherapy and cystectomy in bladder cancer. In: Smith PH, Pavone-Macaluso M, eds. *The Management of Advanced Cancer of the Prostate and Bladder*. New York: Alan R. Liss, 1988: 621–3.

3   Shelfo SW, Brady JD, Soloway MS. Transurethral resection of bladder cancer. *Atlas Urol Clin North Am* 1997; **5**, 2: 1–14.

4   Hall RR, Newling DW, Ramsden PD *et al*. Treatment of invasive bladder cancer by local resection and high dose methotrexate. *Br J Urol* 1984; **56**: 668–74.

5   Gill IS, Wood DP, Jr Taylor RJ. Partial cystectomy in urological cancer. In: Dan D, Crawford D, eds. *Current Genitourinary Cancer Surgery (2)*. Baltimore: Williams & Wilkins, 1996: 380–6.

6   Werf VD, Messing BHP, Menon RS, Hop WDT. Carcinoma of the urinary bladder T2 T3 NX M0 treated by interstitial radium implant. In: Smith PH, Pavone-Macaluso M, eds. *The Management of Advanced Cancer of the Prostate and Bladder*. New York: Alan R. Liss, 1988: 511–24.

7   Koch MO, Smith JA. Radical cystectomy in men. *Atlas Urol Clin North Am* 1997; **5**, 2: 20–36.

8   Thomas PJ, Nurse DE, Delevkotis C, Mundy AR. Cystoprostatectomy and substitution cystoplasty for locally advanced bladder cancer. *Br J Urol* 1992; **70**: 40–2.

9   International Collaboration of Trialists on behalf of the Medical Research Council Advanced Bladder Working Party, EORTC Genitourinary Group, Australian Bladder Cancer Study Group, National Cancer Institute of Canada Clinical Trials Group, Finnbladder Norwegian Bladder Cancer Group and Club Urologico Espanol de Tratamiento Oncologico (CUETO) Group. Neoadjuvant cisplatin, methotrexate, and vinblastine chemotherapy for muscle-invasive bladder cancer: a randomised controlled trial. *Lancet* 1999; **354**: 533–40.

10 Gospodarovicz MK, Quilty PM, Scalliet P *et al*. The place of radiation therapy as definitive treatment of bladder cancer. *Int J Urol* **2** (Suppl. 2): 41–8.

11 Waters WB, Bassi P, Ohi Y *et al*. The role of pelvic lymph node dissection in the management of invasive bladder cancer. *Urol Oncol* 1998; **4**: 168–71.

12 Studer UE, Hautmann RE, Hohenfellner M. Indications for continent diversion after cystectomy and factors affecting long term results. *Urol Oncol* 1998; **4**: 172–82.

13 Stenzl A, Draxl H, Posch B *et al*. The risk of urethral tumours in female bladder cancer; can the urethra be used for orthotopic reconstruction of the lower urinary tract? *J Urol* 1995; **153**: 950–5.

14 Gattegno B, Estrade V. Metabolic consequences of urinary intestinal diversion. *Eur Urol* 1999; **36**, 5 (*Curriculum in Urology* 3–4): 1–6.

6: Chemotherapy and Bladder Cancer

F. Calabrò & C. N. Sternberg

Introduction

Bladder cancer is one of the most common malignancies in Western society. It is the sixth most common cancer in the United States, excluding non-melanoma skin cancers. The American Cancer Society estimated that in 2000 there would be about 53 200 new cases of bladder cancer diagnosed in the United States (about 38 300 men and 14 900 women), and that these would result in about 12 200 deaths (about 8100 men and 4100 women) [1].

The male to female occurrence is three to one. Bladder cancer is primarily a disease of the elderly, with 80% of cases in the 50- to 79-year age groups, and a peak incidence in the seventh decade.

Most bladder cancers are transitional cell carcinomas (TCCs), mostly in the Western world: in fact, squamous cell carcinomas (SCCs) and adenocarcinomas account for only 5% and 2%, respectively. Adenocarcinomas may arise in the dome of the bladder from a primary site in the urachus, but most often occur in the trigone. SCCs are often associated with chronic irritation or infection. SCC of the bilharzial bladder differs from bladder cancer seen in Europe and the United States. SCCs have diverse aetiologies and different biology from TCCs. Rhabdomyosarcoma is a very rare bladder cancer. It usually affects infants and is seldom found in adults. These other histologies merit separate discussion [2].

When bladder cancer is found at a localized stage and appropriately treated, the 5-year relative survival rate is 94%. Some 75% of the cancers are detected this early in the superficial stage, limited to the mucosa, submucosa, or lamina propria. After initial treatment the recurrence rates are 50–80%, with progression to muscle-invading tumour in 10–25%. In muscle-invading bladder cancers, there is a 50% risk of distant metastases. In cases involving regional spread or distant spread, 5-year survival rates are 49% and 6%, respectively.

In most countries, the treatment of choice for muscle-invasive bladder cancer is radical cystectomy and bilateral pelvic lymph node dissection. In a few European Countries and in Canada, radiation therapy has been the traditional treatment. Improvements in surgical techniques, peri-operative care, and early diagnosis have led to an increase in survival, owing to stage migration of 10–20% per stage. In fact tumours are found earlier than in the past and are generally smaller, with fewer deeply invasive tumours. The presence of a palpable mass is less frequent, and the incidence of N+ disease has diminished [3].

Conventional treatments such as surgery and radiotherapy have generally resulted in poor cure rates, and furthermore metastatic disease has frequently developed. Both these occurrences have led to the assumption that occult micrometastases must be present at the time of initial diagnosis.

Despite aggressive locoregional treatment with radical cystectomy and pelvic lymphadenectomy or radical radiotherapy, approximately 50% of all patients with muscle-invasive transitional cell carcinoma develop metastatic disease within two years of cystectomy and subsequently die of the disease. The majority of patients relapse systematically, but pelvic and regional node recurrences may also result in significant morbidity and mortality.

Known prognostic factors for relapse after cystectomy include depth of invasion, involvement of adjacent viscera (perivesicular fat, vascular invasion, prostate and vagina) and presence of nodal metastases. Recurrence is related to stage and nodal status. High-grade, high-stage (pT3–4) tumours are frequently (40–60%) found to have lymph node involvement (pN+) at the time of radical cystectomy. According to current selected studies, patients with nodal metastases have a 15–20% 5-year survival after cystectomy, while for N1 (one microscopic node ipsilateral to tumour) [4] the figure rises to 35–40%. On the other hand, fewer than 10% of patients with direct invasion into adjacent viscera are alive 5 years after diagnosis.

The strongest predictor of risk for later urethral disease is the involvement of the prostate [5]. Other known prognostic factors include histology, grade, presence or absence of ureteral obstruction and the extent of surgical resection [6,7].

Neoadjuvant chemotherapy

The proven chemosensitivity of metastatic transitional cell carcinoma, with response rates of 40–70% with cisplatin-containing combination chemotherapy regimens, has led to the use of chemotherapy, either neoadjuvant or adjuvant, for locally invasive disease in combination with cystectomy or radiotherapy.

Neoadjuvant chemotherapy is directed at possible systemic disease in patients with apparently localized disease. This approach has several advantages over postoperative adjuvant chemotherapy. First, it provides earlier exposure of micrometastases to chemotherapy. Second, the bladder tumour serves as an *in vivo* marker to evaluate response to chemotherapy; this may permit continuation of treatment to maximal response, or discontinuation of ineffective therapy. Third, significant regression of the primary tumour may allow local management to be tailored to the individual patient: surgery may be technically easier, a more conservative surgical procedure may be considered, or radiotherapy may be administered in lieu of surgery. The major disadvantage is that definitive local therapy is delayed.

Non-randomized studies have clearly established the feasibility and safety of giving neoadjuvant chemotherapy. Overall response rates of 60–70%, with complete response rates in the 30% range, have frequently been reported [8]. These trials have demonstrated that neoadjuvant chemotherapy can produce tumour downstaging and have illustrated the problems in interpreting response following neoadjuvant chemotherapy due to inconsistency between clinical and pathological staging. It has been shown that inoperable cases may become operable after neoadjuvant chemotherapy [9].

Whether or not neoadjuvant chemotherapy has an actual effect on survival can be answered only in the context of well-controlled randomized trials. Findings of a number of such trials have been published, and several are ongoing [8] (see Table 6.1). Most trials have been prematurely closed and have failed to show a survival advantage for chemotherapy [10]. All these studies suffer from suboptimal chemotherapy or small sample size. Part of the problem is that a trial with adequate power to detect a 10% survival advantage of one approach over another, for example from 50% 5-year survival to 60%, requires that 1000 patients must be randomized. Four hundred patients are required to detect a 15% difference and 200 to detect a 20% one [11].

The Nordic Cystectomy I trial has suggested a positive trend in survival of patients treated with two cycles of neoadjuvant adriamycin (ADM) and cis-

Table 6.1 Randomized trials of neoadjuvant chemotherapy

Study group	Neoadjuvant arm	Standard arm	*n*	Results
EORTC/MRC [12]	CMV/RT or Cyst	RT or Cyst	976	No difference
Nordic Cyst I [13]	ADM/DDP/RT/Cyst	RT/Cyst	311	15% chemotherapy benefit in T3–T4a
Italy (GUONE) [14]	M-VAC/Cyst	Cyst	206	No difference
USA Intergroup [15]	M-VAC/Cyst	Cyst	298	Closed
Aust/UK [16]	DDP/RT	RT	255	No difference
Canada/NCI [17]	DDP/RT or preop. RT + Cyst	RT or preop. RT + Cyst	99	No difference
Spain (CUETO) [18]	DDP/Cyst	Cyst	121	No difference
Italy (Genoa) [19]	DDP/5-FU/RT/Cyst	Cyst	104	No difference
MGH/RTOG [20]	CMV/DDP/RT	DDP/RT	123	No difference
Nordic Cyst II [21]	MTX/DDP/Cyst	Cyst	317	No difference
Abol-Enein [22]	CarboMV/Cyst	Cyst	194	Chemotherapy benefit

Cyst, cystectomy; RT, radiotherapy. For explanation of other abbreviations see text.

platin (DDP) and 4000 rads for 5 days, followed by cystectomy, vs. radio-therapy (RT) and cystectomy alone [13]. The investigators reported a 20% difference in cancer-specific survival and a 15% ($P = 0.03$) survival benefit at 5 years in the subset of patients with T3a–T4 lesions. No difference was ob-served for patients with T1 and T2 disease. A multivariate analysis showed that chemotherapy and tumour stage were independent prognostic factors for survival.

A subsequent Nordic Cystectomy II trial eliminated the adriamycin and randomized patients to neoadjuvant methotrexate (MTX) and cisplatin with-out RT followed by cystectomy vs. cystectomy alone. No survival difference was detected in 317 patients with muscle-invasive disease [21].

The Medical Research Council (MRC) and European Organization for Research and Treatment of Cancer (EORTC) have completed the largest randomized neoadjuvant chemotherapy trial of cisplatin–methotrexate–vinblastine (CMV) followed by cystectomy or RT vs. immediate cystectomy or RT [12]. This trial was conducted on 976 patients, out of whom 491 were assigned to chemotherapy and 485 to no chemotherapy. The study revealed an 8% difference in the time to progression in treated patients, and a 5.5% dif-ference in absolute 3-year survival (hazard ratio = 0.85; 95% CI 0.71–1.02). The median survival was 44 months for the chemotherapy group and 37.5 months for the no-chemotherapy one. A difference of 6.5 months cannot be considered statistically meaningful, as 3500 patients would need to have been included in this trial for this to be a significant difference. Of note, many pa-tients in the no-chemotherapy group received chemotherapy at relapse. Some 37% received salvage therapy. The pT0 rate was 33% with CMV and 12% without CMV. Chemotherapy demonstrated activity in the primary tumour and may have delayed locoregional and metastatic progression.

An Italian cooperative group randomized patients to four cycles of neoadjuvant methotrexate–vinblastine–adriamycin–cisplatin (M-VAC) fol-lowed by cystectomy vs. cystectomy alone [14]. The study was closed after 206 patients were randomized. The sample size was calculated to detect an improvement in 3-year overall survival of 15%, from 45% to 60%. Survival at 3 years was 62% for the M-VAC arm and 68% for the cystectomy alone arm. Response to M-VAC was the only independent prognostic factor. Of note, 1 in 3 patients received a lower dose intensity of the planned chemotherapy.

The ongoing Southwest Oncology Group trial is evaluating three cycles of M-VAC followed by cystectomy vs. cystectomy alone. This study was closed last year after a very long accrual period [15]. The results are eagerly awaited, and it is hoped that this trial is sufficiently powered.

No significant survival difference was detected examining the results of a meta-analysis from Australia and the UK combined [16], where single agent cisplatin was given prior to RT. Similarly, in a study from the Canadian National Cancer Institute (NCI), patients were treated with neoadjuvant cisplatin and RT or preoperative RT and cystectomy [17]. This randomized trial demonstrated significantly better local control (recurrence rate 40% vs. 59%) by concomitant cisplatin and preoperative RT. However, the initial advantage in overall survival seen at 3 years was not confirmed at 6.5 years.

In another radiation trial, the Massachusetts General Hospital (MGH) and the Radiation Therapy Oncology Group (RTOG) evaluated the combination of two cycles of CMV, cisplatin, RT vs. cisplatin and RT alone [20]. This trial was designed to detect a 20% difference in tumour-free survival, and a 15% difference in disease-free survival. However, the study was prematurely closed because of toxicity. Of 123 patients, no difference in 5-year actuarial survival was observed: 48% and 49%. Five-year survival with a functioning bladder was 38% in the CMV arm and 36% in the RT and cisplatin arm. Two cycles of CMV neoadjuvant chemotherapy were not shown to increase the rate of complete response over standard induction therapy or to increase freedom from metastatic disease. There was no impact on 5-year overall survival.

Although randomized trials have not yet proven a survival benefit with neoadjuvant chemotherapy, response to chemotherapy may be the most important predictor of survival. Data were collected from 147 patients with muscle-infiltrating tumours treated with neoadjuvant chemotherapy and radical or partial cystectomy, in eight centres. Five-year survival was 75% in patients who had downstaging of the primary tumour to pT0 or superficial disease vs. only 20% in patients who had residual muscle-infiltrating disease (> pT2) [23].

These data are similar to our data in Rome, where 87 patients with muscle-invasive TCC of the bladder were evaluated [24]. After three cycles of neoadjuvant M-VAC, 40 patients were T0, 19 had Ta-1 disease, 8 had carcinoma *in situ* (CIS), 12 had T2–3 disease, and 8 refused restaging. Forty-two patients had transurethral resection of the bladder (TURB) alone (including 3 who refused surgery), 13 underwent partial cystectomy, and 32 had radical cystectomy. In those undergoing radical or partial cystectomy P0 was 12/45 (27%). Overall 5-year survival was 67% and 37% with bladder preservation. Five-year survival was 71% for those who were T2–3 post-M-VAC. TURB alone, partial cystectomy and radical cystectomy groups had 5-year survival of 69%, 69% and 53%, respectively. It is clear that response to chemotherapy is an extremely important prognostic factor.

Randomized and non-randomized trials have demonstrated the feasibility of administering neoadjuvant chemotherapy, with an overall response rate of about 70% and pathological complete response of 20–30%. These studies have also shown that approximately 30% of bladder tumours staged as T0 after neoadjuvant chemotherapy will have persistent muscle-invasive disease when cystectomy is performed. The most significant prognostic factor for survival appears to be attainment of P0 status [25]. Response to chemotherapy is a prognostic factor of extreme importance, and should be considered when making clinical decisions. In addition, patients with invasive bladder tumours who achieve T0 status after neoadjuvant M-VAC may preserve their bladders with bladder sparing surgery [26,27].

Neoadjuvant chemotherapy and bladder preservation

There are two major reasons why patients refuse cystectomy: loss of sexual function and loss of the ileal conduit (urostomy). Alternative approaches include bladder substitution and bladder preservation.

Since orthotopic bladder substitution has become available many urologists have preferred this kind of early definitive therapy. But if in selected cases there is the possibility of bladder preservation, this chance should not be dismissed. This approach has been used with success in the treatment of other solid tumours such as breast cancer, anal cancer, laryngeal carcinoma and osteo-sarcoma. Bladder preservation to the patient means less surgery, no need for a urinary diversion and a normal sexual life. These factors are of great importance in determining quality of life.

Bladder preservation is possible with an integrated approach using chemotherapy and RT [28,29]. Table 6.2 outlines some of the most recent studies of combined chemotherapy and RT to achieve bladder preservation. The combination of neoadjuvant chemotherapy and RT can produce 5-year survival rates between 42% and 63%, preserving the organ in approximately 40% of patients.

In the trial from Massachusetts General Hospital, patients were treated with two cycles of CMV chemotherapy followed by cisplatin and RT [28].

Table 6.2 Non-randomized trials of combined chemotherapy and radiotherapy

Series	n	Chemotherapy	5-year survival (%)	5-year survival with intact bladder (%)
Radiation Therapy Oncology Group-1 [30]	42	DDP	52	42
University of Erlangen [31]	139	DDP or Carbo	52	41
Genoa [19]	76	DDP/5-FU	42	Not yet reached
Radiation Therapy Oncology Group-2 [29]	91	CMV	62*	44
Massachusetts General Hospital [28]	106	CMV	52	43
University of Paris [32]	120	DDP/5-FU	63	Not yet reached

*4-year survival data.

Patients who responded received further chemotherapy and RT. Cystectomy was performed on non-responders. Five-year survival was 52%, and 43% of patients retained an intact functioning bladder. Prognostic factors for local curability are small tumour size, absence of hydronephrosis, papillary histology, a visible complete TURB and a complete response to induction chemotherapy. These very interesting results need to be confirmed by randomized trials.

Bladder preservation has recently been reported on by several groups [26–28,33] and has proved to be a feasible alternative. It has also been scrutinized since the advent of neobladders. Bladder preservation remains a controversial topic, and radical cystectomy must still be regarded as the gold standard of treatment for muscle-invasive bladder cancer. However, neoadjuvant chemotherapy/bladder preservation is feasible and may be an effective treatment, particularly in patients with smaller T2–T3a lesions. Other factors such as the presence of CIS in the prostatic urethra, bladder capacity, and general medical condition will affect the decision to employ chemotherapy or immediate surgery. Whether or not RT should be added to bladder preserving treatments is still to be determined.

Attempts at bladder preservation should also evaluate the use and toxicity of these combined modalities. The true success of bladder preserving treatment by chemotherapy and RT will require validation in prospective randomized trials.

Adjuvant chemotherapy

Patients at high risk for relapse after cystectomy are given adjuvant chemotherapy. This approach has led to increases in survival in patients with several solid tumours.

The principal advantage is that the treatment decision can be based on the pathological risk of recurrence and prognostic factors for relapse and/or metastases can be determined, since the cystectomy specimen is available for pathological evaluation. The adjuvant approach also avoids delaying potentially curative surgery. In addition it avoids patient refusal, which may occur when a complete response has been achieved with neoadjuvant chemotherapy [8]. Orthotopic bladder substitutions and the decreased morbidity of cystectomy are reasons to perform cystectomy and use adjuvant chemotherapy.

The major disadvantages of adjuvant chemotherapy are the delay in giving systemic therapy for occult metastases while treatment for the primary tumour is emphasized, and the impossibility of assessing response *in vivo*. Additional disadvantages are that it can be difficult to administer chemotherapy following cystectomy and that clinical trials to define efficacy in the adjuvant setting require large numbers of patients to detect a survival advantage.

Table 6.3 Trials of adjuvant chemotherapy following cystectomy

Reference	Year	Chemotherapy	Chemotherapy (n)	No chemotherapy (n)	Randomized	Results
34, 35	1988	CISCA	62	71	No	Benefit but not randomized
36	1991	CAP	47	44	Yes	Benefit, but too few patients received therapy
37	1992	M-VAC/ M-VEC	23	26	Yes	Benefit, but small patient numbers, premature closure, no treatment at relapse
38	1994	DDP	40	37	Yes	No benefit, single agent therapy probably inadequate
39	1989	CM	48	35	Yes	No benefit for N0M0
40	1996	CMV	25	25	Yes	Benefit in relapse-free survival

In one of the first adjuvant trials, Logothetis *et al.* [34,35] divided patients into three groups: low-risk controls, high-risk controls who had one high-risk pathological finding (refused, not offered or had medical contraindications to adjuvant chemotherapy), and high-risk patients treated with adjuvant chemotherapy. There was clearly a benefit for the 71 patients at high risk who received adjuvant cisplatin, doxorubicin and cyclophosphamide (CISCA) chemotherapy. Although this study is provocative, it is not a randomized trial. These patients were selected for treatment based upon their compliance and general medical condition. This does not substitute for a controlled, randomized trial. However, it may suggest a benefit for adjuvant chemotherapy in highly selected patients.

Five randomized trials have examined adjuvant chemotherapy (Table 6.3). The trials have been difficult to interpret because of problems such as small sample size and early closure. These trials suggest that there may be a benefit for adjuvant chemotherapy, but have not had enough statistical power to prove this.

Two studies that suggested a benefit for chemotherapy over observation alone received considerable attention. The Skinner study [36] was the first randomized prospective trial that showed a significant increase in time to progression and survival in patients who were randomized to receive chemotherapy. Patients with pT3–4 or N+ disease were randomized to either observation or four cycles of cyclophosphamide, doxorubicin and cisplatin (CAP). A significant delay in time to progression was observed for patients who received chemotherapy (70% vs. 46% disease-free survival at 3 years). Median survival time for patients in the chemotherapy group was 4.3 years vs. 2.4 years in the observation group. The single most important variable was the number of involved lymph nodes. This study has been highly criticized by medical oncologists for its retrospective use of subgroup analyses and its statistical methodology. Use of the Wilcoxon test may have provided artificial results in the context of the survival curves, with curves which crossed over with follow-up. While chemotherapy appeared to prolong the median time to recurrence by 14 months, there was no residual advantage at 2 years.

This study demonstrates some of the difficulties in this kind of trial. Of 498 cystectomies, only 229 were pT3–4 or N+. Of 160 eligible patients, only 91 were randomized. Eleven then refused chemotherapy. Only 20/44 (45%) patients received four cycles of chemotherapy as planned.

The other adjuvant study that has been highly noted is by the Mainz group [37]. Patients were randomized to either cystectomy or cystectomy followed by M-VAC or M-VEC. This study treated small numbers of patients with poor risk factors. Sixty per cent had positive nodes and most were stage T4.

The study was closed prematurely after an interim analysis revealed a benefit for those randomized to the chemotherapy arm, with 27% progression in the treated vs. 82% progression in the control, untreated arm. The study was published first in 1992 and updated in 1995. Survival was markedly different between the two arms, as the authors did not treat the patients who relapsed in the observation arm. In an intent to treat analysis, 5-year progression-free survival was 59% after a recommendation to receive chemotherapy vs. 13% after a recommendation of cystectomy alone [41].

Taken together these trials fail to prove that adjuvant chemotherapy provides a survival benefit in muscle-invasive transitional cell carcinoma. The most common problems encountered in the interpretation of results are inadequate numbers, premature closure, deviations from protocol entry, patient selection, subset analysis, and failure to treat at relapse.

Studies have not clearly proven any advantage for adjuvant therapy based upon muscle infiltration alone (pT2). For patients with extravesical extension (pT3), additional therapy may be useful. For patients with nodal metastases (pN+) and direct extension into the adjacent viscera (pT4), there is a suggestion of improved survival with adjuvant chemotherapy [8]. Decisions concerning individual patients must be based on the careful examination of the specimen and knowledge of the relapse rates per pathologic stage. A large international randomized trial coordinated by Dr Cora Sternberg from the EORTC with collaboration of groups throughout the world will prospectively evaluate in more than 1300 patients whether adjuvant chemotherapy must be given immediately to all high risk patients, or can be given at the time of relapse.

Metastatic disease

The only current modality which provides the potential for long-term survival in patients with metastatic disease is systemic chemotherapy. Anti-tumour activity has been demonstrated with several single agents, with only rare improvements in survival. Response rates to single agent chemotherapy are detailed in Table 6.4.

The development of cisplatin-based combination chemotherapy regimens for the treatment of patients with metastatic urothelial cancer was preeminent in the 1980s. M-VAC (methotrexate, vinblastine, adriamycin, cisplatin), CMV (cisplatin, methotrexate, vinblastine), CM (cisplatin, methotrexate), and CISCA/CAP (cyclophosphamide, adriamycin, cisplatin) have been considered among the most active regimens [43–45].

The average duration of survival for single agents varied between 4 and 6 months. Survival with combination regimens, such as methotrexate plus vinblastine or adriamycin plus cisplatin, was 8 months [46].

It has been 15 years since the M-VAC regimen was first developed at Memorial Hospital, New York [47]. In 121 cases with bidimensionally measurable disease, the complete and partial response rate was 72%. Thirty-six per cent of patients attained a complete response (CR). Long-term survival was achieved in patients who attained CR. Patients who achieved a CR to

Table 6.4 Response to single agents in advanced urothelial cancer (modified from Sternberg [42])

Single agent chemotherapy	*n*	CR + PR (%)	95% confidence limits
Methotrexate	236	29	23–35
Cisplatin	578	30	26–34
Adriamycin	269	19	14–24
Vinblastine	42	14	3–25
Cyclophosphamide	26	8	0–10
Ifosfamide	47	21	9–33
Epirubicin	33	15	3–27
Carboplatin	174	13	8–18
Piritrexim	29	38	20–56
Trimetrexate	51	17	7–30
Mitomycin C	42	13	3–23
5-Fluorouracil	75	35	24–46
Gemcitabine	120	28	20–36
Gallium nitrate	66	17	8–26
Taxol	26	42	23–63
Lobaplatin [80]	22	12	0–30
Topotecan [81]	46	10	3–23

CR, complete response; PR, partial response.

chemotherapy plus surgery had twice the survival of patients who had a partial response (PR) alone [43]. Overall survival for the whole group was 13.1
months. Chemotherapy was shown to be more effective against nodal disease
than against visceral metastases [43,48].

These data have been updated by the Memorial group, who have reported
results in 203 patients treated with several different M-VAC regimens. At a
median follow-up of 47 months, 46 patients attained a CR with chemotherapy alone. The 5-year survival rate was 40%. In 30 patients who had a CR
with chemotherapy plus surgery, 5-year survival was 33% at a median follow-
up of 37 months. Post-chemotherapy resection of viable tumour could result
in long-term survival in selected patients [49].

While the optimal chemotherapy combination has not yet been defined,
data from two randomized trials support the assumption that the M-VAC
regimen is the most effective one. The Southeastern Cancer Study Group
studied M-VAC vs. single agent cisplatin. In 239 evaluable patients, a significant difference in overall response rate was observed (11% treated with
cisplatin compared with 36% treated with M-VAC). Eighteen (15%) patients
achieved CR with M-VAC. Median survival for M-VAC treated patients
was 13.5 months compared with 8.2 months in patients given cisplatin
($P = 0.04$) [50].

The second trial at the MD Anderson Cancer Center (Houston, Texas)
compared M-VAC with the three drug regimen cisplatin, doxorubicin and
cyclophosphamide (CISCA). M-VAC was found to be superior to CISCA in
terms of response and survival. The CR + PR rate was 65% with M-VAC and
46% with CISCA ($P < 0.05$). The median survival was 11.2 months after
M-VAC compared with 8.4 months with CISCA [48].

The median survival after M-VAC in these two studies was approximately
one year [48,50], similar to the median survival reported at Memorial (13
months).

Unfortunately, the use of cisplatin-based combination chemotherapy
is associated with significant toxicity and produces long-term survival in
only approximately 15–20% of patients. The median survival duration is
only 13 months, and long-term survival is attained in approximately 15%
of patients with metastases in visceral sites and 30% of those with nodal
disease in the original MSKCC series. In the Intergroup study, only 3.2% of
patients with metastatic lesions treated with M-VAC were alive and free of
disease [51]. Therefore, other therapeutic options and strategies are clearly
needed.

Strategies to increase CR include augmenting the dose of chemotherapy
with haematological growth factor support. When M-VAC was given with
granulocyte colony-stimulating factor (G-CSF), mucositis and myelosuppression were ameliorated [52]. After initial favourable reports of responses in

heavily pretreated patients with escalated M-VAC and growth factors [53], several groups began phase II trials of escalated chemotherapy [6,54,55]. In the United States, this approach has been largely abandoned because of toxicity [54,55].

The EORTC Genitourinary Group trial is the only study which addresses the issue of dose intensity in a randomized trial comparing high-dose M-VAC (HD-M-VAC) with standard M-VAC [56]. With an every 2 weeks schedule plus G-CSF it was possible to deliver twice the dose of DDP and ADM in half the time, with less dose delay and less toxicity. This decrease in toxicity as com- pared with standard M-VAC was most likely attributable to the G-CSF. The overall response rate for both arms was 62%.

Whether or not this approach can lead to an improvement in survival has yet to be determined. Escalated dosage M-VAC cannot be recommended as standard therapy at this time.

The promising early results with new agents such as gemcitabine and paclitaxel has led to the incorporation of these agents into combination regimens.

Gemcitabine

Gemcitabine is a deoxycytidine analogue that inhibits DNA synthesis. When used as a single agent, response rates of 23% to 28% have been obtained in both pretreated patients and those who have not had prior therapy. Single agent studies with gemcitabine are shown in Table 6.5.

Gemcitabine is clearly an active new agent in the treatment of TCC of the urothelium. For patients who have mild renal failure or who have significant underlying poor medical condition, gemcitabine may be considered as a rea- sonable alternative to be used as monotherapy. Combination studies clearly deserve a high priority considering the response rates comparable to that of cisplatin.

Table 6.6 details phase II trials with gemcitabine and cisplatin in advanced bladder cancer. Kaufman evaluated a gemcitabine–cisplatin combination in 47 previously untreated patients. Cisplatin at 100 mg/m^2 was administered on

Table 6.5 Single agent trials with gemcitabine in advanced TCC

Reference	Year	*n*	Prior therapy	Response rate (%)	Gemzar (mg/m^2)
57	1994	15	Yes	27	875–1370
58	1997	39	No	28	1200
59	1997	37	No	24	1200
60	1998	31	Yes	23	1200

Table 6.6 Trials of gemcitabine and cisplatin (DDP) combination regimens in advanced TCC

Reference	Year	n	Prior therapy	Response rate (%)	Gemzar (mg/m²) (day)	DDP (mg/m²) (day)
61	1997	44	No	40	1000 (1, 8, 15)	35 (1, 8, 15)
62	1998	47	No/Yes	66	1000 (1, 8, 15)	100, 75 (1)
63	1998	29	No	59	1000 (1, 8, 15)	70 (2)

day 1 and gemcitabine at 1000 mg/m² on days 1, 8 and 15 of a 28-day cycle [62]. The cisplatin dose was reduced to 75 mg/m² in the last 34 patients because of myelosuppression. Thirteen complete responses and 18 partial responses were noted for an overall response rate of 66% (95% CI 51–79). In this trial myelosuppression was significant.

In a joint Scandinavian, Italian and German study, gemcitabine and cisplatin were given weekly to patients who had had no prior chemotherapy. A 40% response rate was obtained, with a median survival of 12.1 months. Significant myelosuppression, particularly thrombocytopenia, resulted, most likely because of the unusual dosage schedule of cisplatin chemotherapy [61]. Notably, in both of these trials responses were obtained in patients with extra-nodal disease sites including liver and lung.

A more rational dose of gemcitabine and cisplatin was chosen for a randomized international trial in 19 countries, with the majority of patients coming from Denmark, Germany and England [63]. This industry-sponsored study has compared gemcitabine on days 1, 8 and 15 and cisplatin at 70 mg/m² every 4 weeks with M-VAC. Eligibility criteria include patients with T4b, N2, N3 and M1 disease. The trial was designed to detect a difference in survival from 12 months with M-VAC to 16 months with gemcitabine and cisplatin. Almost 400 patients have been entered between October 1996 and September 1998. The results are being analysed in terms of efficacy, survival and toxicity.

Taxoids

The taxoids represent a novel class of antineoplastic drugs. Paclitaxel and docetaxel share a similar mechanism of action: the promotion of microtubule assembly and inhibition of microtubule disassembly. In the Eastern Cooperative Oncology Group trial a 42% response rate (27% CR) was reported in previously untreated patients when a relatively high dose of taxol (250 mg/m²) was administered with G-CSF [64]. Single agent docetaxel produced a 13% response rate in previously treated patients at the Memorial Hospital. However, as first line therapy the regimen produced a 31% response rate. Paclitaxel's significant activity and its renal sparing metabolism make it an

Table 6.7 Single agent trials of paclitaxel or docetaxel in advanced TCC

Reference	Year	n	Prior chemotherapy	Response rate (%)	Dose (mg/m²)	Therapy
64	1994	26	No	42	250 G-CSF	Taxol
65	1997	30	Yes	13	100	Taxotere
66	1998	29	No	31	100	Taxotere

Table 6.8 Trials of taxol and taxotere in combination regimens in advanced TCC

Reference	Year	n	Prior chemotherapy	Response rate (%)	Dose (mg/m²)	Therapy
67	1995	26	Yes	40	200 + G-CSF	Taxol/MTX/DDP
68	1999	34	No	62	135	Taxol/DDP
69	1998	20	No	63	225	Taxol/DDP
70	1999	38	No	63	175	Taxol/CBDCA AUC 5
71	1998	45	Yes/No	37	225	Taxol/CBDCA AUC 6
72	1998	33	No	52	150–225	Taxol/CBDCA AUC 6
73	1999	29	No	14	200	Taxol/CBDCA AUC 5
74	1998	24	No	50	200 + G-CSF	Taxol/CBDCA AUC 5
75	1998	25	No	60	75	Taxotere/DDP

ideal agent to combine with other active drugs in advanced urothelial carcinoma (Table 6.7).

A number of trials have been done on taxol and taxotere combination regimens (Table 6.8). One of the first to use a taxol combination was Tu at MD Anderson. He combined taxol, methotrexate and cisplatin and reported a 40% response rate in patients who had received prior M-VAC [67]. McCaffrey evaluated the combination of ifosfamide, cisplatin and paclitaxel (200 mg/m²). In 44 untreated patients the overall response rate was 68%, with complete response in 23% of the patients. The median survival duration was 20 months but in this study visceral disease was present in only 52% of patients [76]. Vaughn recently reported the results of a phase I/II trial with the combination of taxol and carboplatin; he reported a 52% response rate and time to progression of 6.9 months. Activity of this combination was documented in patients with visceral metastases. Median survival was only 8.5 months [72]. Several other phase II trials have evaluated the combination of taxol and cisplatin [67–69], and of taxol and carboplatin [70–74]. The median duration of survival with taxol and carboplatin has been 9 months. Taxotere has also been combined with cisplatin [75].

Paclitaxel is an active agent in the treatment of patients with advanced urothelial carcinoma. The lack of nephrotoxicity provides potential advantage over the standard cisplatin-based combinations. Paclitaxel-based regimens have been developed and reported. Ongoing cooperative group trials will help to further define the activity and toxicity of these regimens. The role of paclitaxel in the early disease and in a combined modality setting in transitional cell carcinoma remains to be determined.

New combination regimens

Based upon a phase I dose-escalating trial by Rothenberg *et al.* [77], we combined gemcitabine 2500–3000 mg/m^2 and taxol 150 mg/m^2 given every 2 weeks in a trial with patients in Italy and Israel [78]. Of 21 patients with bidimensionally measurable metastatic disease who had failed M-VAC, the overall response rate was 62%. Five (24%) patients attained a complete response and 8 (38%) achieved a partial one. The median duration of response and survival has not yet been reached. Grade 3–4 toxicity consisted of neutropenia in 8 (37%) and neurotoxicity in 1 (4%). Of note, no grade 3–4 thrombocytopenia was observed. This study will be continued until 42 patients have been entered. The combination of gemcitabine and taxol appears to be highly effective for patients with advanced TCC who have failed prior cisplatin-containing chemotherapy.

In a phase II Spanish cooperative group trial, gemcitabine, taxol and cisplatin were combined. Taxol 80 mg/m^2 and gemcitabine 1000 mg/m^2 were given on days 1 and 8, with cisplatin on day 1 [79]. The delivered dose intensity for cisplatin was 100%, and 80–90% for gemcitabine and taxol. Dose reductions occurred in 12 patients on day 1 and in 21 patients on day 8 (48% had dose reductions). G-CSF was given to 18 patients. There was one toxic death. Astenia was a significant problem with this regimen. The overall response rate in 40 patients was extremely high (80%). Ten (25%) attained a CR and 22 (55%) a PR. The median follow-up is only 9.5 months thus far. This regimen will be employed in an upcoming EORTC randomized trial where it will be compared with either M-VAC, HD-M-VAC or gemcitabine and cisplatin.

Conclusion

Transitional cell carcinoma is a chemotherapy-sensitive tumour and patients with metastatic disease are potentially curable with multiagent chemotherapy. A logical consequence of this observation is the use of adjuvant and neoadjuvant chemotherapy to enhance survival in patients with muscle-infiltrating disease. However, thus far trials evaluating preoperative or postoperative chemotherapy in muscle-invasive disease have failed to demonstrate a survival advantage. A major reason is that these studies are flawed by inadequate chemotherapy or insufficient number of patients.

During the last decade several new agents have demonstrated activity in advanced urothelial carcinoma. Although there are now several active combination regimens available, there are no data demonstrating that any of these regimens improve patient survival, produce more durable responses or are less toxic than M-VAC. Therefore, only randomized controlled phase III trials with an endpoint of improving survival can change the gold standard. Consideration must also be given to those regimens that can be administered in an outpatient setting, are relatively cost-effective and have acceptable toxicity. It is to be hoped that improved understanding of the biological predictors of outcome will lead to more effective management of bladder cancer.

References

1   American Cancer Society. What are the key statistics about bladder cancer? Internet Communication. American Cancer Society (GENERIC), 1998.

2   Sternberg CN, Swanson DA. Non transitional cell bladder cancer. In: Raghavan D, Scher HI, Leibel SA, Lange P, eds. *Principles and Practice of Genitourinary Oncology.* Philadelphia: Lippincott-Raven, 1997: 315–30.

3   Herr HW. Staging invasive bladder tumors. *J Surg Oncol* 1992; **51**: 217–20.

4   Vieweg J, Whitmore WF Jr, Herr HW. The role of pelvic lymphadenectomy and radical cystectomy for lymph node positive bladder cancer. *Cancer* 1994; **74**: 3020–8.

5   Montie JE. Follow-up after cystectomy for carcinoma of the bladder. *Urol Clin North Am* 1994; **21**: 639–43.

6   Sternberg CN. The treatment of advanced bladder cancer. *Ann Oncol* 1995; **6**: 113–26.

7   Scher HI. Chemotherapy for invasive bladder tumors. *Prog Clin Biol Res* 1990; **353**: 1–22.

8   Sternberg CN, Raghavan D, Ohi Y. Neo-adjuvant and adjuvant chemotherapy in locally advanced disease: what are the effects on survival and prognosis? *Int J Urol* 1995; **2**: 76–88.

9   Donat SM, Herr HW, Bajorin DF *et al.* Methotrexate, vinblastine, doxorubicin and cisplatin chemotherapy and cystectomy for unresectable bladder cancer. *J Urol* 1996; **156**: 368–71.

10 Advanced Bladder Cancer Overview Collaboration. Does neoadjuvant cisplatin-based chemotherapy improve the survival of patients with locally advanced bladder cancer? A meta-analysis of individual patient data from randomized clinical trials. *Br J Urol* 1995; **75**: 206–13.

11 Parmar MK. Neoadjuvant chemotherapy in invasive bladder cancer: trial design. *Prog Clin Biol Res* 1990; **353**: 115–18.

12 Anonymous. Neoadjuvant cisplatin, methotrexate, and vinblastine chemotherapy for muscle-invasive bladder cancer: a randomised controlled trial. *Lancet* 1999; **354**: 533–40.

13 Malmstrom PU, Rintala E, Wahlqvist R, Hellstrom P, Hellsten S, Hannisdal E. Five year follow-up of a prospective trial of radical cystectomy and neoadjuvant chemotherapy. *J Urol* 1996; **155**: 1903–6.

14 Bassi P, Pagano F, Pappagallo G *et al.* Neo-adjuvant M-VAC of invasive bladder cancer: the G.U.O.N.E. multicenter phase III trial. *Eur Urol* 1998; **33** (Suppl. 1): 142 (Abstract 567).

15 Crawford ED, Natale RB, Burton H. Southwest Oncology Group Study (8710): Trial of cystectomy alone versus neo-adjuvant M-VAC and cystectomy in patients with locally advanced bladder cancer (Intergroup Trial 0080). *Prog Clin Biol Res* 1990; **353**: 111–14.

16 Wallace DM, Raghavan D, Kelly KA *et al.* Neo-adjuvant (pre-emptive) cisplatin therapy in invasive transitional cell carcinoma of the bladder. *Br J Urol* 1991; **67**: 608–15.

17 Coppin CM, Gospodarowicz MK, James K *et al*. Improved local control of invasive bladder cancer by concurrent cisplatin and preoperative or definitive radiation. (The National Cancer Institute of Canada Clinical Trials Group.) *J Clin Oncol* 1996; **14**: 2901–7.

18 Martinez Pineiro JA, Gonzalez Martin M, Arocena F. Neoadjuvant cisplatin chemotherapy before radical cystectomy in invasive transitional cell carcinoma of the bladder: prospective randomized phase III study. *J Urol* 1995; **153**: 964–73.

19 Orsatti M, Curotto A, Canobbio L. Alternating chemo-radiotherapy in bladder cancer: a conservative approach. *Int J Radiation Oncol Biol Phys* 1995; **33**: 173–8.

20 Shipley WU, Winter KA, Kaufman DS *et al*. Phase III trial of neoadjuvant chemotherapy in patients with invasive bladder cancer treated with selective bladder preservation by combined radiation therapy and chemotherapy: initial results of Radiation Therapy Oncology Group 89-03. *J Clin Oncol* 1998; **16**: 3576–83.

21 Malmstrom PU, Rintala E, Wahlqvist R *et al*. Neoadjuvant cisplatin-methotrexate chemotherapy of invasive bladder cancer: Nordic cystectomy trial 2. *Eur Urol* 1999; **35** (Suppl. 2): 60 (Abstract 238).

22 Abol-Enein H, El Makresh M, El Baz M, Ghoneim M. Neo-adjuvant chemotherapy in treatment of invasive transitional bladder cancer: a controlled, prospective randomised study. *Br J Urol* 1997; **80** (Suppl. 2): 49.

23 Splinter TA, Scher HI, Denis L *et al*. The prognostic value of the pathological response to combination chemotherapy before cystectomy in patients with invasive bladder cancer. (European Organization for Research on Treatment of Cancer — Genitourinary Group.) *J Urol* 1992; **147**: 606–8.

24 Sternberg CN, Pansadoro V, Calabrò F *et al*. Neo-adjuvant chemotherapy and bladder preservation in locally advanced transitional cell carcinoma of the bladder. *Ann Oncol* 1999; **10**: 1301–5.

25 Schultz PK, Herr HW, Zhang Z. Neoadjuvant chemotherapy for invasive bladder cancer: prognostic factors for survival of patients with M-VAC with 5 years follow-up. *J Clin Oncol* 1994; **12**: 1394–401.

26 Sternberg CN, Pansadoro V, Lauretti S *et al*. Neo-adjuvant M-VAC (methotrexate, vinblastine, adriamycin and cisplatin) chemotherapy and bladder preservation for muscle infiltrating transitional cell carcinoma of the bladder. *Urol Oncol* 1995; **1**: 127–33.

27 Herr HW, Bajorin DF, Scher HI. Neoadjuvant chemotherapy and bladder sparing surgery for invasive bladder cancer: ten-year outcome. *J Clin Oncol* 1998; **16**: 1298–301.

28 Kachnic LA, Kaufman DS, Heney NM. Bladder preservation by combined modality therapy for invasive bladder cancer. *J Clin Oncol* 1997; **15**: 1022–9.

29 Tester W, Caplan R, Heaney J. Neoadjuvant combined modality program with selective organ preservation for invasive bladder cancer: results of Radiation Therapy Oncology Group phase II trial 8802. *J Clin Oncol* 1996; **14**: 119–26.

30 Tester W, Porter A, Asbell S. Combined modality program with possible organ preservation for invasive bladder carcinoma: results of RTOG protocol 85-12. *Int J Radiation Oncol Biol Phys* 1993; **25**: 783.

31 Sauer R, Birkenhake S, Kühn R *et al*. Muscle-invasive bladder cancer: transurethral resection and radiochemotherapy as an organ-sparing treatment option. In: Petrovich Z, Baert L, Brady LW, eds. *Carcinoma of the Bladder*. Berlin: Springer-Verlag, 1998: 205–14.

32 Housset M, Dufour B, Maulard-Durdux C, Chretien Y, Mejean A. Concomitant fluorouracil (5-FU)-cisplatin (CDDP) and bifractionated split course radiation therapy (BSCRT) for invasive bladder cancer. *Proc Am Soc Clin Oncol* 1997; **16**: 319a (Abstract 139).

33 Sternberg CN, Arena MG, Calabresi F *et al*. Neo-adjuvant M-VAC (methotrexate,

vinblastine, adriamycin and cisplatin) for infiltrating transitional cell carcinoma of the urothelium. *Cancer* 1993; **72**: 1975–82.

34   Logothetis CJ, Johnson DE, Chong C *et al.* Adjuvant chemotherapy of bladder cancer: a preliminary report. *J Urol* 1988; **139**: 1207–11.

35   Logothetis CJ, Johnson DE, Chong C *et al.* Adjuvant cyclophosphamide, doxorubicin, and cisplatin chemotherapy for bladder cancer: an update. *J Clin Oncol* 1988; **6**: 1590–6.

36   Skinner DG, Daniels JR, Russell CA *et al.* The role of adjuvant chemotherapy following cystectomy for invasive bladder cancer: a prospective comparative trial. *J Urol* 1991; **145**: 459–67.

37   Stockle M, Meyenburg W, Wellek S *et al.* Advanced bladder cancer (stages pT3b, pT4a, pN1 and pN2): improved survival after radical cystectomy and 3 adjuvant cycles of chemotherapy — results of a controlled prospective study. *J Urol* 1992; **148**: 302–7.

38   Studer UE, Bacchi M, Biedermann C. Adjuvant cisplatin chemotherapy following cystectomy for bladder cancer: results of a prospective randomized trial. *J Urol* 1994; **152**: 81–4.

39   Bono AV, Benvenuti C, Reali L *et al.* Adjuvant chemotherapy in advanced bladder cancer. (Italian Uro-Oncologic Cooperative Group.) *Prog Clin Biol Res* 1989; **303**: 533–40.

40   Freiha F, Reese J, Torti FM. A randomized trial of radical cystectomy versus radical cystectomy plus cisplatin, vinblastine and methotrexate chemotherapy for muscle invasive bladder cancer. *J Urol* 1996; **155**: 495–9.

41   Stockle M, Meyenburg W, Wellek S. Adjuvant polychemotherapy of nonorgan-confined bladder cancer after radical cystectomy revisited: long term results of a controlled prospective study and further clinical experience. *J Urol* 1995; **153**: 47–52.

42   Sternberg C, Marini L, Calabrò F, Scavina P. Systemic chemotherapy of bladder cancer. In: Skinner DG, Syrigos KN, eds. *Bladder Cancer: Biology and Management.* New York: Oxford University Press, 1999: 299–315.

43   Sternberg CN, Yagoda A, Scher HI *et al.* M-VAC for advanced transitional cell carcinoma of the urothelium: efficacy, patterns of response and relapse. *Cancer* 1989; **64**: 2448–58.

44   Harker W, Meyers FJ, Freiha FS *et al.* Cisplatin, methotrexate, and vinblastine (CMV): an effective chemotherapy regimen for metastatic transitional cell carcinoma of the urinary tract — a Northern California Oncology Group study. *J Clin Oncol* 1985; **3**: 1463–70.

45   Logothetis CJ, Samuels ML, Selig DE, Wallace S, Johnson DE. Combined intravenous and intra-arterial cyclophosphamide, doxorubicin, and cisplatin (CISCA) in the management of select patients with invasive urothelial tumors. *Cancer Treat Report* 1985; **69**: 33–8.

46   Sternberg CN, Scher HI. Management of invasive bladder neoplasms. In: Smith PH, ed. *Combination Therapy in Urological Malignancy.* London: Springer-Verlag, 1989: 95–118.

47   Sternberg CN, Yagoda A, Scher HI *et al.* Preliminary results of methotrexate, vinblastine, adriamycin and cisplatin (M-VAC) in advanced urothelial tumors. *J Urol* 1985; **133**: 403–7.

48   Logothetis CJ, Dexeus F, Sella A *et al.* A prospective randomized trial comparing CISCA to MVAC chemotherapy in advanced metastatic urothelial tumors. *J Clin Oncol* 1990; **8**: 1050–5.

49   Bajorin D, Dodd PM, McCaffrey JA *et al.* M-VAC in transitional cell carcinoma (TCC): prognostic factors and long-term survival in 203 patients (pts). *Proc Am Soc Clin Oncol* 1998; **17**: 311a (Abstract 1198).

50   Loehrer P, Einhorn LH, Elson PJ *et al.* A randomized comparison of cisplatin alone or in combination with methotrexate, vinblastine, and doxorubicin in patients with metastatic urothelial carcinoma: a Cooperative Group study. *J Clin Oncol* 1992; **10**: 1066–73.

51   Saxman SB, Propert KJ, Einhorn LH *et al.* Long-term follow-up of a phase III intergroup study of cisplatin alone or in combination with methotrexate, vinblastine, and doxorubicin

in patients with metastatic urothelial carcinoma: a cooperative group study. *J Clin Oncol* 1997; **15**: 2564–9.

52   Gabrilove JL, Jakubowski A, Scher H *et al*. Effect of granulocyte colony-stimulating factor on neutropenia and associated morbidity due to chemotherapy for transitional-cell carcinoma of the urothelium. *N Engl J Med* 1988; **318**: 1414–22.

53   Logothetis CJ, Dexeus FH, Sella A *et al*. Escalated therapy for refractory urothelial tumors: methotrexate-vinblastine-doxorubicin-cisplatin plus unglycosylated recombinant human granulocyte-macrophage colony-stimulating factor. *J Natl Cancer Inst* 1990; **82**: 667–72.

54   Loehrer PJS, Elson P, Dreicer R *et al*. Escalated dosages of methotrexate, vinblastine, doxorubicin, and cisplatin plus recombinant human granulocyte colony-stimulating factor in advanced urothelial carcinoma: an Eastern Cooperative Oncology Group trial. *J Clin Oncol* 1994; **12**: 483–8.

55   Seidman AD, Scher HI, Gabrilove JL *et al*. Dose-intensification of methotrexate, vinblastine, doxorubicin, and cisplatin with recombinant granulocyte-colony stimulating factor as initial therapy in advanced urothelial cancer. *J Clin Oncol* 1992; **11**: 414–20.

56   Sternberg CN, de Mulder P, Fossa S *et al*. Interim toxicity analysis of a randomized trial in advanced urothelial tract tumors of high-dose intensity M-VAC chemotherapy (HD-MVAC) and recombinant human granulocyte colony stimulating factor (G-CSF) versus classic M-VAC chemotherapy (EORTC 30924). *Proc Am Soc Clin Oncol* 1997; **16**: 320a (Abstract 1140).

57   Pollera CF, Ceribelli A, Crecco M, Calabresi F. Weekly gemcitabine in advanced bladder cancer: a preliminary report from a phase I study. *Ann Oncol* 1994; **5**: 182–4.

58   Stadler WM, Kuzel T, Roth B, Raghavan D, Dorr FA. Phase II study of single-agent gemcitabine in previously untreated patients with metastatic urothelial cancer. *J Clin Oncol* 1997; **15**: 3394–8.

59   Moore MJ, Tannock IF, Ernst DS, Huan S, Murray N. Gemcitabine: a promising new agent in the treatment of advanced urothelial cancer. *J Clin Oncol* 1997; **15**: 3441–5.

60   Lorusso V, Pollera CF, Antimi M *et al*. A phase II study of gemcitabine in patients with transitional cell carcinoma of the urinary tract previously treated with platinum. *Eur J Cancer* 1998; **34**: 1208–12.

61   von der Maase H, Andersen L, Crino L, Weissbach L, Dogliotti L. A phase II study of gemcitabine and cisplatin in patients with transitional cell carcinoma (TCC) of the urothelium. *Proc Am Assoc Cancer Res* 1997; **16**: 324a (Abstract 1155).

62   Kaufman D, Stadler W, Carducci M *et al*. Gemcitabine (GEM) plus cisplatin (CDDP) in metastatic transitional cell carcinoma (TCC): final results of a phase II study. *Proc Am Soc Clin Oncol* 1998; **17**: 320a (Abstract 1235).

63   Moore MJ, Tannock I, Winquist E, Tolcher A, Bennett K, Seymour L. Gemcitabine (G) + cisplatin (C): an active regimen in advanced transitional cell carcinoma (TCC). *Proc Am Soc Clin Oncol* 1998; **17**: 320a (Abstract 1234).

64   Roth BJ, Dreicer R, Einhorn LH. Significant activity of paclitaxel in advanced transitional cell carcinoma of the urothelium: a phase II trial of the Eastern Cooperative Oncology Group. *J Clin Oncol* 1994; **12**: 2264–70.

65   McCaffrey JA, Hilton S, Mazumdar M. Phase II trial of docetaxel in patients with advanced or metastatic transitional cell carcinoma. *J Clin Oncol* 1997; **15**: 1853–7.

66   de Wit R, Kruit WH, Stoter G, de Boer M, Kerger J, Verweij J. Docetaxel (Taxotere): an active agent in metastatic urothelial cancer; results of a phase II study in non-chemotherapy pretreated patients. *Br J Cancer* 1998; **78**: 1342–5.

67   Tu SM, Hossa E, Amato R, Kilbourn R, Logothetis CJ. Paclitaxel, cisplatin and methotrexate combination chemotherapy is active in treatment of refractory urothelial malignancies. *J Urol* 1995; **154**: 1719–22.

68   Burch PA, Richardson RL, Cha SS *et al*. Phase II trial of combination paclitaxel and

cisplatin in advanced urothelial carcinoma (UC). *Proc Am Soc Clin Oncol* 1999; **18**: 329a (Abstract 1266).

69   Dreicer R, Roth B, Lipsitz S, Cohen M, See W, Wilding G. E2895 cisplatin and paclitaxel in advanced carcinoma of the urothelium: a phase II trial of the Eastern Cooperative Oncology Group (ECOG). *Proc Am Soc Clin Oncol* 1998; **17**: 320a (Abstract 1233).

70   Pycha A, Grbovic M, Posch B *et al*. Paclitaxel and carboplatin in patients with metastatic transitional cell cancer of the urinary tract. *Urology* 1999; **53**: 510–15.

71   Droz JP, Mottet N, Prapotrich D *et al*. Phase II study of taxol (Paclitaxel) and carboplatin in patients with advanced transitional cell carcinoma of the urothelium: preliminary results. *Proc Am Soc Clin Oncol* 1998; **17**: 316a (Abstract 1219).

72   Vaughn DJ, Malkowicz SB, Zoltick B *et al*. Paclitaxel plus carboplatin in advanced carcinoma of the urothelium: an active and tolerable outpatient regimen. *J Clin Oncol* 1998; **16**: 255–60.

73   Small EJ, Lew D, Petrylak DP, Crawford ED. Carboplatin and paclitaxel (Carbo/Tax) for advanced transitional cell carcinoma (TCC) of the urothelium. *Proc Am Soc Clin Oncol* 1999; **18**: 333a (Abstract 1280).

74   Meyers FJ, Edelman MJ, Houston J, Lauder I. Phase I/II trial of paclitaxel, carboplatin and methotrexate in advanced transitional cell carcinoma. *Proc Am Soc Clin Oncol* 1998; **17**: 317a (Abstract 1222).

75   Sengelov L, Kamby C, Lund B, Engelholm SA. Docetaxel and cisplatin in metastatic urothelial cancer: a phase II study. *J Clin Oncol* 1998; **16**: 3392–7.

76   McCaffrey JA, Hilton S, Mazumdar M *et al*. A phase II trial of ifosfamide, paclitaxel and cisplatin (TCC). *Proc Am Soc Clin Oncol* 1997; **16**: 324a (Abstract 1154).

77   Rothenberg ML, Sharma A, Weiss GR *et al*. Phase I trial of paclitaxel and gemcitabine administered every two weeks in patients with refractory solid tumors. *Ann Oncol* 1998; **9**: 733–8.

78   Marini L, Sternberg CN, Sella A, Calabrò F, van Rijn A. A new regimen of Gemcitabine and Paclitaxel in previously treated patients with advanced transitional cell carcinoma. *Proc Am Soc Clin Oncol* 1999; **18**: 346a (Abstract 1335).

79   Bellmunt J, Guillem V, Paz-Ares L *et al*. A phase II trial of Paclitaxel, Cisplatin and Gemcitabine (TCG) in patients (pts) with advanced transitional cell carcinoma (TCC). *Proc Am Soc Clin Oncol* 1999; **18**: 332a (Abstract 1279).

80   Sternberg CN, de Mulder P, Fossa S *et al*. Lobaplatin in advanced urothelial tract tumors. (European Organization for Research on Treatment of Cancer — Genitourinary Group.) *Ann Oncol* 1997; **8**: 695–6.

81   Witte RS, Manola J, Burch PA, Kuzel T, Weinshel EL, Loehrer PJ Sr. Topotecan in previously treated advanced urothelial carcinoma: an ECOG phase II trial. *Invest New Drugs* 1998; **16**: 191–5.

7: Treatment Options in Superficial (pTa/pT1/CIS) Bladder Cancer

J. L. Ockrim & P. D. Abel

Introduction

Bladder cancer is the fourth most common cancer in men and the eighth most common cancer in women worldwide and the incidence continues to rise [1]. The management of superficial bladder cancer requires an ever increasing commitment for clinical urologists. In the UK alone 11 000 new cases of bladder cancer per annum will contribute 5% to the national cancer burden [2]. Over 100 000 diagnostic, check and interventional cystoscopies per year will be performed in surveillance protocols in attempting to monitor disease progression. Clinicians are presented with an evolving malignancy requiring a constantly shifting therapeutic dynamic. The difficulties involved in this decision-making process were emphasized in McFarlane's *et al.* [3] interactive seminar in 1996, where considerable divergence of opinion was highlighted amongst clinicians posed with a variety of clinical scenarios.

The purpose of this chapter is to provide an overview of the current rationale behind the therapeutic options available for superficial bladder cancer treatment. In this way, we hope to empower clinicians with a broad sweep of the evidence on which therapy is based.

Current issues in tumour classification

The current system of bladder tumour classification is based on the International Union Against Cancer (UICC) revision of 1997 [4]. Superficial bladder disease is the term used to describe transitional cell carcinomas (TCCs) with histopathological category pTa and pT1 as well as carcinoma *in situ* (CIS). PTa tumours are confined to the urothelium protected by the basement membrane, whereas pT1 tumours have penetrated the lamina propria, invading subepithelial connective tissue but not yet as far as the underlying detrusor muscle. In recent years subcategorization of pT1 tumours has been proposed. The importance of the depth of lamina propria invasion was recognized by several authors [5,6]. Further retrospective analysis of patient cohorts [7,8] has shown significant differences in survival or progression rates when lamina propria invasion was divided into 'up to muscularis mucosae' (pT1a) or 'into muscularis mucosae' (pT1b) and 'beyond muscularis mucosae' (pT1c). By contrast the European Organization for Research and Treatment of Cancer — Genitourinary Group (EORTC-GU) multivariate analysis found little evidence that pT categorization impacted on recurrence or progression rates [9]. This surprising finding contradicts that of many historical series. The controversy is further confounded by the difficulties in obtaining consistent histological reporting from fragmented transurethral specimens [10]. As such the role of pT1 subdivision in deciding on therapy remains a subject for considerable debate, but may yet be an important influence on those proposing radical surgery for pT1 disease. Both vascular and lymphatic invasion have also been suggested as prognostic factors [8,11].

Natural history of superficial bladder cancer

Therapeutic interventions are currently based on clinical and histopathological data. Since the type and timing of adjuvant therapy depend on the prediction of biological change from an indolent to an aggressive phenotype, a good understanding of these prognostic factors is essential for the working practice of urologists and oncologists.

pTa/pT1 disease

STAGE (PT CATEGORY)

Between 70% and 80% of new bladder tumours will be superficial on presentation; 70% pTa and 30% pT1 [12]. Despite an assumption that bladder cancer develops through a logical sequence of biological events from superficial to invasive disease, pTa and pT1 category TCC show substantial differences in their muscle-invasive potential. Several series have shown that progression is nearly always associated with pT1 disease. Early work by Anderstrom *et al.* and Greene *et al.* [5,13] showed 5-year mortality rates of 24% with pT1 disease compared with rates of less than 1% with pTa tumours. The findings of the National Bladder Cancer Collaborative Group (NBCCG) also showed that progression rates are related to tumour stage, with only 3% of pTa disease showing progression compared with 30% of pT1 tumours [14]. Similar differences have been consistently shown in many other series, leading to suggestions for separate protocols for pTa and pT1 surveillance [15] (Figs 7.1 and 7.2).

GRADE

Many series have also shown the importance of tumour grade in rates of recurrence and progression. The NBCCG trials [14] reported progression rates

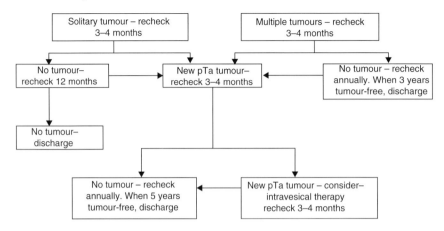

Figure 7.1 Suggested protocol for management of newly diagnosed pTa tumour (Abel [15]).

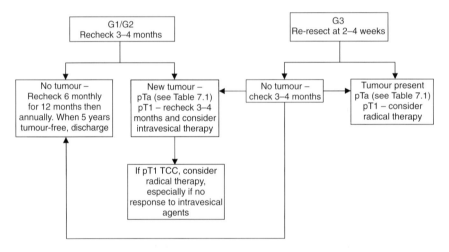

Figure 7.2 Suggested protocol for management of newly diagnosed pT1 tumour (Abel [15]).

for grades I, II and III of 2, 11 and 45%, respectively, figures reflected in similar studies. Other series have shown the importance of assessing grade within pTa/pT1 category [5,16].

FREQUENCY OF RECURRENCE

The interval to recurrence is of vital importance. Recurrence rates steadily decrease with the length of disease-free interval, such that the risk of further disease is less than 10% after 5 years of clear cystoscopic examination [17,18]. Moreover, Fitzpatrick *et al.* [18] demonstrated that the first check cystoscopy also pointed to future tumour activity; 80% of those with a clear 3-month cystoscopy remained disease free, whereas those with recurrent disease at 3 months had only a 10% chance of remaining disease free thereafter. The importance of initial treatment failure as a prognostic factor for long-term outcome has recently been reviewed by the EORTC-GU group [19].

MULTIFOCALITY AND TUMOUR SIZE

Multicentric presentation and tumour volume are also important prognostic factors. At diagnosis, 30% of lesions are multiple [20] and these carry a poorer prognosis than solitary tumours, with shorter disease-free intervals and higher progression rates [21]. In the NBCCG series [14] tumour size greater than 5 cm, and in the more recent EORTC-GU report [9] tumour size greater than 3 cm, correlated with poorer outcome.

RELATIVE RISK OF PROGNOSTIC FACTORS

The factors which predict the biological potential of superficial lesions must be correctly weighted before deciding on future cystoscopic surveillance protocols and interventional therapy. The relative importance of these prognostic factors was measured by multivariate analysis of two Medical Research Council (MRC) trials [22] and two EORTC-GU trials [9]. In the MRC analysis of tumour recurrence rates, tumour number at presentation and tumour recurrence at the first follow-up cystoscopy at 3 months were selected for their statistical strength over other prognostic factors. The certainty of these observations (one or more than one tumour and presence or absence of recurrence at follow-up), compared with the subjective interpretation of other histopathological data, led Hall *et al.* [23] to propose a cystoscopic and adjuvant chemotherapy protocol based on these factors alone (Fig. 7.3). The EORTC-GU analysed the relative risk of disease progression [9]. The greatest risk was for frequent disease recurrence followed by grade and size, respectively. This led to proposals for stratification of pTa/pT1 tumours into three different prognostic groups on which clinicians may decide the necessity of adjuvant therapy (Table 7.1).

Carcinoma *in situ*

The presence of carcinoma *in situ* (CIS) has profound implications for superficial disease prognosis. CIS can be divided into diffuse or focal categories. Diffuse CIS is nearly always reflected in filling (irritative) bladder symptomology and positive urine cytology, whereas focal CIS is frequently a marker for subsequent superficial tumour development. These two subsets of CIS disease have marked differences in invasive potential. In Lamm's [24] review of the CIS literature an overall progression rate of 54% was reported for untreated

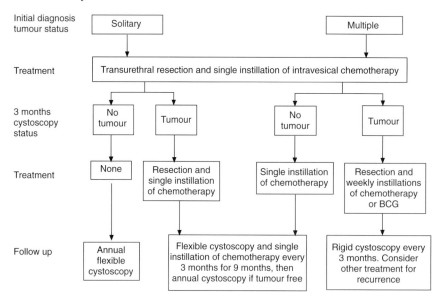

Figure 7.3 Proposed plan of management of patients with Ta or T1 bladder cancer (Hall *et al.* [23]).

Table 7.1 Risk index for patients in various subgroups (adapted from Kurth *et al.* [9]). Each cell gives the risk group

	RR <1			1–3			>3		
Tumour size (cm)	<1.5	1.5–3	>3	<1.5	1.5–3	>3	<1.5	1.5–3	>3
Grade									
G1	1	1	1	1	2	2	2	2	3
G2	1	2	2	2	2	3	3	3	3
G3	2	2	2	2	3	3	3	3	3

RR, recurrence rate per year.
Risk index estimated from the Cox model including only three factors: tumour size, G grade and RR. The estimated Cox models are: for invasion, $0.51RR + 0.84G + 0.48TS$; for death, $0.89RR + 0.73G + 0.44TS$.

CIS. Riddle *et al.* [25] showed muscle invasion occurring in 58% of those with diffuse disease compared with 8% of those with focal urothelial abnormalities. Association with papillary tumours increases this risk. Series reported by Althausen *et al.* and Herr *et al.* [26,27] showed progression rates of 83% and 71% when CIS and papillary tumour were noted together. Moreover, with diffuse CIS occult disease of the distal ureters and prostatic urethra may be present in as many as 60% [28]. This multicentric nature limits the use of transurethral extirpation in CIS treatment.

Role of transurethral surveillance and tumour resection

Cystoscopic visualization of the bladder remains the primary modality of diagnosis, surveillance and treatment of superficial bladder tumours. Attention to and accurate documentation of relevant clinical prognostic factors are essential components for future therapeutic decisions. This should include estimation of tumour number, size, position and configuration and intervals of recurrence. CIS is most commonly seen as 'velvety erythematous elevation' though it may also mimic the thickened white squamous metaplasia of catheter reaction or trigonitis. Tissue sampling by transurethral surveillance from all the affected areas is advocated to document the worst stage and tumour grade. The presence of muscle in the biopsy specimen is essential to maximize correct pT stage and should be documented in the histopathology report. In cases of suspected CIS, sampling of the prostatic urethra around the verumontanum is suggested, especially if cystectomy or cystoprostatectomy is proposed. The role of random biopsies of macroscopically normal urothelium to identify dysplasia has recently been thrown into doubt as less than 10% of normal appearing urothelium in either pTa or pT1 disease will show an abnormality [29]. Moreover, significant variations in the interpretation of histological samples may in fact hinder rather than benefit therapeutic decisions [30].

Recurrence vs. new occurrence

It is assumed that the incidence of local recurrence is low following cystoscopic extirpation of tumour, and that most treatment failure is a result of 'new occurrences' in remote areas of *de novo* urothelial dysplasia. The overall new occurrence rate following transurethral tumour ablation is approximately 50–70%. This rate is substantially affected by clinical response, with over 75% of those with rapidly recurrent lesions developing subsequent recurrences.

Inadequate resection may, however, be more common than expected. In one series of pT1 TCC [31], recurrent tumour was detected in 43% of those subjected to repeat biopsy of the original resection site. Although rates of this local recurrence may be reduced with laser ablation [32] there is no evidence to suggest that either modality is better than the other for reducing the rate of overall recurrence.

TRANSURETHRAL RESECTION VS. LASER ABLATION

Ablation of visible lesions may be achieved using diathermy or laser techniques. Resection allows the advantage of concomitant tissue sampling.

Whereas small pedunculated tumours may be removed in entirety, resection of larger or sessile areas should be achieved in layers to expose and sample the underlying muscle fibres. In lesions where invasive disease is a possibility, a separate biopsy of the tumour base is mandatory.

Laser therapy has the advantage of reducing the risk of postoperative bleeding. Most experience has been documented with Nd:Yag lasers. As the depth of penetration is largely dependent on the duration of tissue exposure, laser therapy is most suitable for small papillary tumours, although more extensive sessile tumours may also be treated if they are of limited thickness. The risk of bladder and adjacent visceral perforation is small if the laser is used within recommended power parameters [33], although caution should be used with lesions at the bladder dome, especially in women, where the bladder wall is most thin.

Role of intravesical therapy in tumour prophylaxis and CIS disease

Adjuvant intravesical therapy has been in use since the early 1970s. Its purpose is threefold: to eradicate residual tumour or CIS disease, to reduce the rate of recurrence and to reduce the risk of tumour progression. Differences are measured against treatment with transurethral tumour extirpation alone. Tumour response is dependent on the clinical status of the tumour and critically disease stage and grade. At present, four agents—doxorubicin, epirubicin, mitomycin C (MMC) and bacille Calmette-Guérin (BCG)—are in common use.

Intravesical cytotoxic chemotherapy

MECHANISMS, SIDE-EFFECTS AND DOSE REGIMES

Doxorubicin and epirubicin are anthracyclines, causing their cytotoxic effect by intercalating DNA base pairs, interrupting DNA and protein synthesis [34]. Their high molecular weight prevents systemic absorption and systemic side-effects, although self-limiting urgency and filling bladder symptoms are seen in up to 20% of cases [35]. Anthracycline chemotherapy has been tried in doses varying from 30 to 90 mg in induction and in maintenance schedules up to 1 year.

MMC is an alkylating agent, derived from *Streptomyces caespitosus*, which alkylates DNA causing strand breakage during replication [36]. Like the anthracyclines, high molecular weight limits systemic complications, and local side-effects such as bladder irritation do not pose a significant problem.

Cutaneous reactions often involving the genitalia and palms have been noted in up to 9% of patients exposed to multiple intravesical dosing. This is most likely caused by a delayed hypersensitivity response [37] and has seldom resulted in treatment termination. The typical regime for MMC is 20–40 mg given weekly for 6 weeks. Monthly maintenance regimes have also been tried for up to 1 year [38].

EFFICACY

Many series have shown significant reductions in short-term tumour recurrence rates with intravesical chemotherapy, with an average complete tumour regression rate of 33% for anthracyclines [38] and 33–50% for mitomycin C [39]. These rates are notably affected by tumour stage and grade with most efficacy apparent with low-grade, low-stage tumours [40]. The meta-analysis of Traynelis & Lamm [41] and subsequently the EORTC-GU and MRC trials [42] have indicated that intravesical chemotherapy increases the duration of disease-free interval. The influential study of the MRC showed that immediate instillation of MMC within 24 h of transurethral resection decreased recurrence rates and increased disease-free interval [43]. Although no apparent superiority of one chemotherapy agent over another has emerged, the trials comparing chemotherapy agents directly with BCG immunotherapy have shown a clear advantage of BCG over the anthracyclines. The superiority of BCG over mitomycin C is, however, less clear cut.

Unfortunately the long-term benefits of intravesical chemotherapy are less convincing. In a review of 2861 patients enrolled in controlled studies, Lamm [39] demonstrated that overall reduction in tumour recurrence averaged only 17% when extrapolated for estimated 5-year rates. Indeed, in those followed 5 years or more, the recurrence rate had reached that achieved using transurethral resection alone [44]. Neither has this figure been improved significantly by protracted maintenance therapy [45,46]. Even more disappointing is the failure of chemotherapy to affect overall survival rates. The EORTC-GU/MRC analysis [42] has shown that intravesical chemotherapy has no impact on either stage progression or survival statistics. No trial to date has demonstrated a significant improvement in these parameters.

MITOMYCIN C VS. BCG

Trials comparing MMC directly with BCG have been inconsistent in outcome. Inter- and cross-trial differences of inclusion criteria for therapy and interpretation of clinical and pathological factors have compounded the problems of analysis. At least three studies [47–49] have suggested that MMC could be equal to or better than certain BCG strains at reducing tumour recurrence. In each of these series, however, the BCG schedules used suboptimal maintenance regimen. The balance of evidence still suggests an advantage for BCG immunotherapy. Series reported by the Finnbladder Group [50] and Lundholm *et al.* [51] showed short-term response rates of 65% and 49% for BCG compared with 38% and 34% for MMC. The Southwest Oncology Group (SWOG) trials also showed superior BCG effect, with the SWOG 8795 trial [52] comparing MMC and BCG Ta/T1 tumour prophylaxis being terminated due to the significant advantage of BCG. In the meta-analysis of over 2000 patients treated in chemotherapy or immunotherapy trials (see above) Lamm [39] found recurrence rates at 5 years to be reduced only in the immunotherapy group. Thus, it appears that the therapeutic effect of BCG in prophylaxis is more durable than that of chemotherapy and tumours respond better to BCG especially at higher stage (pT1) and grade (2 and 3), although this improved response rate occurs at a cost of increased toxicity.

ROLE OF INTRAVESICAL CHEMOTHERAPY IN
TUMOUR PROPHYLAXIS

Intravesical chemotherapy is indicated for use following transurethral ablation of superficial tumours to reduce the rate of recurrence. Although no definitive evidence of improved efficacy of one agent over another exists, MMC use has rather superseded the anthracyclines in most countries. The balance of efficacy vs. toxicity dictates their selection over BCG immunotherapy. Tumours of low grade and pTa stage seem more susceptible to chemotherapy, and response rates are more similar to BCG. In such cases where there is a tendency for repeat tumour recurrences but limited potential to progress, the low toxicity of chemotherapeutic agents suggests their use over BCG. Others have advocated MMC at the time of initial transurethral resection as a prophylaxis against recurrence [43]. With lesions of more aggressive potential or those patients in whom tumours recur in spite of chemotherapy, BCG is indicated.

Intravesical immunotherapy

MECHANISM AND TOXICITY

The antitumour effect of BCG was noted as early as 1929. Its mechanism of action, however, is not yet fully understood. Mycobacterial particles attach to the urothelial lining via fibronectin, a component of the extracellular matrix [53]. Internalization of these particles leaves bacterial components on the cell membrane capable of antigen presentation to the immune system [53] and up-regulation of cytokine synthesis. Cytokine cascades including IL-1, 2 and 6, TNF and IFN induce MHC class II expression by urothelial epithelium and stimulate the migration of wide-ranging immune cells. Significant increases in CD4 helper T cells, CD8 cytotoxic T cells and lymphokine-activated killer (LAK) cells have been reported in the lamina propria, persisting 3 months after BCG instillation [54]. This non-specific immune activation results in tumour cell destruction. Elevation of urinary levels of various cytokines has been proposed to monitor response to intravesical BCG therapy [55].

The risk of adverse side-effects to intravesical BCG immunotherapy is low but significant. Most common are self-limiting local reactions of urinary frequency, haematuria and bladder irritation reflecting the topical immune stimulation. In patients with more severe filling symptoms, mild fever or malaise, isoniazid can be used until symptoms resolve as well as prophylactically prior to subsequent installations. Serious systemic reactions to BCG fortunately occur in less than 1% [56] and could be further reduced by avoiding therapy during episodes of cystitis, immediately after cystoscopy and after traumatic catheterization which predispose to systemic absorption. Typical features of systemic BCG infection such as intermittent high-grade fever, malaise or weight loss should be treated with a high index of suspicion, and antituberculous therapy initiated for at least 3 months. In the rare cases of life-threatening septic reactions prednisolone should also be added.

DOSE SCHEDULE AND EFFICACY

BCG immunotherapy reduces tumour recurrence rates by approximately 40%. However, the optimal BCG treatment schedule remains a matter of some debate. Most urologists continue with the single induction course of six consecutive weekly BCG installations as first proposed by Morales *et al.* [57]. This regimen gives complete response rates of 60–100% at 1 year, 55–75% after 2 years and mean recurrence-free intervals of 10–22.5 months [58]. More recent data suggest that the single induction course may be suboptimal. A review of 13 trials [59] showed that response rates were maximized with additional BCG courses and led to a durable long-term advantage over single induction regimens. Better response rates have been reported with continued weekly, biweekly and monthly instillations [60] as well as longer induction regimens [61]. However, these therapeutic advantages were compromised by significant increases in toxicity. This has led some groups to propose a second 'three or six week regime' for those failing a single induction course [62]. Trials by Catalona *et al.* and Haaf *et al.* [63,64] have shown improved response rates from 60% to 80% with this second dosing schedule, without significant increases in toxicity.

Role of intravesical BCG immunotherapy in prevention of tumour progression and tumour prophylaxis

BCG may also impact on disease progression, with a trend towards prolonged survival. Randomized, controlled trials have been limited and a cumulative analysis analogous to that of intravesical chemotherapy has not yet been possible. Nevertheless at least three randomized, controlled trials consisting of a total of 335 patients have suggested a statistically significant reduction in either stage progression or improvement in overall survival rates [65–67]. It is interesting to note, however, that a recently published EORTC-GU trial comparing mitomycin C with BCG showed little difference in progression rates in the two groups [68].

Although BCG offers the only potential for decreasing the risk of disease progression, this advantage must be titrated against the potential for toxicity. Since the potential toxicity of BCG is impossible to predict on an individual basis, BCG immunotherapy should be restricted to those who are at high risk of stage progression (Fig. 7.3) or intractable recurrences. These include patients with pT1, multifocal or high-grade disease. Patients with more indolent lesions should have intravesical chemotherapy as a first line treatment if tumour prophylaxis for continued recurrence is indicated.

Role of BCG in CIS treatment

BCG remains the treatment of choice for CIS disease. Although cytotoxic chemotherapy agents have shown initial response rates as good as 48% with anthracyclines and 53% with mitomycin C, most series have demonstrated that this response is time limited, with fewer than 20% remaining disease free at 5 years [69]. This apparent chemoresistance may well reflect the high grade of CIS disease, whereas high grade may imply greater antigenicity and therefore susceptibility to immunotherapy. BCG therapy gives complete response rates greater than 70% with a median duration of action beyond 3 years and projected 5-year response of 45% [70]. This durability of response may be improved with maintenance therapy. Further maintenance, 3-weekly regimen at 3- then 6-monthly intervals have increased long-term disease-free status from 70% to over 80% [69,71] at 3 years. As such, BCG induction and maintenance therapy is the first line treatment for CIS. Patients must be continually and closely monitored for disease recurrence, especially at extravesical sites of urothelium. Radical cystectomy is reserved for those who fail to respond to initial therapy or become resistant to maintenance courses.

Treatment options in G3pT1 disease

Most urologists would agree that G3pT1 tumours are a watershed for therapeutic intervention, but the ideal treatment remains controversial. Treatment with transurethral resection alone is inadequate, with recurrence rates between 70% and 80% and progression rates ranging from 29% to 50% [72]. In Birch and Harland's review [73] 40% of G3pT1 cases followed beyond 24 months developed muscle-invasive disease. Therefore choosing conservative (bladder-sparing) treatment obligates the use of adjuvant therapy. The adjuvant therapy of choice is BCG immunotherapy. However, the impact of BCG immunotherapy on G3pT1 tumours has been difficult to assess. This is due in part to the limited number of patients with G3pT1 disease available for study, but also to the interdependence of other factors such as concomitant CIS, multifocality, tumour size and previous recurrence rates. Non-standardization of BCG treatment protocols has also limited direct comparison of data. As such, reports of response rates following BCG therapy have varied from 25% to 75% for recurrence and from 7% to 54% for progression [74–76]. Important differences have, however, been noted. In Herr's series [74], where progression rates were high (54%), all selected cases had previous multiple tumour recurrences. By contrast, Cookson's & Sarodsdy's series [75], where post-BCG progression rates were lower (19%), the selected patients had only a 30% prior recurrence prevalence. In Seretta *et al.*'s series [76] G3pT1 patients were treated with various chemotherapy and combination agents. In this trial all patients with other clinical prognostic indicators of poor response were excluded, resulting in progression rates of only 12%. The lack of a randomized control throws open the question of whether this apparent success was due to the chemotherapy or the patient selection process.

It is clear that adjuvant (BCG) therapy will benefit a certain percentage of those with G3pT1 disease and delay (or possibly prevent) disease progression. Despite this, the biological potential of an individual's disease remains difficult to predict. An initial 'complete' transurethral resection followed by BCG therapy is advocated for most patients with G3pT1 bladder cancer. Other poor prognostic factors may indicate a subset of patients in whom this therapy is less likely to succeed. Failure of this first line of therapy (reappearance of tumour or positive urine cytology) is an indication for more aggressive therapy. In these patients radical cystectomy, or cystoprostatectomy for those with prostatic urethral involvement, appears to be indicated.

Role of alternative therapies

Other immunomodulators

The relative success of BCG has stimulated interest in other immuno-modulators for use as antitumour agents. Interferons are key components of the cytokine response, causing increased expression of MHC antigens on transitional cells, activating T cells, LAK cells and natural killer (NK) cells. Of the interferons, intravesical IFN-α2b has demonstrated the most activity against bladder cancer. Several phase I and II clinical trials assessing IFN-α2b have now been completed [77,78]. The results have shown moderate tumour response with a variety of dose schedules, although these responses and relapse rates are inferior to those with BCG. Only one trial to date has compared IFN-α2b directly with MMC [79]. With short follow-up, this has also shown a significant advantage of MMC compared with IFN-α2b. Of note, however, is the positive response of several patient groups who had previously been BCG-resistant. Although it is clear that MMC and BCG are generally superior, these results have encouraged the use of IFN-α2b as a second line agent, especially following intolerance or treatment failure of first line therapy. Interferons may also find a role as a supplement to BCG or chemotherapy [80]. Studies have already shown synergistic action of IFN-α2b with epirubicin [81], MMC [82] and BCG [83]. However, the numbers in these preliminary studies have been small and follow-up limited. Further large-scale trials are awaited.

Keyhole limpet haemocyanin (KLH) is a protein derived from the mollusc *Megathura crenulata*, which has been used for many years to stimulate delayed-type hypersensitivity reactions. Its ability to reduce bladder tumour recurrence rates was first noted incidentally by Olsson *et al.* [84] in 1974. Although its antitumour activity has been confirmed on several animal models, substantial clinical trials have been limited. Jurinic *et al.* [85] demonstrated that combination intradermal and intravesical KLH was better than MMC in prevention of tumour recurrence, although this result was achieved on small patient numbers. A second study, by Flamm *et al.* [86], compared KLH with ethoglucid. Remission rates were similar for the two groups, at 50%.

Although KLH and other immunostimulating agents such as bropirimine are active against superficial bladder cancer, their role in the treatment of the disease is as yet undefined and large multicentre trials are required to establish their potential.

Photofrin-mediated photodynamic therapy

Phototherapy is the use of visible laser light to destroy living tissue sensitized by the prior administration of a photosensitizing compound. The self-contained nature of the bladder and the superficial nature of early bladder cancer make topical light application a viable option. Systemic sensitization is achieved by the intravenous administration of porphyrins and laser light is applied via a double balloon catheter filled with a light-scattering medium [87]. The cytotoxic mechanisms involve production of singlet oxygen and superoxide radicals, inducing endothelial damage and intense local inflammation. The technique is thus limited by dose-dependent cystitis and the risk of permanent bladder contracture, reported in 4–24% of patients [87]. In addition, systemic porphyrins induce skin photosensitization and solar isolation is required up to 6 weeks following injection. Phototherapy has been proposed for prophylaxis of recurrent superficial disease and refractory CIS. As yet, clinical trials have been limited by small numbers and short-term follow-up. Response rates of 50% for tumour prophylaxis and 50–80% for resistant CIS have been reported [88] but the use of this technique will require further study before it is applied to significant numbers of patients.

Conclusion

Many patients with bladder cancer are elderly, with extensive co-morbidity, and a careful approach to their treatment is necessary. Attention to and accurate documentation of relevant clinical and histopathological prognostic factors allow stratification of the risk of tumour recurrence and critically tumour progression into low-, intermediate- and high-risk groups. Diffuse carcinoma *in situ* is considered a separate and aggressive disease category. The timing of future surveillance cystoscopy and interventional adjuvant therapy are dependent on these criteria. A change in risk classification should prompt a re-evaluation of patient status.

   In all patients, the initial approach is to attempt cystoscopic tumour ablation. Adjuvant intravesical therapy is decided by the prognostic status and the dynamic of stage change. For those with low- or intermediate-risk lesions, with early or repeated recurrences intravesical chemotherapy is probably the first choice. High-risk lesions including carcinoma *in situ* should be treated with intravesical BCG immunotherapy. Maintenance regimens confer better efficacy but at a cost of increased risk of toxicity. Treatment failure or increasing resistance to adjuvant therapy should prompt consideration of open surgical intervention.

   Further randomized, controlled trials are necessary to assess the impact of different dose and combination protocols. The role of new therapies is promising, although their potential is dependent on further large-scale study.

References

1 Napalkov P, Maisonneuve P, Boyle P. Epidemiology of bladder cancer. In: Pagano F, Fair WR, eds. *Superficial Bladder Cancer*. Oxford: ISIS Medical Media, 1997: 1–23.

2 Population and Health Monitor. *MB96/1*. London: Office for National Statistics, 1996.

3 McFarlane JP, Ellis BW, Harland SJ. The management of superficial bladder cancer: an interactive seminar. *Br J Urol* 1996; **78**: 372–8.

4 International Union Against Cancer. Urinary bladder. In: Sobin LH, Wittekind C, eds. *TNM Classification of Malignant Tumours*, 5th edn. New York: Wiley-Liss, 1997: 187–90.

5 Anderstrom C, Johansson S, Nilsson S. The significance of lamina propria invasion on the prognosis of patients with bladder tumors. *J Urol* 1980; **124**: 23–6.

6 Abel PD, Hall RR, Williams G. Should pT1 transitional cell cancers of the bladder still be classified as superficial? *Br J Urol* 1988; **62**: 235–9.

7 Angulo JC, Lopez JL, Grignon DJ *et al*. Muscularis mucosa differentiates two populations with different prognosis in stage T1 bladder cancer. *Urology* 1995; **45**: 47–53.

8 Smits G, Schaafsma E, Kiemeney L, Caris C, Debruyne F, Witjes JA. Microstaging of pT1 transitional cell carcinoma of the bladder: identification of subgroups with distinct risks of progression. *Urology* 1998; **52**: 1009–14.

9 Kurth KH, Denis L, Bouffioux C *et al*. Factors affecting recurrence and progression in superficial bladder tumours. *Eur J Cancer* 1995; **31**: 1840–6.

10 Abel PD, Henderson D, Bennett MK *et al*. Differing interpretations by pathologists of the pT category and grade of transitional cell cancer of the bladder. *Br J Urol* 1988; **62**: 339–42.

11 Lopez JL, Angulo JC. The prognostic significance of vascular invasion in stage T1 bladder cancer. *Histopathology* 1995; **27**: 27–33.

12 Ro JY, Staerkel GA, Ayala AG. Cytologic and histopathologic features of superficial bladder cancer. *Urol Clin North Am* 1992; **19**: 435–49.

13 Greene LF, Hanash KA, Farrow GM. Benign papilloma or papillary carcinoma of the bladder? *J Urol* 1973; **110**: 205–7.

14 Heney NM, Ahmed S, Flanagan MJ *et al*. for National Bladder Cancer Collaborative Group A. Superficial bladder cancer: progression and recurrence. *J Urol* 1983; **130**: 1083–6.

15 Abel PD. Follow-up of patients with 'superficial' transitional cell carcinoma of the bladder: the case for a change in policy. *Br J Urol* 1993; **72**: 135–42.

16 Malmstrom PU, Busch C, Norlen BJ. Recurrence, progression and survival in bladder cancer. *Scand J Urol Nephrol* 1987; **21**: 185–95.

17 Prout GR Jr, Barton BA, Griffin PP, Friedel GH. Treated history of noninvasive grade 1 transitional cell carcinoma. (The National Bladder Cancer Group.) *J Urol* 1992; **148**: 1413–19.

18 Fitzpatrick JM, West AB, Butler MR *et al*. Superficial bladder tumors (stage pTa, grade I and II): the importance of recurrence pattern following initial resection. *J Urol* 1986; **135**: 920–2.

19 Collette L, Sylvester R, Denis LJ *et al*. The three-month recurrence rate as a prognostic factor for the long term outcome of TaT1 bladder cancer. *Eur J Cancer* 1999; **35** (Suppl. 4): 342 (Abstract 1382).

20 Heney NM, Proppe K, Prout GR *et al*. Invasive bladder cancer: tumor configuration, lymphatic invasion and survival. *J Urol* 1983; **130**: 895–7.

21 Dalesio O, Schulman CC, Sylvester R *et al*. Prognostic factors in superficial bladder tumors: A study of the European Organization for Research on Treatment of Cancer: Genitourinary Tract Cancer Cooperative Group. *J Urol* 1983; **129**: 730–3.

22 Parmar MKB, Freedman LS, Hargreave TB, Tolley DA. Prognostic factors for recurrence

and follow up policies in the treatment of superficial bladder cancer: report from the British Medical Research Council subgroup on superficial bladder cancer (Urological Cancer Working Party). *J Urol* 1989; **142**: 284–8.

23 Hall RR, Parmar MKB, Richards AB, Smith PH. Proposal for changes in cystoscopic follow up of patients with bladder cancer and adjuvant intravesical chemotherapy. *Br Med J* 1994; **308**: 257–60.

24 Lamm DL. Carcinoma in situ. [Review.] *Urol Clin North Am* 1992; **19**: 499–508.

25 Riddle PR, Chisholm GD, Trott PA, Pugh PC. Flat carcinoma in situ of bladder. *Br J Urol* 1976; **47**: 829–33.

26 Althausen AF, Prout GR, Daly JJ. Noninvasive papillary carcinoma of the bladder associated with carcinoma in situ. *J Urol* 1976; **116**: 575–80.

27 Herr HW, Warttinger DD, Fair WF, Oettgen HF. Bacillus Calmette-Guerin therapy for superficial bladder cancer: a 10 year follow-up. *J Urol* 1993; **149**: 318–21.

28 Utz DC, Farrow DM. Carcinoma in situ of the urinary tract. *Urol Clin North Am* 1992; **19**: 499–508.

29 Van der Meijden A, Oosterlinck W, Brausi M, Kurth K, Sylvester R, de Balincourt C, Members of the EORTC-GU Group Superficial Bladder Cancer Committee. Significance of bladder biopsies in TaT1 bladder tumors: a report from the EORTC Genito-Urinary Tract Cancer Cooperative Group. *Eur Urol* 1999; **35**: 267–71.

30 Richards B, Parmar MKB, Anderson CK *et al*. Interpretation of biopsies of 'normal' urothelium in patients with superficial bladder cancer. *Br J Urol* 1991; **67**: 369–75.

31 Klan R, Loy V, Huland H. Residual tumour discovered in routine second transurethral resection in patients with stage T1 transitional cell carcinoma of the bladder. *J Urol* 1991; **46**: 316–18.

32 Beisland HO, Seland P. A prospective randomized study on neodinium: YAG laser irradiation versus TUR in the treatment of urinary bladder cancer. *Scand J Urol Nephrol* 1986; **20**: 209–12.

33 Sander S, Beisland HO. Lasers in urologic surgery. In: Smith JA, ed. *Superficial Bladder Cancer*. St Louis, MO: Mosby Year-Book, 1994: 126–34.

34 Di Marco A, Zunino F, Silvestrini R *et al*. Interaction of some daunomycin derivatives with deoxyribonucleic acid and their biological activity. *Biochem Pharmacol* 1971; **20**: 1323–8.

35 Thrasher JB, Crawford ED. Complications of intravesical chemotherapy. *Urol Clin North Am* 1992; **19**: 529–39.

36 Badalament RA, Farah RN. Treatment of superficial bladder cancer with intravesical chemotherapy. *Semin Surg Oncol* 1997; **13**: 335–41.

37 De Groot AC, Van der Meijden APM, Conemans JMH, Maibach HI. Frequency and nature of cutaneous reactions to intravesical instillation of mitomycin C for superficial bladder cancer. *Urology* 1992; **31** (Suppl. 40): 16–19.

38 Ritchie JP. Intravesical chemotherapy: treatment, selection, techniques and results. *Urol Clin North Am* 1992; **19**: 521–7.

39 Lamm DL. Long-term results of intravesical therapy for superficial bladder cancer. *Urol Clin North Am* 1992; **19**: 573–80.

40 Mishina T, Oda K, Murata S *et al*. Mitomycin C bladder instillation therapy for bladder tumours. *J Urol* 1975; **114**: 217–19.

41 Traynelis CL, Lamm DL. Current status of intravesical therapy for bladder cancer. In: Rous SN, ed. *Urology Annual*, 8. New York: WW Norton, 1994: 113–43.

42 Pawinski A, Sylvester R, Kurth KH *et al*. for the members of the European Organization for Research and Treatment of Cancer Genitourinary Tract Cancer Cooperative Group and the Medical Research Council Working Party on Superficial Bladder Cancer. A combined analysis of European Organization for Research and Treatment of Cancer, and Medical

Research Council randomized clinical trials for the prophylactic treatment of stage TaT1 bladder cancer. *J Urol* 1996; **156**: 1934–41.

43   Tolley DA, Parmar MKB, Grigor KM, Lallemand G, the Medical Research Council Superficial Bladder Cancer Working Party. The effect of intravesical mitomycin C on recurrence of newly diagnosed superficial bladder cancer: a further report with 7 years of follow up. *J Urol* 1996; **155**: 1233–8.

44   Lamm DL, Torti FM. Bladder cancer 1996. *CA Cancer J Clin* 1996; **46**: 93–112.

45   Flamm J. Long-term versus short-term doxorubicin hydrochloride instillation after transurethral resection of superficial bladder cancer. *Eur Urol* 1990; **17**: 119–24.

46   Hulland H, Kloppel G, Fedderson F *et al*. Comparison of different schedules of cytostatic intravesical instillations in patients with superficial bladder carcinoma: final evaluation of prospective multicenter study with 419 patients. *J Urol* 1990; **144**: 68.

47   Debruyne FMJ, Van der Meijden APM, Geboers AD *et al*. BCG-RIVM treatment in pTapT1 papillary carcinoma and carcinoma in situ of the bladder. *J Urol* 1985; **153** (Suppl. 3): 20–25.

48   Krege S, Otto T, Rubben H *et al*. Final report on a randomized multi-centre trial on adjuvant therapy in superficial bladder cancer: TUR only versus TUR and mitomycin versus TUR and bacillus Calmette-Guerin. *J Urol* 1996; **155**: 494a (Abstract 734).

49   Vegt PDJ, Witjes JA, Witjes WPJ *et al*. A randomized study of intravesical mitomycin C, bacillus Calmette-Guerin Tice and bacillus Calmette-Guerin RIVM treatment in pTapT1 papillary carcinoma and carcinoma in situ of the bladder. *J Urol* 1995; **153**: 929–33.

50   Jauhiainen K, Rintala E, Alfthan O, the Finnbladder Group. Immunotherapy (BCG) versus chemotherapy (MMC) in intravesical treatment of superficial urinary bladder cancer. In: deKernion JB, ed. *Immunotherapy of Urological Tumors*. Edinburgh: Churchill Livingstone, 1990: 13–26.

51   Lundholm C, Norlen BJ, Ekman P *et al*. A randomized prospective study comparing long-term intravesical instillations of mitomycin C and bacillus Calmette-Guerin in patients with superficial bladder carcinoma. *J Urol* 1996; **156**: 372–6.

52   Lamm DL, Crawford ED, Blumenstein B *et al*. SWOG 8795: a randomized comparison of bacillus Calmette-Guerin and mitomycin C prophylaxis in stage Ta and T1 transitional cell carcinoma of the bladder. *J Urol* 1993; **149**: 275–82.

53   Kavousi LR, Brown EJ, Ritchey JK, Ratliff TL. Fibronectin mediated bacillus Calmette-Guerin attachment to murine bladder mucosa: requirement for expression of an antitumor response. *J Clin Invest* 1990; **85**: 62–8.

54   Prescott S, James K, Hargreave TB, Chisholm GD, Smyth JF. Intravesical Evans strain of BCG therapy: quantitative immunohistochemical analysis of the immunoresponse within the bladder wall. *J Urol* 1995; **154**: 269–74.

55   De Reijke TM, de Boer EC, Kurth KH, Schamhart DHJ. Urinary cytokines during intravesical bacillus Calmette-Guerin for superficial bladder cancer: processing, stability and prognostic value. *J Urol* 1996; **155**: 477–82.

56   Lamm DL. Overview on bacillus Calmette-Guerin. In: Pagano F, Fair WR, eds. *Superficial Bladder Cancer*. Oxford: ISIS Medical Media, 1997: 120–6.

57   Morales A, Eidinger D, Bruce AW. Intracavity bacillus Calmette-Guerin in the treatment of superficial bladder tumors. *J Urol* 1976; **116**: 180–3.

58   Mungan KA, Witjes JA. Bacille Calmette-Guerin in superficial transitional cell carcinoma. [Review.] *Br J Urol* 1998; **82**: 213–23.

59   Khana OP, Son DL, Mazer H. Multicentre study of superficial bladder cancer treated with intravesical bacillus Calmette-Guerin or adriamycin. *Urology* 1990; **35**: 101–8.

60   Brosman SA. Experience with bacillus Calmette-Guerin in patients with superficial bladder carcinoma. *J Urol* 1982; **128**: 27–34.

61   Gruenwald IE, Stein A, Rascovitsky R, Shifroni G, Leuri A. A 12 week versus 6 week course

of bacillus Calmette-Guerin prophylaxis for the treatment of high risk superficial bladder cancer. *J Urol* 1997; **157**: 487–91.

62 Lamm DL. Optimal BCG treatment of superficial bladder cancer as defined by American trials. [Review.] *Eur Urol* 1992; **21** (Suppl. 2): 12–16.

63 Catalona WJ, Hudson MA, Gillen DP *et al*. Risk and benefits of repeated courses of intravesical bacillus Calmette-Guerin therapy for superficial bladder cancer. *J Urol* 1987; **137**: 220–4.

64 Haaf EO, Dresner SM, Ratliff TL. Two courses of bacillus Calmette-Guerin for transitional cell carcinoma of bladder. *J Urol* 1986; **136**: 820–4.

65 Herr HW, Laudone VP, Badalament RA *et al*. Bacillus Calmette-Guerin therapy alters the progression of superficial bladder cancer. *J Clin Oncol* 1988; **6**: 1450–5.

66 Lamm DL, Crissman J, Blumenstein B *et al*. Adriamycin versus BCG in superficial bladder cancer: a Southwest Oncology Group study. *Prog Clin Biol Res* 1989; **310**: 263–70.

67 Pagano F, Bassi P, Milani C *et al*. A low dose bacillus Calmette–Guerin regimen in superficial bladder cancer therapy: Is it effective? *J Urol* 1991; **146**: 32–5.

68 Witjes JA, van der Meijden APM, Collette L *et al*. and the EORTC GU Group and the Dutch South East Cooperative Group. Long term follow-up of an EORTC randomized prospective trial comparing intravesical bacille Calmette-Guerin-RIVM and Mitomycin C in superficial bladder cancer. *Urology* 1998; **52**: 403–10.

69 Lamm DL. BCG immunotherapy for transitional-cell carcinoma in situ of the bladder. *Oncology* 1995; **9**: 947–65.

70 Lamm DL, Blumenstein BA, Crawford ED *et al*. A randomized trial of intravesical doxorubicin and immunotherapy with bacille Calmette-Guerin for transitional-cell carcinoma of the bladder. *New Engl J Med* 1991; **325**: 1205–9.

71 Lamm DL, Crawford ED, Blumenstein B *et al*. Maintenance BCG immunotherapy of superficial bladder cancer: a randomized prospective Southwest Oncology Group study. *J Urol* 1992; **147**: 274a, 242.

72 Pham HT, Soloway MS. High-risk superficial bladder cancer: intravesical therapy for T1G3 transitional cell carcinoma of the urinary bladder. *Semin Urol Oncol* 1997; **15**: 147–53.

73 Birch BRP, Harland SJ. The pT1G3 bladder tumour. *Br J Urol* 1989; **64**: 109–16.

74 Herr HW. Progression of stage T1 bladder tumors after intravesical bacillus Calmette-Guerin. *J Urol* 1991; **145**: 40–4.

75 Cookson MS, Sarodsdy MF. Management of T1 superficial bladder cancer with intravesical bacillus Calmette-Guerin therapy. *J Urol* 1992; **148**: 797–801.

76 Seretta V, Piazza S, Pavone C *et al*. Results of conservative treatment (transurethral resection plus adjuvant intravesical chemotherapy) in patients with primary T1G3 transitional cell carcinoma of the bladder. *Urology* 1996; **47**: 647–51.

77 Torti FM, Shortliffe LD, Williams RD *et al*. Alpha-interferon in superficial bladder cancer: a Northern Californian Oncology Group Study. *J Clin Oncol* 1988; **6**: 476–83.

78 Glashan RW. A randomized control study of intravesical a-2b-interferon in carcinoma in situ of the bladder. *J Urol* 1990; **144**: 658–61.

79 Boccardo F, Cannata D, Rubagotti A *et al*. Prophylaxis of superficial bladder cancer with mitomycin or interferon alpha-2b: results of a multicentric Italian study. *J Clin Oncol* 1994; **12**: 7–13.

80 Belldegrun AS, Franklin JR, O'Donnell MA *et al*. Superficial bladder cancer; the role of interferon-alpha. *J Urol* 1998; **159**: 1793–801.

81 Ferrari P, Castagnetti G, Pollastri CA *et al*. Chemoimmunotherapy for prophylaxis of recurrence in superficial bladder cancer: interferon-alpha 2b versus interferon-alpha 2b with epirubicin. *Anticancer Drugs* 1992; **25** (Suppl. 1): 25–7.

82 Engelman U, Knopf HJ, Graff J. Interferon-alpha 2b instillation prophylaxis in superficial

bladder cancer—a prospective, controlled three-armed trial. (Project Group Bochum-interferon and superficial bladder cancer.) *Anticancer Drugs* 1992; **25** (Suppl. 1): 33–7.

83   Stricker P, Pryor K, Nicholson T *et al*. Bacillus Calmette-Guerin plus intravesical interferon-alpha-2b in patients with superficial bladder cancer. *Urology* 1996; **48**: 957–61.

84   Olsson C, Chute R, Rao C. Immunologic reduction of bladder cancer recurrence rate. *J Urol* 1974; **111**: 173–6.

85   Jurinic CD, Engelman V, Gasch J *et al*. Immunotherapy in bladder cancer with keyhole-limpet haemocyanin: a randomized study. *J Urol* 1988; **139**: 723.

86   Flamm J, Donner G, Bucher A *et al*. Topical immunotherapy (KLH) vs chemotherapy (Ethoglucid) in prevention of recurrence of superficial bladder cancer: a prospective randomized study. *Urologe-Ausgabe A* 1994; **33**: 138–43.

87   Jocham D. Photodynamic therapy of bladder carcinoma. In: Pagano F, Fair WR, eds. *Superficial Bladder Cancer*. Oxford: ISIS Medical Media, 1997: 145–57.

88   Nseyo UO, Crawford ED, Shumaker BP, Hoodin AO, Marcus SL, Dugan MH. A phase II multicentre trial of photodynamic therapy as treatment for refractory carcinoma in situ. *J Urol* 1993; **149**: 281.

Bladder Cancer: Commentary

J. Waxman

Bladder cancer is a significant cause of morbidity and death. Over the last decade we have seen an improvement in our understanding of the molecular biology of this condition, with the identification of new molecular markers for this disease. It is likely that if one looked to the future in the next decade we will see the development of treatments targeting these molecular markers.

These changes are most likely to be seen in superficial bladder cancer, where the accessibility of a tumour target makes drug delivery more straight-forward than in other solid tumours. The chapter by Keegan, Neal and Lunec highlights the changes in our understanding of the science of bladder cancer, and points to the development of new ways of looking at prognosis in this condition, as defined by molecular markers. Ockrim and Abel present an algorithm that helps us in our understanding of superficial bladder cancer and point to the significance of carcinoma *in situ* and the poorly differentiated superficial tumour. The impact on health economics of superficial bladder cancer is clearly described in this chapter.

Surgery remains a common therapeutic approach in the treatment of invasive bladder cancer. However, despite the refinements in technique described by Newling, it is clear that only 30% of all patients with this condition will survive 5 years. Other approaches need to be considered for invasive bladder cancer: over the last 20 years combination chemotherapy has emerged as one alternative. Cures may be obtained in localized tumours. It is of interest that bladder cancer is so chemosensitive, and in recent times new chemotherapeutic options have emerged, as described by Calabrò and Sternberg.

Part 3
Prostate Cancer

8: The Molecular Biology of Prostate Cancer

J. Wang & J. Waxman

Introduction

Prostate cancer is the most common cancer diagnosed in men, and is the second most common cause of cancer death in the Western world. In the United States in 1999 approximately 180 000 men were expected to develop prostate cancer, and 37 000 to die from the disease [1]. In England and Wales, the ratio of incidence to mortality is higher, with 17 000 cases diagnosed and nearly 9000 deaths annually [2].

Relatively little is known of the pathogenesis of prostate cancer, as compared with other malignancies, and this may be because of limited numbers of human immortalized cell lines available for study. It is hoped that recent advances in molecular biology techniques will improve our understanding of this condition. In recent years there has been a significant increase in interest in prostate cancer biology, a relatively neglected subject in the previous two decades. This chapter describes the current status of research into the molecular biology of prostate cancer.

Epidemiology of prostate cancer

There are clues from the epidemiology of prostate cancer that may throw light on its aetiology. For example, the incidence of prostate cancer increases with age. Yet clinically diagnosed disease is only the tip of the iceberg, as autopsy studies show. In the Western world, it is estimated that up to 30% of men over 50 years have undetectable cancer, with the incidence rising with age [3]. Racial differences in its incidence are also recognized, with African–American men in the United States having higher incidences and mortality from prostate cancer than Caucasians [4]. The differences may be due to genetic factors. Alternatively, environmental factors may be at play, as shown by much higher death rates in Japanese men who migrated to America, compared with those in Japan [5]. The most significant environmental factors are dietary [4] (Table 8.1).

Prostate cancer has a familial component but the relationship is weaker than for breast or colon cancer. Just as in breast and colon cancer, the familial relationship appears to be more significant in disease of early onset and the

Possible/likely risk factors
Age
Race
Premalignant lesions (prostatic intraepithelial neoplasia)
Affected relatives
Carnivorous diet
Dietary fat
Vitamin D
Sexual habits
Controversial/disproven risk factors
Benign prostatic hypertrophy
Sexually transmitted diseases
Cigarette smoking
Alcohol intake
Cadmium exposure

Table 8.1 Proposed risk factors for prostate cancer. (From Morton [4])

Table 8.2 Risk of prostate cancer in families with prostate cancer. (From Carter *et al.* [7])

Risk factor	Odds ratio	95% confidence interval
Three relatives affected	10.9	2.7–43.1
Two relatives	4.9	2.0–12.3
One relative	2.2	1.4–3.5
Two relatives (first and second degree) affected	8.8	2.8–28.1
One first-degree relative	2.0	1.2–3.3
One second-degree relative	1.7	1.0–2.9

number of relatives affected (Table 8.2). The relative risk for developing prostate cancer, for example, is 1.9, 1.4 and 1.0 for a relative of a patient who is 50, 60 or 70 years old, respectively, at diagnosis [6]. The mode of inheritance and the gene involved have yet to be determined. It is suggested that a single gene Mendelian mode of inheritance is implicated in just 9% of all prostate cancers [7].

Oncogenes

There have been many candidate oncogenes and tumour-suppressor genes whose roles have been examined in prostate cancer. As in other areas of research, initial positive reports of relationships between tumour expression and biology have been refuted by later observations.

Ras

Mutations in the *ras* family of oncogenes are common in cancers. The *ras* oncogene family encodes for cell membrane proteins involved in signal transduction via GTP/GDP binding. Binding leads to changes in the control of cell growth. Viola *et al.* [8] first analysed ras expression by immunohistochemistry using the RAP-5 murine monoclonal antibody comparing seven benign prostatic hypertrophy specimens and 29 carcinomas. Ras expression was present only in cancer cells and correlated with the grade of prostate cancer. Later studies showed that changes in ras oncogenes were infrequent. *Ras* oncogenes are commonly mutated at codons 12, 13 or 61, and analysis of these mutations showed mutations in less than 5% of cases [9].

Myc

The *myc* proto-oncogene family encodes for nuclear phosphoproteins, which control DNA replication, cell cycle regulation and differentiation. C-*myc* expression was found to be inhibited by androgens in the hormone sensitive LNCaP cell line [10]. An early study of c-*myc* expression by Northern blotting, of two normal, 11 hyperplastic and seven carcinoma specimens, suggested that levels of transcription were higher in prostate cancer than in normal tissues or benign hypertrophy [11]. *In situ* hybridization, however, failed to show a relationship between c-*myc* expression and prostate cancer biology [12].

Erb-B2/HER-2/neu

This oncogene codes for a transmembrane tyrosine kinase growth factor, similar to the epidermal growth factor (EGF) receptor. Translational research has been of significance for this family of oncogenes in breast cancer, with therapeutic advances coming from the use of herceptin, a monoclonal antibody targeting the gene product. Unlike in breast cancer, studies of gene mutation or amplification in prostate cancer by means of immunohistochemistry have produced conflicting results. While some groups have reported increased expression in prostate cancer [13], others have shown no difference between cancer and benign hypertrophy [14].

Bcl-2

Changes in this oncogene were initially described in association with the t[14:18] chromosome translocation in follicular lymphoma. The *bcl*-2 proto-oncogene codes for a protein that inhibits apoptosis. Although *bcl*-2 overexpression is infrequent in early prostate cancer, expression is increased in the tumours of patients with recurrence [15].

Other oncogenes

The *sis*, *fos*, *abl*, *myb* and *fms* oncogene families have not been studied in detail in prostate cancer. Using cell lines, high levels of *sis* and *fos*, as well as *ras* and *myc*, have been reported [12]. However, this is not reflected in the Dunning rat model nor in human specimens.

Tumour-suppressor genes (TSGs)

p53

Discovered in 1969, on chromosome 17, the p53 gene encodes a 53-kDa phosphoprotein crucial in regulating cell proliferation and determining apoptosis. Mutations of p53 are present in up to 50% of most cancers, with loss of heterozygosity (LOH) in 80% of breast, lung and colon cancers. Mutations of p53 are not commonly seen in benign prostatic hypertrophy [13]. In prostate cancer, the incidence of p53 mutation and LOH ranges from 0% to 80% [16]. This incidence varies with the patient age and grade and stage of disease. Localized, untreated cancer specimens have an approximate incidence of p53 mutations of 20%, which reaches 50–75% in metastatic or treatment-resistant samples [17]. This suggests that mutations of the p53 gene may be a late phenomenon in the natural history of the progression of prostate cancer.

The reported incidence of p53 mutation varies widely. This may be due to a true variation but also to the heterogeneity of tumours where p53 expression varies between cells. It may also be that different methodologies for assessing p53 expression lead to different results [18]. Despite these reservations, the consensus is that p53 mutations are a late phenomenon, with adverse prognostic implications.

Retinoblastoma (Rb)

The retinoblastoma gene is located at 13p, and encodes for a 110-kDa protein involved in the cell cycle pathway. Abnormal Rb protein expression in one of three different cell lines was reported by Bookstein *et al.* [19]. Transfection of the Rb gene led to changes in malignant potential [19]. LOH studies suggest alteration of Rb gene expression in up to 60% of prostate cancers [20], with absence of Rb protein also found in a similar proportion of prostate cancers by immunohistochemistry. In addition, by single-stranded conformation polymorphism analysis, mutations of Rb were found in 16% of prostate cancer biopsies [21]. However, Rb changes are also found in benign prostatic hypertrophy [20]. The wide range in the incidence of Rb mutation can be attributed to the factors ascribed to p53 in the previous section. Opinions are divided as to whether changes in Rb expression are causal or a non-specific finding in prostate cancer.

BRCA-1

BRCA-1 mutations were initially linked to familial clustering of breast and ovarian cancers. Subsequently, BRCA-1 carriers were also found to have increased incidences of a variety of malignancies, among which prostate cancer was found to be one of the commonest. The relative risk of prostate cancer in carriers was 2.95 compared with the general population [22] (Table 8.3). Although it would appear that BRCA-1 mutations are important in the relatively uncommon forms of prostate cancer, the role of BRCA-1 in sporadic disease is unclear.

Loss of heterozygosity and comparative genomic hybridization

Up to 54% of primary cancers and 100% of metastatic tumours have loss of heterozygosity occurring in at least one chromosome. The commonly noted loci include 3p, 7q, 8p, 9q, 10p, 10q, 11p, 13q, 16p, 16q, 17p and 18q. The technique of comparative genomic hybridization has been used to confirm observations made by fluorescence *in situ* hybridization. This technique can demonstrate chromosomal gain as well as loss and has shown regional gains

Table 8.3 The sites of elevated risk of developing cancer, other than breast and ovarian, in BRCA1 carriers. (From Ford *et al.* [22])

Site of cancer	Relative risk	Significance (*P*)
Liver	5.12	NS
Colon	3.30	<0.01
Bone	3.25	NS
Prostate	2.95	<0.01
Cervix	2.74	NS
Brain	2.08	NS
Kidney	2.02	NS
Connective tissue	1.70	NS
Larynx	1.58	NS
Melanoma	1.18	NS
Stomach	1.11	NS
Unknown site	3.97	<0.01

NS, not significant.

[23]. Such is the extent of loss and gain of chromosomes that it is likely that there may be tumour-suppressor and new proto-oncogenes awaiting identification or that the changes are non-specific.

The androgen receptor

Androgen deprivation results in responses in 50–80% of patients. This response is short lived, with prostate-specific antigen (PSA) progression demonstrable after a median period of 13 months from starting treatment. It is only recently that the molecular effects of androgen deprivation have become understood. The potential for translational research that has come from these discoveries has yet to be realized.

The androgen receptor and androgen synthesis

The development and maintenance of the male phenotype is under the influence of androgens. Testosterone is the most significant circulating androgen and is produced by Leydig cells under the influence of the pituitary hormones luteinizing hormone (LH) and follicle-stimulating hormone (FSH) (Fig. 8.1). Ninety per cent of testosterone is converted intracellularly by the enzyme 5α-reductase to dihydrotestosterone (DHT) in target organs, such as the prostate. DHT has 100 times more relative androgenicity than testosterone. Both

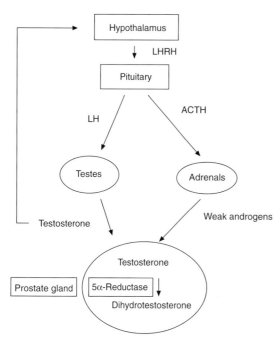

Figure 8.1 The hypothalamic–pituitary–gonadal endocrine axis. ACTH, adrenocorticotrophic hormone. For explanation of all other abbreviations see text.

testosterone and DHT bind to the androgen receptor, which has higher affinity for DHT than for testosterone.

The androgen receptor is a member of a superfamily of steroid receptors, which bind oestrogens, retinoids and vitamin D. There is a strong dietary basis to prostate cancer and it is relevant to note that it has been suggested that the vitamin D receptor mediates the protective effects of some diets against the development of prostate cancer [24]. The androgen receptor binds to heat shock protein when it is in its inactivated state. On binding with DHT or testosterone, the androgen receptor dissociates from heat shock protein, dimerizes and then binds to specific DNA sequences, known as androgen response elements, which are located in the promoter regions of androgen target genes (Fig. 8.2). In this way the androgen receptor acts as a transcription factor. Downstream target genes which are regulated in this fashion include those encoding PSA, insulin-like growth factor-1 (IGF-1), keratinocyte growth factor (KGF) and vascular endothelial growth factor (VEGF). These are important genes involved in differentiation, angiogenesis and metastasis.

This description of androgen receptor activation and binding is simplistic. This process is actually most complex. Other factors, termed co-activators and co-repressors, either upregulate or downregulate the activity of androgen receptor leading to chromatin remodelling and RNA polymerase binding.

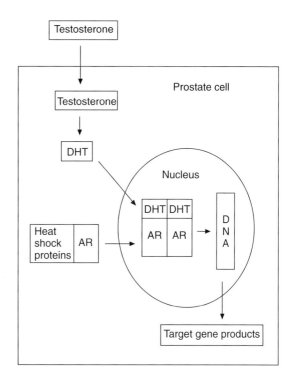

Figure 8.2 The intracellular action of the androgen receptor (AR). DHT, dihydrotestosterone; DNA, deoxyribonucleic acid.

There are very many co-activators and co-repressors that have been described. Other hormones and cytokines have also been shown to interact with the androgen receptor and to be involved in the process of transcription [25]. These include peptide growth factors such as IGF-1, KGF, EGF and possibly luteinizing hormone-releasing hormone (LHRH). The last may be clinically relevant, as LHRH agonists are used as treatments for prostate cancer.

The androgen receptor in differentiation

The androgen receptor is initially expressed in mesenchymal tissue in the early development of the prostate gland [26]. Epithelium and mesenchyme are in close conjunction during development. In later development, both mesenchymal and epithelial cells express androgen receptor and in the adult prostate gland, stromal–epithelial interactions remain significant. These interactions may be through growth factors released into local environments, such as KGF, IGF-1 and -2, transforming growth factor-alpha and -beta (TGF-α and -β) and fibroblast growth factor (FGF) [25]. Overall, there are probably complex paracrine and autocrine interactions involved in the growth and development of the prostate gland, as shown in Fig. 8.3. It may be that imbalances of these factors cause prostate cancer and benign prostatic hypertrophy.

Treatment resistance

Currently patients are treated with an LHRH agonist and an anti-androgen which may be given in the short or long term. LHRH agonists were traditionally thought to exert their effects by inhibiting LH and FSH secretion from the pituitary, thereby blocking androgen production from the testicles. There is evidence that LHRH may also act locally in the prostate [27].

Hormonal manipulation inevitably fails, with biochemical evidence of disease relapse occurring at a median of 13 months from the institution of treatment. This is thought to be due to adaptation by cancer cells to low androgen environments by amplification or mutation of the androgen receptor or through co-activator or co-repressor activity. Investigations in experimental models have shown that even in early stage tumours cancer is heterogeneous and contains androgen sensitive and independent cells [28]. The adaptation of the tumour to hormone independence under the evolutionary pressure of treatment may involve a selection process. This results in the tumour possibly depending for its growth on agents used to treat it.

There may be other mechanisms for treatment resistance operating involving overexpression and loss of control of growth factors (see later in this

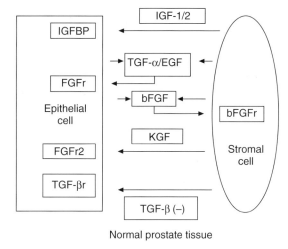

Figure 8.3 Possible epithelial–stromal interactions in normal prostate glands and prostate cancer. For explanation of abbreviations see text.

chapter). Androgen resistance might also involve the *bcl*-2 oncogene induced through androgen deprivation [15]. As a result of hormonal therapy, androgen receptor expression may be entirely lost either at gene or RNA or protein level. This phenomenon is reported in cultured cell lines [29].

The androgen receptor may adapt to androgen deprivation through gene amplification or mutation. In one study 28% of specimens from hormone-resistant patients had amplification of the androgen receptor gene, compared with none in specimens which were treatment naive. These patients with androgen receptor amplification had a better prognosis than those with receptor mutation [30].

The incidence of mutations of the androgen receptor gene has been variably reported and they occur following the development of hormone-resistant disease [31]. Point mutations have been observed in a variety of different regions. The most clinically relevant of these are mutations which affect the ligand-binding domain of the androgen receptor gene. The first of such mutations, in which the threonine at position 877 is replaced by alanine, was reported initially in the LNCaP cell line [32]. This mutation allows the androgen receptor to be activated by oestrogens, progestogens, adrenal androgens and anti-androgens. Similar mutations have been subsequently reported in human cancer specimens [33].

The activation of androgen receptor by one anti-androgen, flutamide, is clinically important, as it explains how some patients with disease progression respond to withdrawal of flutamide [34]. Such mutations may be specific to flutamide, rather than anti-androgens as a class, since responses to bicalutamide following progression after flutamide withdrawal are observed [35].

Other possibilities for the molecular basis for the development of androgen insensitivity include the development of mutations rendering the androgen receptor constitutionally activated.

Trinucleotide repeats

The severity of a number of neuromuscular degenerative disorders such as Kennedy's disease is linked to the number of X chromosome-associated CAG and GGC trinucleotide repeats. Attempts have been made to link this phenomenon with prostate cancer biology [36]. Some researchers have found that a shorter glutamine repeat coded by the CAG sequence in the N-terminal region results in increased AR activity. This in turn predicts for a higher grade and more advanced disease at diagnosis [37]. Other studies, however, failed to show that the CAG length affects AR transcriptional activity [38]. These observations may be clinically relevant, explaining the racial differences seen in prostate cancer. African–Americans generally have shorter CAG repeats than Caucasians and Asians, and this may reflect on malignant potential [39].

5α-Reductase activity

How do mutations of the androgen receptor confer survival advantages on malignant cells? It is possible that mutations confer a significant selection advantage on tumour cells prior to hormonal therapy, by allowing them to adapt to lower levels of 5α-reductase enzyme levels found in tumours [40]. In one study of mutation rates in the different races it was found that in specimens from clinically evident cancer patients no mutations were seen in both American and Japanese men [41]. However, 18 of 79 specimens of clinically silent disease obtained at autopsy from Japanese men dying of causes other than prostate cancer showed androgen receptor mutations, whereas none of the 43 specimens from corresponding American men showed any mutation. The result of this only serves to confound the issue further.

It is of interest that 5α-reductase activity correlates with race, and that African–Americans and Caucasians have higher levels of activity than Japanese men [42]. This may relate to polymorphisms in the two genes coding for the enzyme, SRD5A1 and 2. 5α-reductase hydroxylates testosterone to dihydrotestosterone but it is arguable whether or not androgen levels vary with race. One study has shown that testosterone levels were higher in African–American men than in Caucasian Americans but the difference diminishes with age [43]. Finally, the enzyme 3β-hydroxylsteroid dehydrogenase 2, which is involved with the breakdown of DHT, has been shown to exhibit polymorphism in its coding gene [44]. It remains to be seen whether polymorphism in this gene correlates with prostate cancer behaviour or incidence.

Tumour–environment interactions

Several observations have suggested that the interaction between prostate cancer and its local environment plays an important part in tumour progression. In the process of embryogenesis the prostate gland shows a close interaction between the epithelial and mesenchymal elements. This continues in the adult, where the stroma, via a variety of paracrine influences, maintains the differentiation of the glandular structure of the epithelium. This may explain the pattern of tumour spread which is unique to prostate cancer. The tumour disseminates to bone where there is marked sclerosis. This suggests that the bone stroma may also be a fertile ground for prostate cancer cell growth because of a pattern of growth factor production that has similarities with that in the local environment of the prostate.

This observation is supported by the results of co-culture experiments where different organ-specific fibroblasts co-inoculated with the prostate cell line LNCaP into mice were shown to promote cancer growth. It is well known that fibroblasts produce a variety of growth factors, and the actions of many of these have been characterized.

Growth factors

There are many growth factors thought to interact with the androgen receptor. The involvement of these growth factors with prostatic cancer is summarized in Table 8.4.

EGF and TGF-α are related peptide factors produced in normal and cancerous prostate cells and levels are increased in many cancers [45]. EGF/TGF-α levels in prostate cancer specimens correlate with tissue testosterone levels, suggesting that they may have significance [45]. In human cancer specimens, compared with benign hypertrophy specimens the levels of EGF receptors (EGFr) have been variably reported as elevated [46] or equivalent [13]. At present it remains unclear whether EGF or TGF-α has any important role in normal or malignant prostate growth (Fig. 8.3).

The transforming growth factors are a family of peptides, including TGF-β, that regulate cell growth and differentiation. TGF-β is implicated in angiogenesis and remodelling of the extracellular matrix. Its role in prostate cancer is complex, as it both inhibits epithelial growth and enhances cell motility through its stromal effects [47]. TGF-β is produced in both stromal and epithelial cells, and its expression is downregulated by androgens [48]. *In vitro* and animal studies have consistently failed to show that TGF-β has any tumour-suppressor effect, and it has been reported in some studies to stimulate tumour growth [48].

The fibroblast growth factors (FGFs) are a family of at least 14 members. Of these, FGF-1 (acidic FGF, aFGF), FGF-2 (basic FGF, bFGF) and FGF-7 and FGF-8 have been examined in prostate cancer. Acidic FGF is expressed in the mesenchyme of the Dunning rat tumours, but it does not appear to be expressed in human prostate [49]. Basic FGF is found in both normal and cancerous prostate tissues, and is expressed by both stromal and epithelial components [49]. Basic FGF stimulates cell proliferation and angiogenesis and may be of significance in prostate cancer. In human prostatic specimens, normal or benign hypertrophy samples show expression of basic FGF in stromal cells, but not epithelial cells, while in cancer cells the opposite is observed [50].

FGF-7 was initially found to stimulate the growth of the Dunning cell line [51]. Fibroblast growth factor receptor (FGFr) is found in normal epithelial cells, suggesting a paracrine action in normal tissues [52]. It may therefore be a mediator of androgen function, inducing growth and differentiation. In advanced cancer, however, FGFr-2 expression is lost [53]. Loss of this pathway may therefore be a means whereby androgen independence develops.

FGF-8 is probably the most relevant member of this family in prostatic cancer, because its expression is androgen induced. We have examined FGF-8 expression in tumours and benign hypertrophy and found a correlation between expression as assessed by *in situ* hybridization and differentiation [54].

Table 8.4 The possible role for growth factors in normal prostate development and in prostate cancer

Growth factor	Activities reported	Expression in normal/benign tissues	Expression in prostate cancer
EGF	Stimulates replication of epithelial/fibroblast cell lines Stimulates invasion of cells	Present in prostatic fluid/epithelial cells Stimulated by androgens EGFr on epithelial cells	Increased by epithelial cells Increased further in androgen-independent cell lines EGFr expression increased?
TGF-α	Binds to EGFr; ? similar function	Produced usually in stroma Stimulated by androgens Receptor, EGFr on epithelial cells	Produced by epithelial cells Increased in androgen-independent cell lines c-erb-b2, EGFr expression increased
TGF-β	Inhibits epithelial growth *in vitro* Stimulates angiogenesis, stromal growth, cell adhesion	Expressed by epithelium and stroma Downregulated by androgens	Increased with tumour progression ? Change in receptor responsiveness with loss of inhibitory effect
aFGF	Not defined	Produced by stroma in developing rat prostate, not in humans Receptor present in stroma/epithelium	Produced by rat epithelial tumour cells in aggressive lines
bFGF	Strongly angiogenic Regulates matrix enzymes	Produced by epithelium/stroma Increased by androgens bFGF receptor only in stroma	Production independent of androgens Receptor produced by epithelial cells
KGF (FGF-7)	Mitogen for normal and tumour cells	Produced by stroma, stimulated by androgens Receptor, bFGFr-2 in epithelial cells	Produced by epithelial cells in androgen-independent tumours Increased receptor levels, lost in androgen-independent
IGF-1/2	Mitogenic for epithelial cells	Produced by stroma IGFrs and IGFBP present in epithelial cells	IGFBP expression altered in cell lines May affect release of stored IGF from epithelial cells

Another family of growth factors which may prove to be important in the development or progression of prostate cancer is the insulin-like growth factors, IGF-1 and -2. IGFs are mitogenic for prostate epithelial cells [55]. It has been argued whether these growth factors are synthesized by epithelial cells but it is agreed that IGF-binding proteins (IGFBP) are [56]. These binding proteins are significant in prostate metabolism, as they are regulated in part by androgens [57]. Attempts have been made to correlate serum levels with prostate biology but no relationship has been found [58]. In Fig. 8.3 we summarize the interaction of the various growth factors with prostate cancer cells and their surrounding stroma.

Other cellular–matrix interactions

E-cadherin is a protein involved in cell–cell recognition and adhesion, thereby maintaining the normal phenotype. Inhibition of E-cadherin expression leads to disruption of normal contact inhibition of growth, and an invasive phenotype [59]. The E-cadherin gene is located on chromosome 16q, a region associated with LOH in prostate cancer. Decreased E-cadherin expression has been correlated with increased tumour grade and stage at diagnosis [60]. E-cadherin associates with members of the catenin family of proteins. These cadherin–catenin complexes influence junctional activity and affect cell phenotype. α-Catenin is encoded by chromosome 5q, another site of LOH in prostate cancer [61].

Yet another site of loss of heterozygosity is chromosome 11p. Linkage studies have isolated two genes on chromosome 11 that affect cell-matrix interactions. The KAI1 gene, located at loci 11p11.2 [62], codes for what is thought possibly to be a transmembrane protein of uncertain function. Transfection of the KAI1 gene into the Dunning rat model inhibits metastasis. KAI1 underexpression is found to be present in a large proportion of both primary and metastatic cancer specimens [63]. The second gene lost at chromosome 11 encodes for CD44, part of the family of CD cell surface glycoproteins. This glycoprotein is expressed in many different tumours and functions as a receptor for hyaluronic acid, collagen and fibronectin. It also alters the intracellular cytoskeleton, and hence has implications in affecting malignant phenotype. Downregulation of the CD44 protein increases the incidence of metastases in the Dunning rat model [64]. The CD44 protein exists in various isoforms, and the expression of some variants has been found in both prostate cancer and benign hypertrophy, and prostatic intraepithelial neoplasm [65].

The *PTEN/MMAC1* gene, located on chromosome 10q, and which may also be subject to LOH, codes for a protein that has a tyrosine phosphatase function and a homology to elements of the cytoskeleton, tensin and auxillin. The role of this protein is not certain, but it may be involved in signalling. LOH

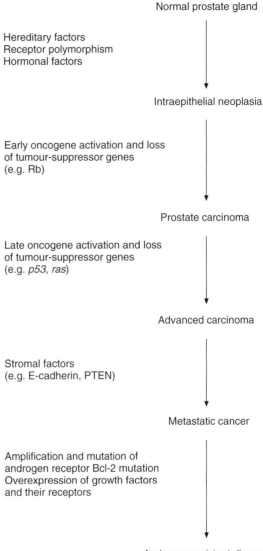

Normal prostate gland

Hereditary factors
Receptor polymorphism
Hormonal factors

Intraepithelial neoplasia

Early oncogene activation and loss
of tumour-suppressor genes
(e.g. Rb)

Prostate carcinoma

Late oncogene activation and loss
of tumour-suppressor genes
(e.g. *p53, ras*)

Advanced carcinoma

Stromal factors
(e.g. E-cadherin, PTEN)

Metastatic cancer

Amplification and mutation of
androgen receptor Bcl-2 mutation
Overexpression of growth factors
and their receptors

Androgen-resistant disease

Figure 8.4 A possible pathway
for the pathogenesis and
progression of prostate cancer.

at this region has been found in 18% (11 of 60) of specimens from patients with localized disease, and in 60% (12 of 20) of specimens from patients with pelvic metastases [66].

The tissue metalloproteinases are a group of enzymes thought to be involved in the facilitation of local invasion and metastasis. The metalloproteinases are proteases and are involved in normal physiological regulation, controlling cytoskeletal structure and normal cellular processes such as placental development. These enzymes are regulated by non-specific proteins such as albumin and specific regulatory proteins termed tissue inhibitors of metalloproteinases. In prostate cancer, there is increased tissue expression of metalloproteinases compared with controls [67] and serum levels of both the metalloproteinases and tissue inhibitors of metalloproteinases distinguish those patients who have metastases from those who do not and predicate for relapse [68].

Conclusion

We hope we have shown that research into prostate cancer, once neglected, has accelerated at a great pace. It is clear that at present we catch only a glimpse of the complex interactions between cells, steroidogenesis, and genes affecting growth and metastasis. Several models for the accumulation of mutations and changes which characterize the pathogenesis of prostate cancer have been proposed (e.g. Fig. 8.4), but none has been universally accepted. Specialization has led to an individual understanding of single complex molecules but to no overview of the big picture.

Nevertheless, it is hoped that such research will lead to diagnostic and therapeutic applications. Apart from the current interest in gene and immune therapy, the understanding of the biology of prostate cancer will also enable us to improve on our hormonal and chemotherapy options.

References

1   Landis SH, Murray T, Bolden S, Wingo PA. Cancer statistics 1999. *CA Cancer J Clin* 1999; **49**: 8–31.
2   Chamberlain J, Melia J, Moss S, Brown J. The diagnosis, management, treatment and costs of prostate cancer in England and Wales. *Health Technol Assess* 1997; **1**: 1–53.
3   Holund B. Latent prostatic cancer in a consecutive autopsy series. *Scand J Urol Nephrol* 1980; **14**: 29–35.
4   Morton RA. Racial differences in adenocarcinoma of the prostate in North American men. *Urology* 1994; **44**: 637–45.
5   Haenzel W, Kurihara M. Studies of Japanese migrants: 1. Mortality from cancer and other diseases among Japanese in the United States. *J Natl Cancer Inst* 1968; **40**: 43–68.
6   Carter BS, Bova GS, Beaty TH *et al.* Hereditary prostate carcinoma: epidemiologic and clinical features. *J Urol* 1993; **150**: 797–802.
7   Carter BS, Beaty TH, Steinberg GD, Childs B, Walsh PC. Mendelian inheritance of familial prostate cancer. *Proc Natl Acad Sci USA* 1992; **89**: 3367–71.
8   Viola MV, Fromowitz F, Oravez S *et al.* Expression of ras oncogene p21 in prostate cancer. *N Engl J Med* 1986; **314**: 133–7.
9   Carter BS, Epstein JI, Isaacs WB. Ras gene mutations in human prostate carcinoma. *Cancer Res* 1990; **50**: 6830–2.
10 Wolf DA, Kohlhuber F, Schulz P, Fittler F, Eick D. Transcriptional down-regulation of c-myc in human prostate carcinoma cells by the synthetic androgen mibolerone. *Br J Cancer* 1992; **65**: 376–82.
11 Fleming WH, Hamel A, MacDonald R *et al.* Expression of the c-myc protooncogene in human prostatic carcinoma and benign prostatic hyperplasia. *Cancer Res* 1986; **46**: 1535–8.

12 Funa K, Nordgren H, Nilsson S. In situ expression of mRNA for proto-oncogenes in benign prostatic hyperplasia and in prostatic carcinoma. *Scand J Urol Nephrol* 1991; **25**: 95–100.

13 Mellon K, Thompson S, Charlton RG *et al.* P53, c-erbB-2 and the epidermal growth factor receptor in the benign and malignant prostate. *J Urol* 1992; **147**: 496–9.

14 Giri DK, Wadhwa SM, Upadhaya SN, Talwar GP. Expression of NEU/HER-2 oncoprotein (p185neu) in prostate tumors: an immunohistochemical study. *Prostate* 1993; **23**: 329–36.

15 Furuya Y, Krajewski S, Epstein JI, Reed JC, Isaacs JT. Expression of bcl-2 and progression of human and rodent prostate cancers. *Clin Cancer Res* 1996; **2**: 389–98.

16 Heidenberg HB, Bauber JJ, McLeod DG, Moul JW, Srivastava S. The role of p53 tumor suppressor gene in prostate cancer: a possible biomarker? *Urology* 1996; **48**: 971–9.

17 Heidenberg HB, Sesterhenn I, Gaddipati J *et al.* Alteration of the tumor suppressor gene p53 in a high fraction of treatment-resistant prostate cancer. *J Urol* 1995; **153**: 414–21.

18 Ruijter E, van de Kaa CA, Aalders T *et al.* Heterogeneous expression of E-cadherin and p53 in prostate cancer: clinical implications. (The BIOMED-II MPC study group.) *Mod Pathol* 1998; **11**: 276–81.

19 Bookstein R, Rio P, Medreperia SA *et al.* Promoter deletion and loss of retinoblastoma gene expression in human prostate carcinoma. *Proc Natl Acad Sci USA* 1990; **87**: 7762–6.

20 Phillips SM, Barton CM, Lee SJ *et al.* Loss of the retinoblastoma susceptibility gene (RB1) is a frequent and early event in prostatic tumorigenesis. *Br J Cancer* 1994; **70**: 1252–7.

21 Kutoba Y, Fujinami K, Uemura H *et al.* Retinoblastoma gene mutations in primary human prostate cancer. *Prostate* 1995; **27**: 314–20.

22 Ford D, Easton DF, Bishop DT, Marod SA, Goldga DE. Risks of cancer in BRCA1 mutations carriers. (Breast Cancer Linkage Consortium.) *Lancet* 1994; **343**: 692–5.

23 Bova GS, Isaacs B. Review of allelic loss and gain in prostate cancer. *World J Urol* 1996; **14**: 338–46.

24 Hedlund TE, Moffatt KA, Millet GJ. Stable expression of the nuclear vitamin D receptor in the human prostatic carcinoma cell line JCA-1: evidence that the antiproliferative effects of $1\alpha,25$-dihydroxyvitamin D_3 are mediated exclusively through the genomic signalling pathway. *Endocrinology* 1996; **137**: 1554–61.

25 Russell PJ, Bennett S, Stricker P. Growth factor involvement in progression of prostate cancer. *Clin Chem* 1998; **44**: 705–23.

26 Cooke PS, Young P, Cunha GR. Androgen receptor expression in developing male reproductive organs. *Endocrinology* 1991; **128**: 2867–73.

27 Culig Z, Hobisch A, Hittmair A *et al.* Synergistic activation of androgen receptor by androgen and luteinizing hormone-releasing hormone in prostatic carcinoma cells. *Prostate* 1997; **32**: 106–14.

28 Issacs JT, Heston WD, Weissman RM, Coffey DS. Animal models of the hormone-sensitive and insensitive prostatic adenocarcinomas, Dunning R-3327-H, R-3327-H1 and R-3327-AT. *Cancer Res* 1978; **38**: 4353–9.

29 Tilley WD, Wilson CM, Marcelli M, McPhaul MJ. Androgen receptor gene expression in human prostate carcinoma cell lines. *Cancer Res* 1990; **50**: 5382–6.

30 Koivisto P, Kononen J, Palmberg C *et al.* Androgen receptor gene amplification: a possible molecular mechanism for androgen deprivation therapy failure in prostate cancer. *Cancer Res* 1997; **57**: 314–19.

31 Bentel JM, Tilley WD. Androgen receptors in prostate cancers. *J Endocrinol* 1996; **151**: 1–11.

32 Veldscholte J, Ris-Stalpers C, Kuiper GG *et al.* A mutation in the ligand binding domain of the androgen receptor of human LNCaP cells affects steroid binding characteristics and response to anti-androgens. *Biochem Biophys Res Commun* 1990; **173**: 534–40.

33 Gaddipati JP, McLeod DG, Heidenberg HB *et al.* Frequent detection of codon 877 mutation in the androgen receptor gene in advanced prostate cancers. *Cancer Res* 1994; **54**: 2861–4.

34   Kemppainen JA, Wilson EM. Agonist and antagonist activities of hydroxylflutamide and Casodex relate to androgen receptor stabilization. *Urology* 1996; **48**: 157–62.

35   Culig Z, Hoffmann J, Erdel M *et al.* Switch from antagonist to agonist of the androgen receptor bicalutamide is associated with prostate tumour progression in a new model system. *Br J Cancer* 1999; **81**: 242–51.

36   Irvine RA, Yu MC, Ross RK *et al.* The CAG and GGC microsatellites of the androgen receptor gene are in linkage disequilibrium in men with prostate cancer. *Cancer Res* 1995; **55**: 1937–40.

37   Kantoff P, Giovannucci E, Brown M. The androgen receptor CAG repeat polymorphism and its relationship to prostate cancer. *Biochim Biophys Acta* 1998; **1378**: C1–C5.

38   Neuschmid Kaspar F, Gast A, Peterziel H *et al.* CAG-repeat expansions in androgen receptor in Kennedy's disease is not a loss of function mutation. *Mol Cell Endocrinol* 1996; **117**: 148–56.

39   Edwards A, Hammond HA, Jin L, Caskey CT, Chakraborty R. Genetic variation at five trimeric and tetrameric tandem repeat loci in four human population groups. *Genomics* 1992; **12**: 241–53.

40   Tilley WD, Buchanan G, Hickey TE, Bentel JM. Mutations in the androgen receptor gene are associated with progression of human prostate carcinoma to androgen independence. *Clin Cancer Res* 1996; **2**: 277–85.

41   Takahashi H, Furusato M, Allsbrook WC *et al.* Prevalence of androgen receptor gene mutations in latent prostatic carcinomas from Japanese men. *Cancer Res* 1995; **55**: 1621–4.

42   Ross RK, Bernstein L, Lobo RA *et al.* 5α-reductase activity and risk of prostate cancer among Japanese and US white and black males. *Lancet* 1992; **339**: 887–9.

43   Ellis L, Nybord H. Racial/ethnic variations in male testosterone levels: a probable contributor to group differences in health. *Steroids* 1992; **57**: 72–5.

44   Devgan SA, Henderson BE, Yu MC *et al.* Genetic variation of 3 beta-hydroxysteroid dehydrogenase type II in three racial/ethnic groups: implications for prostate cancer risk. *Prostate* 1997; **33**: 9–12.

45   Yang Y, Chisholm GD, Habib FK. Epidermal growth factor and transforming growth factor α concentration in benign hypertrophy and cancer of the prostate: their relationships with tissue androgen levels. *Br J Cancer* 1993; **67**: 152–5.

46   Glynne-Jones E, Goddard L, Harper ME. Comparative analysis of mRNA and protein expression for epidermal growth factor receptor and ligands relative to the proliferative index in human prostate tissue. *Hum Pathol* 1996; **27**: 688–94.

47   Barrack ER. TGF beta in prostate cancer: a growth inhibitor that can enhance tumorigenicity. *Prostate* 1997; **31**: 61–70.

48   Steiner MS, Barrack ER. Transforming growth factor-beta 1 overproduction in prostate cancer: effects on growth in vivo and in vitro. *Mol Endocrinol* 1992; **6**: 15–25.

49   Story MT. Regulation of prostate growth by fibroblast growth factors. *World J Urol* 1995; **13**: 297–305.

50   Sherwood ER, Fong CY, Lee C, Kozlowski JM. Basic fibroblast growth factor: a potential mediator of stromal growth in the human prostate. *Endocrinology* 1992; **130**: 2955–63.

51   Yan G, Fukabori Y, Nikolaropoulos S, Wang F, McKeehan WL. Heparin binding keratinocyte growth factor is a candidate stromal to epithelial cell andromedin. *Mol Endocrinol* 1992; **6**: 2123–8.

52   Planz B, Wang Q, Kirley SD, Lin CW, McDougal WS. Androgen responsiveness of stromal cells of the human prostate: regulation of cell proliferation and keratinocyte growth factor by androgen. *J Urol* 1998; **160**: 1850–5.

53 Matsubura A, Kan M, Feng S, McKeehan WL. Inhibition of growth of malignant rate prostate tumor cells by restoration of fibroblast growth factor receptor 2. *Cancer Res* 1998; **58**: 1509–14.

54 Wang Q, Stamp GWH, Powell S *et al.* Correlation between androgen receptor expression and FGF8 mRNA levels in patients with prostate cancer and benign prostatic hypertrophy. *J Clin Pathol* 1999; **52**: 29–39.

55 Iwamura M, Sluss PM, Casamento JB, Cockett ATK. Insulin-like growth factor I: action and receptor characterization in human prostate cancer cell lines. *Prostate* 1993; **22**: 243–52.

56 Cohen P, Peehl DM, Lamson G, Rosenfeld RG. Insulin-like growth factors (IGFs), IGF receptors, and IGF binding proteins in primary cultures of prostate epithelial cells. *J Clin Endocrinol Metab* 1991; **73**: 401–7.

57 Gregory CW, Hamil KG, Kim D *et al.* Androgen receptor expression in androgen-independent prostate cancer is associated with increased expression of androgen-regulated genes. *Cancer Res* 1998; **58**: 5718–24.

58 Kurek R, Tunn UW, Eckrt O, Aumüller G, Wong J, Renneberg H. The significance of serum levels of insulin-like growth factor-1 in patients with prostate cancer. *BJU Int* 2000; **85**: 125–9.

59 Behrens J, Mareel MM, Van Roy FM, Birchmeier W. Dissecting tumor cell invasion: epithelial cells acquire invasive properties after the loss of uvomorulin-mediated cell–cell adhesion. *J Cell Biol* 1989; **108**: 2435–47.

60 Richmond PJ, Karayiannakis AJ, Nagafuchi A, Kaisary AB, Pignatelli M. Aberrant E-cadherin and α-catenin expression in prostatic cancer: correlation with patient survival. *Cancer Res* 1997; **57**: 3189–93.

61 McPherson JD, Morton RA, Ewing CM *et al.* Assignment of the human α-catenin gene (CTNNA1) to chromosome 5q21-q22. *Genomics* 1994; **19**: 188–90.

62 Dong JT, Lamb PW, Rinker-Schaeffer CW *et al.* KAI1, a metastasis suppressor gene for prostate cancer on human chromosome 11p11.2. *Science* 1995; **268**: 884–6.

63 Dong JT, Suzuki H, Pin SS *et al.* Down-regulation of the KAI1 metastasis suppressor gene during the progression of human prostatic cancer infrequently involves gene mutation of allelic loss. *Cancer Res* 1996; **56**: 4387–90.

64 Gunthert U, Hoffmann M, Rudy W *et al.* A new variant of glycoprotein CD44 confers metastatic potential to rat carcinoma cells. *Cells* 1991; **65**: 13–24.

65 Iczkowski HA, Pantazis CG, Collins J. The loss of expression of CD44 standard and variant isoforms is related to prostatic carcinoma development and tumor progression. *J Urol Pathol* 1997; **6**: 119–29.

66 Suzuki H, Freije D, Nusskern DR *et al.* Interfocal heterogeneity of PTEN/MMAC1 gene alterations in multiple metastatic prostate cancer tissues. *Cancer Res* 1998; **58**: 204–9.

67 Lein M, Nowak L, Jung K *et al.* Metalloproteinases and tissue inhibitors of matrix-metalloproteinases in plasma of patients with prostate cancer and in prostate cancer tissue. *Ann N Y Acad Sci* 1999; **878**: 544–6.

68 Baker T, Tickle S, Wasan H, Docherty A, Isenberg D, Waxman J. Serum metalloproteinases and their inhibitors: markers for malignant potential. *Br J Cancer* 1994; **70**: 506–12.

9: Surgical Pathology of Prostate Cancer

C. S. Foster

Introduction

Even the smallest tissue specimen from the prostate, whether fine-needle aspirate, biopsy, transurethral resection or radical prostatectomy, contains a wealth of clinically useful information. To complement conventional morphological features, interesting observations are constantly being made with respect to a wide range of cellular components including morphometric parameters, protein expression and nucleic acid content. Despite the fascination of such findings, few have proven to be of practical value in the clinical assessment or management of an individual patient with prostate cancer. The relative ease with which such studies can be performed outside the surgical pathology laboratory, the small numbers of cases described, lack of standardization and failure to relate tissue findings to parameters of clinical outcome (either survival or response to therapy) have rendered many of these data valueless. Such disparity negates the utility of any observation until standardization occurs at all levels, so that valid interlaboratory comparison may be made. The actualité of the diagnostic information abstracted from patient tissue samples is that clinically relevant data require to be collected accurately, efficiently and according to a rationality based upon biological relevance. No technique or information will find clinical utility unless it can be performed or obtained quickly and has proven benefit to clinical management. Laborious procedures, however interesting or important to research, find little acceptance in the diagnostic laboratory.

It is the primary remit of diagnostic surgical pathologists to identify approaches which will optimally provide the most valuable data on individual prostate cancers. Clarity around difficult or contentious issues such as grading, staging and borderline lesions remains of paramount importance. It is imperative that high-quality, investigative research is performed on clinically derived tissues with outcome analyses that are relevant to the clinical situation. The objective of this type of research should be to make diagnosis and treatment patient (tumour) specific. In the meantime, the 'gold standard' of prostate cancer diagnosis remains accurate and detailed morphology using consensus-agreed criteria performed to a consistently high standard.

Cancer grade

Grade prior to radical prostatectomy

Grade is one of the strongest predictors of biological behaviour in prostate cancer, including invasiveness and metastatic potential, but is not sufficiently reliable when used alone for predicting pathological stage or patient outcome for individual patients. Grade is an invariable component of most clinical nomograms in prostate cancer. The subjective nature of grading precludes absolute precision, irrespective of the care with which an individual system is defined. However, the significant correlation between prostate cancer grade and virtually every outcome measure attests to the predictive strength and utility of accurate grading. The Gleason score is a scalar measurement which combines discrete primary and secondary patterns [1] into a total of nine discrete groups (Table 9.1). Inter- and intraobserver variability have been reported with the Gleason grading system and other grading systems [2,3]. Gleason noted exact reproducibility of scores in 50% of needle biopsies and of one score in 85%.

Needle core biopsy underestimates tumour grade in up to 45% of cases and overestimates grade in up to 32% [4–6]. Exact correlation is present in about one-third of biopsies and within one Gleason unit in another third. Grading errors are common in biopsies with small amounts of tumour or with low-grade tumour, and are probably due to tissue sampling variation, tumour heterogeneity and undergrading of needle biopsies [7]. Accuracy of biopsy is highest for the primary Gleason pattern, but the secondary pattern also provides useful predictive information, particularly when combined with the primary pattern, to create the Gleason score. Nevertheless, Gleason grading should be attempted for all needle biopsies [8], even those with small amounts of tumour.

On average, there are 2.7 (range 1–5) different Gleason primary patterns (Fig. 9.1) in prostate cancers received during radical prostatectomy. More than 50% of these cancers contain at least three different grades. The number of grades increases with greater cancer volume, the most common finding being high-grade cancer within the centre of a larger well- or moderately differentiated cancer, occurring in some 53% of cases. Reproducibility of this system has been reported to be a problem in some laboratories. In 35 of the 46 cases (about 70%) there was consensus among the urological pathologists. Interobserver consensus among general pathologists was overall at the low end of the moderate range (kappa = 0.435). There was consistent undergrading of Gleason scores 5–6 (47%), 7 (47%) and to lesser extent 8–10 (25%) among general pathologists [9].

Outside the US, the WHO grading system (Table 9.2) is used widely. This

Table 9.1 Gleason grading system (see Foster & Bostwick [1])

Pattern	Peripheral borders of tumour	Stromal invasion	Appearance of glands	Size of glands	Architecture of glands	Cytoplasm
1	Circumscribed, pushing, expansile	Minimal	Simple, round, monotonously replicated	Medium, regular	Closely packed, rounded masses	Similar to benign epithelium
2	Less circumscribed, early infiltration	Mild, with definite separation of glands by stroma	Simple, round, some variability in shape	Medium, less regular	Loosely packed, rounded masses	Similar to benign epithelium
3a	Infiltration	Marked	Angular, with variation in shape	Medium to large	Variably packed, irregular masses	More basophilic than patterns 1 and 2
3b	Infiltration	Marked	Angular, with variation in shape	Small	Variably packed, irregular masses	More basophilic than patterns 1 and 2
3c	Smooth, rounded	Marked	Papillary and cribriform	Irregular	Round to elongate masses	More basophilic than patterns 1 and 2
4a	Ragged infiltration	Marked	Microacinar, papillary and cribriform	Irregular	Fused, with chains and cords	Dark
4b	Ragged infiltration	Marked	Microacinar, papillary and cribriform	Irregular	Fused, with chains and cords	Clear (hypernephroid)
5a	Smooth, rounded	Marked	Comedocarcinoma	Irregular	Round to elongate masses	Variable
5b	Ragged infiltration	Marked	Difficult to identify gland lumina	Sheets of glands	Fused sheets and masses	Variable

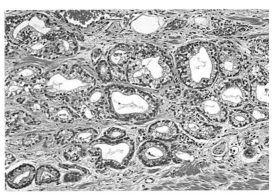

Figure 9.1 Carcinoma, well differentiated, Gleason pattern 3. Simple neoplastic glands are irregular in morphology, formed by cells with mild nuclear anaplasia. The malignant glands are infiltrating between pre-existing benign glands. Their nuclei are homogeneous in appearance (WHO nuclear grade I) and basal cells are absent, emphasizing, although not pathognomonic of, their malignant status. H+E × 60. (Shown in colour, Plate 1, facing p. 178.)

Table 9.2 WHO grading system (see Mostofi *et al.* [10])

Feature	Characteristic	Individual score	Summative score
Tumour grade	100% of the tumour forms well-defined glands	0	0–4
	Tumour is not entirely well differentiated but there are no poorly differentiated glands	1	
	Poorly differentiated component constitues 1–15% of total	2	
	Poorly differentiated component constitutes 16–25% of total	3	
	Poorly differentiated component constitutes >25% of total	4	
Nuclear anaplasia	Slight	1	1–3
	Moderate	2	
	Marked	3	

system takes into account glandular differentiation and nuclear anaplasia [10]. Glandular differentiation score is based on the relative proportion of tumour glands that can be classified into categories of well, moderately and poorly differentiated. Nuclear anaplasia is scored as 1, 2 and 3, corresponding to slight, moderate and marked nuclear changes, respectively (Fig. 9.2). Combination of the two scores into a single measure occurs to indicate increasingly poorer prognosis. An additive scale resulting in overall scores which range between 1 and 7, with all categories represented, has been suggested (Table 9.2). For the purposes of prognostication, the association (correlation) of death rate from cancer of the prostate with the prognostic score was very similar to that shown using the Gleason score in a range of 2–10. The prognosis of the WHO score 3 was very similar to that seen for the Gleason score 7,

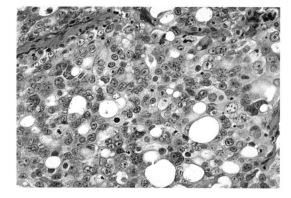

Figure 9.2 Carcinoma, poorly differentiated, Gleason pattern 5. The tumour consists of solid sheets of cells with enlarged prominent nucleoli, variation in nuclear size and frequent mitoses (WHO nuclear grade III). H+E × 200. (Shown in colour, Plate 2, facing p. 178.)

and according to Gleason's own scoring of these tumours. In these two groups, the death rate was nearly identical, with 6 deaths per 1000 months from prostate cancer [11].

Nuclear anaplasia also provides information which is additional to that given by glandular differentiation as determined by either Gleason grading or the proposed differentiation scoring system. When patients are scored by Gleason grade, the additional classification by 'marked' vs. 'moderate' nuclear anaplasia further separates patients into two groups with distinctly different prognoses. For Gleason grades 6 through 10, this difference was approximately 5 prostate cancer deaths per 1000 months. A similar pattern is observed when considering nuclear anaplasia in addition to the new 0–4 score for glandular differentiation. This increase in cancer death rate is 5 for marked anaplasia when compared to moderate anaplasia. This consistent effect was also observed for the tumours that had poorly differentiated glands and fell into the three high-score categories. In the proposed system, the score of 1 identifies patients with prognosis similar to Gleason system 2–5.

Present guidelines recommend that pathologists report both Gleason score and WHO nuclear grade for all prostate specimens. The relative percentage or proportion of high-grade cancer (Gleason primary patterns 4 and 5) should be included. Nuclear grade is based on the predominant nuclear grade, but there may also be value in reporting the highest nuclear grade. For the entirety of multiple biopsies containing cancer a global Gleason score should be given in addition to individual specimen grading.

Transrectal needle biopsy

Transrectal needle biopsy of the prostate is now so common that standardization of specimen handling and reporting is mandatory. Irrespective of whether specimens are single, sextant or octant (including transition zone biopsies), specimen cores from individual zones, and from each lobe of the prostate, should be kept separate in distinctly labelled containers and processed separately into different wax blocks. One histological section (haematoxylin and eosin stained) from each specimen core is inadequate to exclude the presence of small focal lesions. Therefore, routine step-sectioning at three levels of each individual specimen core is recommended. This practice takes cognizance of the potential multiplicity of primary neoplasms occurring simultaneously within a single prostate, and their potentially distinct phenotype with respect to behaviour and treatment response.

When assigning Gleason grades to needle biopsies or to small tissue samples, current convention records the two highest grades to limit sampling errors. If only one small focus is present, then one grade only is recorded. Undergrading of needle biopsy specimens is the most common problem and tends to occur in low-grade cancers. An approach to grading a needle biopsy accepted by the WHO Consensus Panel is:

1   If the specimen contains well-formed malignant glands showing a variation in size, then this is regarded as being an element of Gleason grade 3. If that is the only pattern in the sample, the grade is given as '3 + 3'.

2   When glands start to fuse, in addition to appearing discrete and well formed, such tumours are defined as Gleason grade '3 + 4' or '4 + 3', depending on the relative amounts of each pattern.

3   In carcinomas where well-formed neoplastic glands are composed of pale-staining tumour cells infiltrating benign prostate glands, the tumour is then graded as Gleason Grade 3.

Throughout the past decade, the amount of core biopsy tissue available for pathological examination has decreased because traditional 14-gauge biopsy needles have been replaced by 18-gauge ones. Also, more biopsies contain smaller amounts of tumour than were formerly identified because of the dramatic success of efforts made during recent years to detect smaller tumours at an earlier stage.

Since underdiagnosis of carcinoma in needle biopsy material containing only small amounts of tumour is a relatively frequent occurrence, the primary consideration is to confirm the presence of cancer. If small foci of cancer are missed on needle biopsy, the chance that a subsequent repeat biopsy will also be negative is greater than 20%. Recognition of prostate cancer in fine-needle biopsy specimens rests on identification of architectural and cytological abnormalities.

It is important to survey the entire needle biopsy specimen at low power, in order to appreciate the distribution of the non-neoplastic prostate glands and to identify glands that do not correspond with the appearance of non-neoplastic glands. The following criteria are recommended to diagnose limited amounts of gland-forming carcinoma on needle biopsy:

1 *Abnormal architecture*: The primary step is identification of glands that are smaller than normal and that may be found infiltrating and occupying the stroma between benign glands. After recognizing, on low power, that some glands are suspicious, evaluation of cytological details can be made at higher magnification.

2 *Cytoplasm*: The gland-forming carcinomas found on needle biopsy are usually of intermediate grade and have a more granular amphophilic cytoplasm than the surrounding benign glands. Against a background of atrophic non-neoplastic glands, infiltrating prostate carcinoma may stand out as glands with distinctly pale cytoplasm. The observation that the cells comprising such glands contain enlarged nuclei with prominent nucleoli is common in prostate carcinomas of intermediate grade.

3 *Nuclear details*: Intermediate gland-forming tumours also contain atypical nuclear features, most frequently enlarged nuclei, often with small nucleoli. However, such nuclear features are frequently found in benign glands with associated intense inflammation. The appropriate abnormal architectural pattern is a co-requisite before assigning the diagnosis of carcinoma through recognition of cytological features such as prominent nucleoli.

4 *Basal cell layer*: An unequivocal lack of a basal cell layer is the hallmark of carcinoma. Application of monoclonal antibody 34β-E12 makes it possible to selectively stain basal cells of normal and hyperplastic prostate [12]. While negative immunohistochemical staining for basal cells should not be used as the sole determinant for malignancy, strategic use of this feature in conjunction with other morphological criteria may add significant weight to the diagnosis of prostate cancer.

5 *Other features*: Two morphological features formerly considered of assistance in distinguishing benign from malignant prostate tissue are perineural invasion with malignant glands encircling nerve and the presence of apparently specific microcrystalline structures within malignant acini and/or in adjacent benign glands. The former is a difficult criterion to apply, particularly in small samples, since perineural infiltration by epithelium has been identified in benign prostatic disease in a manner analogous to that of mammary epithelium occurring in benign fibroadenomatous disease of the human breast. Nevertheless, when applied judiciously, the observation of perineural invasion may be helpful in confirming the diagnosis of prostate cancer. The glands in question should completely encircle the nerve (Fig. 9.3), thus distinguishing the appearance from that of the perineural infiltration that has been reported in benign disease [13]. The second feature, microcrystalline structures, can be a useful adjunctive indicator of the presence of malignancy. However, this is not a reliable diagnostic feature, nor is the presence of crystals in grading or prognosticating the likely behaviour of confirmed prostate cancer. Nevertheless, the presence of intraluminal crystalloids should significantly heighten

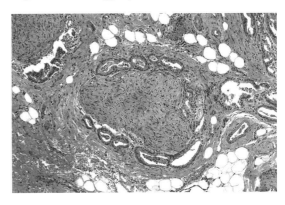

Figure 9.3 Perineural invasion. There is unresolved controversy as to whether a prognostic distribution should be made between tumour in perineural lymphatics and that which is truly intraneural. H+E × 150. (Shown in colour, Plate 3, facing p. 178.)

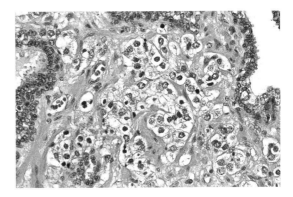

Figure 9.4 Androgen ablation effect: infiltrative prostatic carcinoma cells are employed with hydropic and vacuolated cytoplasm. Nuclei are variably hyperchromatic. Adjacent non-neoplastic epithelium is relatively unaffected. H+E × 350. (Shown in colour, Plate 4, facing p. 178.)

suspicion of associated malignancy, and this possibility must be investigated by a detailed evaluation of all adjacent tissues [14].

Grade after radiation therapy

The merit of histological grading of prostate cancer after radiation therapy is controversial. Histological changes induced by radiation therapy (Fig. 9.4) are well recognized, and a trend towards higher Gleason score after radiation therapy has been reported [15]. The frequent reporting of high-grade cancer in post-irradiation prostatic biopsies may be related to clonal evolution which results in apparent cancer progression and tumour dedifferentiation [16]. Sampling variation in pre-irradiation biopsies and preferential progression of high-grade cancer may also account for this observation.

Pathological examination of salvage prostatectomy specimens showed that only 33% of patients had organ-confined cancer at the time of surgery. Of these, 76% had non-diploid DNA content, which indicated that this group of patients had worse prognostic features than patients treated primarily with prostatectomy. Ahlering *et al.* [15] reported a series of 35 patients who underwent salvage surgery and in which 11 (32%) had Gleason grade 8 and 12 (34%) had organ-confined cancer. Higher Gleason scores observed in salvage prostatectomy series may reflect selection bias resulting from the increased risk of progression of these tumours after initial management. Radiorecurrent cancer may be at the aggressive end of a biological continuum which parallels the advanced pathological stage seen in these patients.

When grading radiated prostates, the most important consideration is whether or not the biopsy shows any treatment effect and, if so, how much. The only portion that can be graded using current criteria is the part which shows no treatment effect. Biological behaviour may not correlate with the degree of regression. Biopsy evaluation of treatment results is unreliable before 9–12 months after treatment unless there is clinical evidence of progression.

Grade after androgen deprivation therapy

Following androgen deprivation therapy, distinctive changes occur to prostate cancer morphology. Schenken *et al.* [17] first reported that oestrogen therapy for prostate cancer reduced nuclear size by 56% as compared with untreated controls. Loss of recognizable nucleoli, condensation of chromatin, nuclear pyknosis and cytoplasmic vacuolation were all identified as features characteristic of androgen deprivation. It is essential that pathologists are aware of these changes, because of the reliance on nuclear and nucleolar size as reliable criteria when identifying prostate cancer, particularly in small biopsy specimens or in lymph node metastases.

Murphy *et al.* [18] found a substantial increase in the Gleason grade for cases treated by androgen deprivation therapy. Their independent observations raise the question: 'Does high grade reflect aggressive androgen-insensitive clones or merely the collapse of cancer of low viability?' Murphy suggested that the apparent increase in grade might have two possible explanations. Apparent change in grade could be the result of incomplete sampling, by core needle biopsy, of a widely distributed tumour having foci of different grades, or could relate to gland shrinkage with apparent loss of lumina and increased peri-glandular connective tissue. In this latter situation, pathologists might be prompted by one absence of gland lumina to regard neoplasms as being poorly differentiated when in fact they were responding favourably to treatment. Measurements of gland density, together with a decrease in serum prostate-specific antigen (PSA) or prostatic acid phosphatase (PAP) levels after treatment, tend to support this hypothesis. DNA ploidy analysis has revealed no difference between treated and untreated cases but also that treated prostate cancer retains its immunophenotype, although the clinical importance of high grade remains uncertain.

Location of cancer

The site of origin of cancer within an individual prostate gland is a significant prognostic factor. When cancer arises in the transition zone, it is apparently less aggressive than typical acinar adenocarcinoma arising in the peripheral zone. The majority of transition zone cancers occur adjacent to hyperplastic nodules, and one-third actually originate within nodules. Such adenocarcinomas are better differentiated than those in the peripheral zone, accounting for the majority of Gleason primary grade 1 and 2 tumours. The volume of low-grade tumours tends to be smaller than that of those arising in the peripheral zone, although frequent exceptions are seen. The confinement of transition zone adenocarcinoma to its anatomical site of origin may account, in part, for the favourable prognosis of clinical stage T1 tumours. The transition zone boundary may act as a relative barrier to tumour extension, since malignant acini frequently appear to fan out along this boundary before invading the peripheral and central zones.

Prostate cancer is frequently multifocal and bilateral. These individual cancers are likely to be both genotypically and phenotypically distinct, with respect to their behaviour and their response to therapy. Therefore, all prostate biopsy specimens should be submitted separately, with the anatomical origin of each specimen being individually recorded. Pathologists should report each specimen separately. Thus, the anatomical site(s) of carcinoma within each prostate biopsy can be included in the pathology report and identified in the anatomical area specified by the urologist. Whenever possible, the anatomical location of carcinoma within total prostatectomy specimens should also be specified in the pathology report.

Cancer volume

Biopsy cancer volume depends upon multiple factors, including prostate volume, cancer volume, cancer distribution, number of biopsy cores obtained, the cohort of patients being evaluated and the technical competence of the investigator. The combined results from multiple studies indicate that the biopsy extent of tumour provides some predictive value for extent in radical prostatectomy specimens and should probably be reported, although its predictive value for an individual patient is limited [19]. Reliance upon this measure alone may often be misleading. Consequently, the volume of cancer in the needle biopsy should not significantly influence therapeutic decisions.

Small biopsies

There is a fair to good correlation between amount of cancer reported in biopsies and that subsequently found in radical prostatectomy specimens [19]. This correlation is greatest for large cancers. High cancer burden on needle biopsy is strongly suggestive of large-volume high-stage cancer [19]. In one study, lymph node metastases were identified in 52 of 57 patients (91% specificity) and 10 of 14 patients (71% sensitivity) when adenocarcinoma replaced two core biopsies, and 80% of a third from the sextant sample.

Unfortunately, low tumour burden on needle biopsy does not necessarily indicate low-volume or low-stage cancer. Patients with less than 30% of needle cores replaced by cancer have a mean volume in the radical prostatectomy of $6.1\,cm^3$ (range $0.19–16.8\,cm^3$), indicating that the amount of tumour on transrectal needle biopsy is not a good predictor of tumour volume. Patients with less than 10% cancer in the biopsy have a 30% risk of positive surgical margins, 27% risk of extraprostatic extension and 22% risk of PSA biochemical progression; these risks are higher in patients with more than 10% cancer. Patients with less than 3 mm cancer and Gleason score 6 or less on needle biopsy have a 59% risk of cancer volume exceeding $0.5\,cm^3$. Those with less than 2 mm of cancer have a 26% risk of extraprostatic cancer, and those with less than 3 mm have a 52% risk.

With respect to the most appropriate methods for measuring and reporting the volume of cancer in the needle biopsy, cancer volume has been assessed in four different ways:
1   percentage of biopsy cores involved;
2   percentage of cancer area in each biopsy specimen;
3   millimetres of adenocarcinoma in the entire biopsy;
4   millimetres of adenocarcinoma per core [20].
All measures were essentially equivalent in their predictive value for cancer volume in the prostatectomy. Consequently, the current recommendation is use of the percentage of cancer area because of its ease of application and likely acceptance by most pathologists, similarly to the method for quantitating cancer volume in transurethral resection specimens.

Radical prostatectomies

Measurement of cancer volume may become an adjunct to digital rectal examination-based staging of prostatic adenocarcinoma because of its powerful prognostic capability [21]. This approach may become feasible following improvements in imaging techniques such as transrectal ultrasonography (TRUS). A cancer volume-based prognostic index has been proposed, based on evidence linking adenocarcinoma volume with patterns of progression (extraprostatic extension, seminal vesicle invasion and lymph node metastases). For organ-confined cancer, three main categories are suggested: V1, cancer lesions smaller than 1 cm^3; V2a, cancer 1–5 cm^3; and V2b, tumour larger than 5 cm^3. The goal of the proposed prognostic index is to achieve greater precision in predicting outcome for individual patients [21].

A positive correlation between cancer volume and serum PSA concentration suggests that PSA can serve as a surrogate of volume [22]. However, the additive and compounding effect of nodular hyperplasia limits the power of PSA in estimating preoperative cancer size and extent. As adenocarcinoma enlarges, it usually becomes less differentiated and may lose some of its capacity for PSA production. Although PSA concentration increases with increasing Gleason grade, PSA decreases when tumour volume is held constant (PSA concentration declines as Gleason grade increases). This finding results from production of less PSA per cell in poorly differentiated tumours when compared with well- and moderately differentiated ones [22].

No accepted standard exists for reporting cancer volume in prostatectomy specimens. The most practical approach is to estimate the percentage of cancer in the entire specimen. After accounting for pathological stage, tumour volume may not provide significant additional prognostic information, but this observation has not been confirmed.

When constructing reports, pathologists should include the total percentage of cancer in the total number of needle biopsy segments. Conversely, although the volume of cancer in radical prostatectomy specimens has been shown to have predictive value in only some studies, also including this determination may be of value until more reliable predictive features become available. There is currently no agreement or recommendation as to the specific method of quantifying volume in these specimens.

Surgical margins

A 'positive surgical margin' is defined as the occurrence of cancer cells touching the inked surface of the prostate (Fig. 9.5). Care must be taken to avoid interpreting ink within tissue crevices created by postoperative handling of the specimen as positive margins. Careful handling of the specimen and awareness of this potential problem are usually sufficient. Surgical margins are not currently included in pathological staging. However, many studies have erroneously equated positive margins with extraprostatic extension, particularly when the surgeon has cut into the prostate and penetrated intraprostatic cancer. The 1996 Mayo Clinic consensus conference emphasized this distinction and called on investigators to carefully describe surgical margin status separately from extraprostatic extension [23]. Confusion may persist in interpretation of prostatectomy specimens in which there is focally no

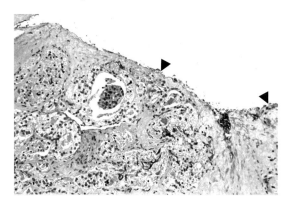

Figure 9.5 Positive surgical resection margin in which foci of cancer cells (arrows) abut the inked margin (green). Elsewhere, there is a rim of stromal tissue which is free from invasion. The vertical crack (right field) is an artefact and should not be misinterpreted or considered as part of the surgical margin. H+E × 250. (Shown in colour, Plate 5, facing p. 178.)

extraprostatic tissue for examination. At such sites, the surgical resection margin corresponds exactly with the outer surface of the prostate or cuts into the prostatic capsule or parenchyma. If the surgical margin at this site contains cancer, does this represent extraprostatic extension? Participants at the 1996 consensus conference agreed that these foci should be considered T2(+) rather than T3. The 'plus' sign is a 'telescopic ramification' of the TNM staging system that is added to emphasize that the available evidence indicates T2 cancer but there may be cancer outside of the prostate that cannot be evaluated in the specimen submitted [23].

Prevalence of positive surgical margins has steadily declined in the past decade, probably as a result of refinements in surgical techniques and earlier detection of cancer of smaller volumes. Ohori and colleagues found positive surgical margins in 24% of whole-mount radical prostatectomy specimens obtained at their hospital before 1987, usually in the posterolateral region near the neurovascular bundles. By modifying surgery to approach the neurovascular bundles laterally and to widely dissect the apex of the prostate, by 1993 they observed a positive surgical margin rate of only 8% [24], despite similar volumes, grades and pathological stages of cancer. Earlier reports noted frequencies of positive surgical margins of 33%, 46% and 57%, with no difference in specimens from nerve-sparing and non-nerve-sparing operations. Positive surgical margins are strongly correlated with cancer volume [24,25] and number of needle biopsies containing cancer. Most positive surgical margins in prostates with cancer smaller than 4 cm^3 are caused by surgical incision [26].

Positive margins are variously located at the apex (48%), rectal and lateral surfaces (24%), bladder neck (16%) and superior pedicles (10%). The clinical significance of positive surgical margins in patients treated by prostatectomy is unclear. Patients with organ-confined cancer and positive surgical margins have a 60% chance of dying from cancer, a risk significantly greater than the 30% possibility for patients without positive surgical margins. Also, surgical margin status is the only predictor of cancer progression other than Gleason score in patients without seminal vesicle invasion or lymph node metastases. Conversely, Ohori and colleagues [24] found that positive surgical margins had no effect on prognosis. Currently, there is no consensus on the utility of postoperative adjuvant therapy in patients with positive surgical margins, probably because of uncertainty about the clinical significance of this finding [27].

When reporting, pathologists should describe the presence, extent and location of all surgical margins. However, there is no current agreement or recommendation as to the specific method of quantifying the amount of cancer in these locations. Further, pathologists should routinely report the presence of benign prostate glands in the surgical resection margin to alert clinicians to the possible retention of residual PSA-producing tissue after surgery.

Pathological stage

Current clinical and pathological staging of early prostatic adenocarcinoma separates patients into two groups, those with palpable and impalpable tumours [8,28]. Reliance on palpability of the tumour, as determined by digital rectal examination, is unique among organ-staging systems and is hampered by the low sensitivity, low specificity and low positive predictive value of digital rectal examination. Recent refinements in staging have led to the introduction of a new stage of non-palpable adenocarcinoma, detected by elevated serum PSA level and referred to as 'stage T1c'; however, this new stage was introduced without supportive clinical evidence, and studies show that it does not identify a distinct group of patients. The question remains whether patients who will benefit from early detection and intervention can be separated from those who will not. The two principal clinical staging systems currently in widespread use are the TNM system and the American system (modified Whitmore–Jewett). These two systems are similar, although the TNM system contains a greater number of subdivisions for most stages. Also, the TNM system includes stage groupings, which consist of combined clinical stage and tumour grade.

TNM staging system

The TNM (tumour–node–metastasis) classification for prostatic adeno-carcinoma was first published by the American Joint Committee on Cancer (AJCC) and the Union Internationale Contre le Cancer (UICC) in 1978, but their definitions at that time contained significant differences [28]. By 1987, these differences had been resolved, but the resulting classification was criticized by the European Organization for Research and Treatment of Cancer (EORTC) Genitourinary Group and others, particularly for the T (primary tumour) category and the proposed stage groupings. A consensus conference held to resolve discrepancies included representatives from the AJCC, UICC, EORTC Genitourinary Group and American Urological Association. A consequence of this meeting was the revised and uniform TNM classification published in 1992 [11]. The 1992 revision of the TNM system is currently the international standard for staging of prostatic adenocarcinoma [8,28,29]. Efforts directed towards standardization of staging, including guidelines for pathological evaluation of specimens, are useful in allowing comparison of results from different centres [30].

The 1992 revision included four significant changes compared with the 1987 version. First, a new category (T1c) was introduced to recognize non-palpable, invisible adenocarcinomas identified by random biopsy following detection of elevated serum PSA level. Second, palpable adenocarcinoma confined to the prostate (T2) was subdivided into three groups rather than two, based on the relative involvement of the prostate (involvement of half a lobe or less, more than half a lobe but not both lobes, or both lobes) instead of absolute tumour size as determined by digital rectal examination. Third, adenocarcinoma with local extraprostatic extension (T3) was subdivided into three groups rather than two, based on laterality and seminal vesicle invasion (unilateral, bilateral and seminal vesicle invasion). Finally, the concept of 'telescopic ramification' was introduced, to allow introduction of additional prognostic factors without altering existing categories.

American (modified Whitmore–Jewett) staging system

The American staging system, introduced by Whitmore in 1956, consists of letters A though D to denote stages. It was modified by Jewett to allow substaging of stage B. He and others noted that patients with a palpably discrete nodule (B1 nodule, 'Jewett nodule') had longer cancer-free survival time. Recently, the American system was modified to accommodate PSA-detected adenocarcinoma [28]. The current stage divisions are similar to those of the TNM system, but do not include tumour grade except to separate stages A1 and A2.

Limitations of current staging systems

Current staging systems are limited by several factors:
1 clinical understaging with transurethral resection;
2 clinical understaging with digital rectal examination;

3   limited ability of imaging studies to evaluate the presence and extent of prostatic adenocarcinoma;
4   heterogeneity of stage T1c adenocarcinoma;
5   variability in pathological staging of stage T1 adenocarcinoma; and
6   variability in examination of radical prostatectomy specimens.

CLINICAL UNDERSTAGING WITH DIGITAL RECTAL EXAMINATION

Current staging of palpable organ-confined adenocarcinoma relies on digital rectal examination to separate unilateral tumours from bilateral ones or small tumours from large ones (less than half of one lobe, between one-half and one lobe, and more than one lobe). There is, however, a high level of inaccuracy and interobserver variability in determining tumour size and pathological stage by digital rectal examination. Prostatic adenocarcinoma staging is unique among organ-staging systems because it relies on the presence or absence of palpability and substage T2 adenocarcinoma based on the proportion of prostatic induration identified.

Bostwick identified clinical understaging in 59% of cases and clinical overstaging in 5% in a series of 311 serially sectioned radical retropubic prostatectomies removed for clinically localized prostatic adenocarcinoma (excluding stages T1a, T1b and T1c). There is no equivalent pathological stage for clinical stage T1c, so this group will always be restaged pathologically. These results were similar to those reported by others who have also undertaken careful pathological sectioning of prostatectomy specimens. This substantial error rate must be accounted for when evaluating recurrence and survival rates, especially when comparing studies of clinically staged patients followed with active surveillance and surgically (pathologically) staged patients. There was considerable overlap in the volume of adenocarcinoma in clinical stages T2a+b and T2c, with tumours measuring up to 41 and 43 cm^3, respectively. These data indicate that digital rectal examination is inaccurate for preoperative assessment of tumour volume. Imaging studies to assess tumour volume and extent would be invaluable in clinical staging. Unfortunately, current accuracy of such methods is insufficient to be reliable for all patients. The accuracy of correctly identifying extraprostatic extension is 63% with TRUS [31], 71% with body-coil magnetic resonance imaging (MRI) and 83% with endorectal and surface-coil MRI.

PATHOLOGY OF PSA-DETECTED ADENOCARCINOMA

Before clinical use of PSA became widespread, most organ-confined adenocarcinoma was discovered by digital rectal examination (clinical stage T2) or at the time of transurethral resection (clinical stage T1). Routine use of serum

PSA increased the detection rate of prostatic adenocarcinoma and uncovered some adenocarcinomas that would not have been detected by digital rectal examination [32]. There was a sevenfold increase (14 to 118 cases, respectively) in PSA-detected adenocarcinomas at the Mayo Clinic in the 3-year period from 1988 to 1991.

There is no pathological stage equivalent for clinical stage T1c, and such tumours are invariably 'upstaged' at surgery, usually to pathological stage T2 or T3. Oesterling and colleagues found that clinical stage T1c adenocarcinoma and clinical stage T2a+b adenocarcinoma had similar maximum tumour diameters, frequencies of multifocality, tumour grades, DNA content results, pathological stages and tumour locations. Interestingly, they had different serum PSA values, tumour volumes, rates of positive surgical margins and prostate gland sizes, the T1c tumours having higher values for each feature. These findings indicate that PSA detects adenocarcinoma which is clinically important and potentially curable. Also, PSA-detected tumours that are visible on TRUS have pathological features similar to those of lesions that are not visible. Further long-term follow-up of PSA-detected prostatic adenocarcinoma is necessary to establish the prognosis of these tumours and determine whether a separate staging category is warranted for them.

PROBLEMS WITH TNM STAGING (1992 REVISION) OF RADICAL
PROSTATECTOMY SPECIMENS

Three practical problems have been described for pathological staging using the TNM system for radical prostatectomy specimens. First, separation of substages T2a (less than half of one lobe) and T2b (more than half of one lobe) is difficult, particularly in specimens that are partially sampled rather than whole mounted. This problem is resolved by reporting such cases as T2a+b, an approach that necessarily compresses data. Second, the pathologist rarely (if ever) has access to clinical information pertaining to distant metastases at the time of histological evaluation of the prostatectomy specimen and thus cannot accurately report the M of TNM. This problem is resolved by reporting all cases as 'Mx', with a brief qualification that refers to the clinical record. The third problem is pathological 'upstaging' of adenocarcinoma, which usually occurs with prostatectomy following transurethral resection; as noted above, transurethral resection-detected adenocarcinomas are T1a and T1b, yet additional adenocarcinoma identified on prostatectomy frequently results in upstaging to T2 and T3. This problem is resolved by reporting both TNM stages (transurethral resection and prostatectomy) with a brief note describing this issue. Alternatively, it may be better to exclude the T1 category from pathological staging of radical prostatectomy specimens.

It is now recommended that all pathologists routinely employ the pathological classifications of TNM to report radical prostatectomy specimens. This includes evaluation of the presence of extraprostatic extension and the amount. Although there is no current agreement or recommendation as to a specific method for quantifying extraprostatic extension in these specimens, a recent WHO Consensus Panel [33] recommended adoption of the decision of the 1995 UICC/AJCC consensus meeting as a working methodology. If the amount of extraprostatic tumour is equal to, or less than, two high-power microscopic fields (40× objective with 10× eyepiece), then the amount of extraprostatic extension should be considered as focal. Any amount in excess of two high-power fields is considered to be either non-focal or extensive.

Perineural invasion

Perineural invasion is common in adenocarcinoma, being present in up to 38% of biopsies [33], and may be the only evidence of malignancy in a needle core. This finding is strong presumptive evidence of cancer, but is not pathognomonic because it occurs rarely with benign acini [13]. Initially, prostatic epithelial cells enter minor lymphatic channels surrounding neural bundles (Fig. 9.3). These structures are usually inconspicuous, although demonstrable using antibodies to thrombomodulin. However, complete circumferential growth, intraneural invasion and ganglionic invasion are found only with cancer. Perineural invasion usually indicates tumour spread along the path of least resistance, and does not necessarily predict iliac lymph node invasion. Only half of patients with intraprostatic perineural invasion on biopsy have extraprostatic extension. In univariate analysis, perineural invasion was predictive of extraprostatic extension, seminal vesicle invasion and pathological stage in patients treated by radical prostatectomy [33]. However, in multivariate analysis, perineural invasion had no predictive value after consideration of Gleason grade, serum PSA and amount of cancer on biopsy. It has limited utility as a diagnostic test for the prediction of extraprostatic extension, with a sensitivity of only 51%, specificity of 71% and positive predictive value of 49%. The negative predictive value was 71%, indicating that the absence of perineural invasion was associated with extraprostatic extension in 29% of cases. Utility of perineural invasion on biopsy as a diagnostic test for the prediction of seminal vesicle invasion was even worse.

Perineural invasion was a significant independent predictive factor for adverse outcome at 3 years for patients treated by external beam radiation therapy. However, its value was associated only with a pretreatment PSA of less than 20 ng/mL, indicating that poor prognosis associated with high PSA overrides any additional information that perineural invasion may provide. These findings suggest that there is no value in routinely reporting perineural invasion in biopsy specimens.

Vascular/lymphatic invasion

Microvascular invasion consists of tumour cells within endothelial-lined spaces. The presence of a cellular reaction by or within the adjacent stroma is not a prerequisite for diagnosis. Hitherto, differentiation between vascular and lymphatic channels has not been required because of the difficulty and lack of reproducibility among different observers attempting to make this distinction by unaided light microscopic examination. Microvascular invasion may be confused with perineural invasion and fixation-associated retraction artefacts of acini.

Microvascular invasion is present in 38% of radical prostatectomy specimens. It is commonly associated with extraprostatic extension and lymph node metastases (62% and 67% of cases, respectively), and its presence correlates with histological grade [34]. Microvascular invasion appears to be an important predictor of outcome, and carries a fourfold greater risk of tumour progression and death. However, it is not an independent predictor of progression when stage and grade are included in the analysis.

The Cancer Committee of the College of American Pathologists [30] recommends reporting microvascular invasion in all prostatic specimens, using routine morphological (H+E) microscopic examination. Despite this recommendation, this finding is not evaluated in prostatic biopsies by many laboratories. Immunohistochemical stains directed against endothelial cells such as Factor VIII-related, antigen *Ulex europaeus* or thrombomodulin may increase the detection rate [34]. However, these identify different endothelial phenotypes and there is no consensus agreement on their use, either individually or combined.

Morphometric markers

Morphometric markers provide useful predictive information in prostate cancer, but are still considered research modalities. Morphometric studies should employ objective, quantitative techniques which are preferably computer-assisted. The College of American Pathologists [35] and a recent WHO Consensus Panel [36] recognized that there are no accepted standards for morphometric studies, and this is considered an important and significant area for investigation.

The variety of different potential problems encountered in quantitative digital image analysis are summarized as in Table 9.3. Variables should be controlled and standardized with respect to an interlaboratory convention in order to minimize variance in digital image analysis and thus provide a framework within which to obtain meaningful comparative data (Table 9.4). Roundness refers to approximation of a nucleus to a circle, deviations from

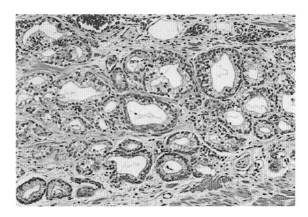

Plate 1 Carcinoma, well differentiated, Gleason pattern 3. Simple neoplastic glands are irregular in morphology, formed by cells with mild nuclear anaplasia. The malignant glands are infiltrating between pre-existing benign glands. Their nuclei are homogeneous in appearance (WHO nuclear grade I) and basal cells are absent, emphasizing, although not pathognomonic of, their malignant status. H+E × 60.

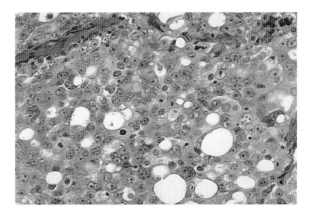

Plate 2 Carcinoma, poorly differentiated, Gleason pattern 5. The tumour consists of solid sheets of cells with enlarged prominent nucleoli, variation in nuclear size and frequent mitoses (WHO nuclear grade III). H+E × 200.

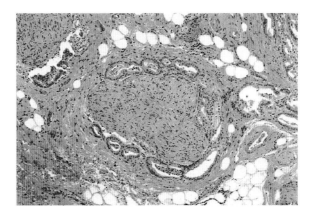

Plate 3 Perineural invasion. There is unresolved controversy as to whether a prognostic distribution should be made between tumour in perineural lymphatics and that which is truly intraneural. H+E × 150.

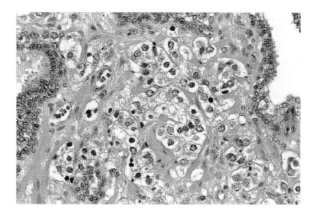

Plate 4 Androgen ablation effect: infiltrative prostatic carcinoma cells are employed with hydropic and vacuolated cytoplasm. Nuclei are variably hyperchromatic. Adjacent non-neoplastic epithelium is relatively unaffected. H+E × 350.

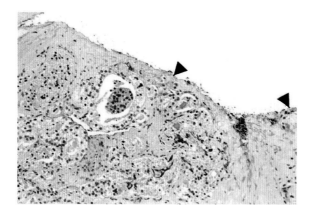

Plate 5 Positive surgical resection margin in which foci of cancer cells (arrows) abut the inked margin (green). Elsewhere, there is a rim of stromal tissue which is free from invasion. The vertical crack (right field) is an artefact and should not be misinterpreted or considered as part of the surgical margin. H+E × 250.

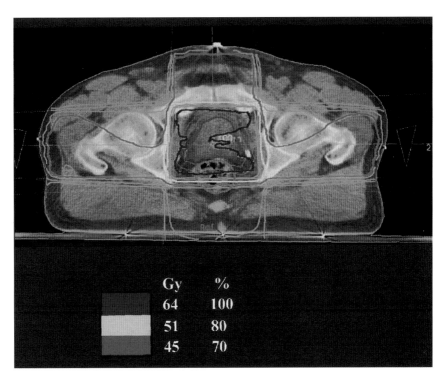

Gy	%
64	100
51	80
45	70

Plate 6 CT planning scan illustrating irradiation of the prostate gland with three 10 MV photon fields.

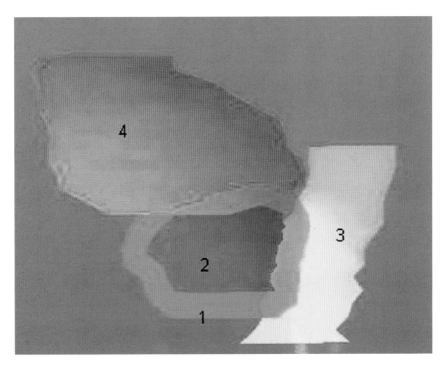

Plate 7 Three-dimensional computer reconstruction of conformal prostate radiotherapy showing (1) planning target volume, (2) clinical target volume, (3) rectum and (4) bladder.

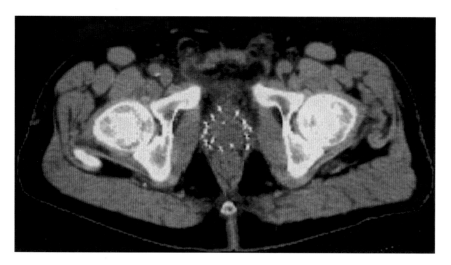

Plate 8 Post-brachytherapy implant CT scan illustrating multiple palladium-103 seeds within the prostate gland.

(c)

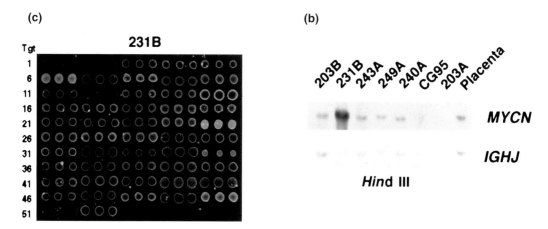

(b)

Plate 9 Microarray hybridization of 51 genes with GCT 231B DNA. The image obtained for the microarray hybridization with control placenta DNA (red) and GCT 231B DNA (green) is shown (a). Each gene is arrayed three times, and in this case the target gene showing excess green signal is *MYCN*. Amplification of *MYCN* in GCT 231B was confirmed by Southern hybridization (b). *IGHJ* was used to control for DNA loading.

Table 9.3 Problems of quantitative digital image analysis

Reproducibility by different analytical modalities
High intra- and interobserver variability
High cost of equipment and personnel
User-dependence on equipment
Subjectivity in selection of cases, fields to analyse, etc.
Lack of standardized methods
Discrepant results with prostate cancer
Unproven clinical utility

Table 9.4 Standardized features for quantitative digital image analysis

Intact, non-overlapping and well-focused nuclei
At least 150 nuclei per case
Consistent tissue processing and preparation
Internal age- and procedure-matched controls
Rigorous definitions for classifying data
Sufficiently large population groups to perform valid
   comparative statistical analyses

roundness indicating more aggressive cancer. Many of the initial reports predicting favourable survival from nuclear roundness emanated from one institution were limited by small sample size (fewer than 30 patients), required expenditure of a large amount of time for analysis (approximately 4h per case), used the same patient cohort in multiple publications, failed to describe the morphological variations and nuclear roundness extremes and were beset with patient selection bias.

Significant problems of reproducibility in nuclear roundness measurement have been described, and the results with different digitizing instruments are not comparable. A comparative study of digital image analysis and video planimetry with manual nuclear tracing found a lower level of intra- and interobserver variability with planimetry. Blom *et al.* [37] were unable to reproduce the positive results from an earlier study at another institution, despite use of identical equipment and examination of the same cases. They found that intraobserver variation was low, but interobserver variation was high. There was no correlation of nuclear roundness and patient survival. Nuclear roundness measurements were not reliable in needle biopsy specimens. Further, multivariate analyses correlating nuclear morphometry and nuclear grade with pathological stage at radical prostatectomy demonstrated little additional predictive value for nuclear roundness when compared with Gleason grade. Virtually all measures of nuclear morphology revealed the same similarity between high-grade prostatic intraepithelial neoplasia (PIN) and cancer, in contrast with either normal or hyperplastic epithelium [38,39].

Mean nuclear volume data showed a wide range of values in prostate cancer, varying from 81 to 782 μm^3, which may or may not correlate with cancer grade and clinical stage. Nucleolar size is a significant diagnostic factor in prostate cancer, and is a major determinant of nuclear grade. 'Prominent' nucleoli in cancer have been variously defined as a diameter greater than 1.0–3.0 μm. The presence of two or more nucleoli in an individual cell usually indicates carcinoma [40]. In routine practice, nucleolar size is not objectively measured, and differences in tissue preparation and staining limit comparability of this factor in morphometric studies.

Proliferation and apoptotic markers

Mitotic figures

Mitotic figures are rarely found in tissue sections in normal or hyperplastic prostatic epithelium. Therefore, S-phase markers are commonly employed as surrogate markers for estimating proliferation rates. Cells in the DNA synthetic phase of the cell cycle incorporate thymidine analogue bromodeoxyuridine (BRdU) into newly synthesized DNA and also express both proliferating cell nuclear antigen (PCNA) and Ki-67 antigens. One study of BRdU, PCNA and Ki-67 labelling in prostatic tissues demonstrated that the three methods are strongly correlated with each other [41]. In most studies, the number of mitotic figures increased progressively from benign epithelium through PIN to cancer [42]. Adenocarcinoma with a cribriform growth pattern and those composed of solid areas of undifferentiated tumour cells contained most mitotic figures. Additionally, the number of mitotic figures correlated with cancer stage and grade [41,43], and also with progression and progression-free survival [42]. Androgen deprivation therapy results in a dramatic decline in the number of mitotic figures in prostate cancer, whereas normal prostatic epithelium undergoes apoptosis-mediated involution [44]. Thus it appears that elevation in epithelial cell proliferation parallels cancer progression and that determinants of elevated cellular proliferation have significant potential value as prognostic markers.

Proliferating cell nuclear antigen

Proliferating cell nuclear antigen (PCNA) is an auxiliary protein for DNA polymerase which reaches maximal expression during the S phase of the cell cycle. Hence, PCNA has been widely used as an index of the proliferative activity of cancers. However, PCNA also measures DNA repair in non-dividing cells and hence is not an accurate method for assessing proliferation.

The PCNA labelling index is reported to be lowest in benign normal prostatic epithelium and organ-confined cancer but to increase progressively from well-through poorly differentiated invasive prostate cancer, although there is wide variance [45]. The correlation between PCNA index and cancer stage is strong. Hence, a high PCNA labelling index may be an independent prognostic indicator and may indicate progression of prostate cancer. Nonetheless, this factor is not currently recommended for routine clinical use.

Ki-67 and MIB-1

Ki-67 is a non-histone nuclear protein expressed by non-proliferating cells in the G0 phase of the cell cycle. Antibodies to either Ki-67 or MIB-1 may be used interchangeably depending on the form of tissue preparation. Ki-67 and MIB-1 labelling indices correlate with cancer [46]. However, in prostate cancer, a high proliferation index for either antibody appears to add little predictive information for patient outcome above the traditional indicators of Gleason score, pathological stage and DNA ploidy [47]. Nevertheless, the Ki-67 labelling index may discriminate between organ-confined and metastatic cancer [41]. Hence, elevation in the proliferation indices of Ki-67/MIB-1 appears to reflect progression. This is further reflected in an association between expression of Ki-67 and the epidermal growth factor receptor, mutant p53, particular chromosomal aberrations and perineural invasion. Taken together, all of these findings suggest that Ki-67 expression may be a weak prognostic indicator of recurrence, progression and survival.

Apoptosis and apoptotic bodies

Apoptosis is a genetically programmed active mode of cell death which involves activation of multiple signalling pathways. It is widely believed that apoptosis is an effective, intrinsic anti-cancer mechanism, through which tissues discard transformed cells. Thus, suppression of apoptosis, specifically development of resistance to inductive signals, may favour accumulation of initiated cells and contribute to the establishment of early neoplastic lesions. Furthermore, as neoplasm develops, it often exhibits additional phenotypes of apoptotic deregulation. An imbalance in rates of cell proliferation and death contributes to clonal expansion and augments net cancer growth rate. Acquisition of independence of tissue-specific survival factors and/or apoptotic regulators allows metastatic cancer cells to survive and grow at sites distinct from their tissue of origin.

Apoptotic bodies are present throughout all normal prostatic ductular and acinar epithelium. They are usually present in intercellular spaces and occasionally within the cytoplasm of epithelial cells, the latter being observed more often in PIN and carcinoma than in benign epithelium. In non-neoplastic prostatic tissues the greatest frequency is invariably in the basal cell layer. In carcinoma the apoptotic process occurs in cells at the periphery of the malignant glands adjacent to the stroma. These trends are virtually identical to those seen with PCNA immunoreactivity. The percentage of apoptotic bodies has been estimated to be progressively higher in low-grade PIN, high-grade PIN and adenocarcinoma than in benign prostate hyperplasia (0.68%, 0.75% and 0.92–2.10% vs. 0.26%, respectively), but with no apparent correlation between the numbers of mitotic figures and apoptotic bodies.

Derangement of apoptosis appears to play a critical role in the pathogenesis of prostate cancer [48,49]. There is downregulation of apoptotic rates and upregulation of proliferative indices in localized prostatic cancer when compared with adjacent normal tissues [50]. In localized cancer, expression of bcl-2, an intracellular antagonist of apoptosis, was markedly elevated, suggesting that inhibition of apoptosis may be an early event in transformation. Conversely, metastatic prostate cancer exhibited significantly higher levels of bcl-2 with concomitant marked elevation of proliferative index than in primary cancer. Cell proliferation rates were higher than apoptotic rates, resulting in a net gain in cell number in localized and metastatic carcinoma. The apoptotic rate of an individual prostatic carcinoma provided more accurate prognostic information than the proliferation rate. There was a significant elevation in apoptotic count in high-grade cancer and those with aggressive progression profiles [48,51]. Cancer with perineural invasion has a lower apoptotic rate than that without invasion, perhaps accounting for the frequent tumour spread through perineural spaces. The molecular mechanisms underlying lower apoptotic rate in carcinomas with perineural invasion appeared to be due not to overexpression of bcl-2 [52] but to an unidentified nerve-derived factor(s), since the apoptotic rates were negatively correlated with the diameter of the nerves. This finding suggests that the microenvironment influences apoptotic activity, and hence the growth potential of carcinomas, which in turn controls tumour progression and metastasis. Androgen deprivation therapy increased the apoptotic rate in prostate cancer [53].

Microvessel density

Microvessel density analysis offers promise for predicting pathological stage and patient outcome in prostate cancer. The microvessels associated with prostate cancer are shorter than those in benign or hyperplastic prostatic tissue, with more undulating vessel walls [54]. The cumulative evidence suggests that there is an important role for microvessel density analysis in management of selected patients with prostate cancer.

Microvessel density and prediction of pathological stage

At least 12 different studies have investigated the relationship of microvessel density (MVD) and cancer stage [34,55,56]. Most compared MVD in prostatectomy specimens with pathological stage, probably because of the ease of evaluation and abundance of available tissue. Two assessed MVD in contemporary needle biopsies and correlated it with pathological stage at prostatectomy [55]. Two others compared MVD in transurethral resections from patients undergoing irradiation or predominantly watchful waiting with clinical stage; however, clinical stage is prone to serious staging error when compared with pathological stage, so these findings should be interpreted with caution.

Most of the prostatectomy studies found a positive correlation of MVD with pathological stage. In one study, the important difference in MVD between stage pT2 and pT3 was observed only among low-grade cancer, although this finding was not substantiated in a subsequent report. Silberman *et al.* [56] found no correlation between MVD and stage, but limited study to only patients with Gleason scores 6 and 7; then, surprisingly, the authors combined this cohort with another that had different selection criteria.

MVD in cancer on biopsy showed a positive correlation with matched prostatectomies, and was an independent predictor of extraprostatic extension [55]. When optimized MVD was added to the Gleason score and serum PSA concentration, the predictive value of these measures for stage increased significantly. Microvascular invasion also correlated with stage, grade, and other parameters. Microvessel density greater than 90, when analysed as a dichotomous variable, shows a trend to be related to a higher proliferative index as determined by immunohistochemistry (MIB-1). Although the MVD increases with higher tumour grade and stage, the that surrounding benign prostatic glands and PIN in the same section does not increase. The bulk of evidence favours the relationship of MVD and cancer stage, although variance exists between methods and patient cohorts.

Microvessel density and prediction of cancer recurrence and survival

There is generally good agreement about prediction of cancer recurrence based on MVD [57]. In studies in which patients were treated by surgery or external beam radiation therapy, MVD and microvascular invasion predicted biochemical (PSA) failure. However, in patients treated with radiation therapy, MVD was not analysed independently of grade. When most patients were treated only with palliative hormonal manipulation, MVD did not predict progression independent of grade. MVD did not correlate with biochemical failure after controlling for stage (pT2) and grade (Gleason grade

6 and higher) in patients treated by radical prostatectomy. Other studies which have addressed the potential of MVD or microvascular invasion to predict cancer-specific survival have found no independent predictive value. The predictive value on univariate analysis was negated by inclusion of grade or stage.

Vascular endothelial growth factors and receptors

Vascular endothelial growth factor (VEGF) promotes angiogenesis in a wide

Table 9.5 Consensus features (WHO) of reporting prostatic adenocarcinoma

---

Category 1
Factors established to be of demonstrable predictive value on evidence collected from multiple studies over a long period of time, and which should be considered essential in making clinical decisions
　　Clinical stage
　　Serum PSA
　　Gleason score and WHO nuclear grade
　　Pathological stage
　　Surgical margins
　　Pathological effects of treatment
　　Location of the cancer

Category 2
Factors which show promise as predictive factors based upon evidence from multiple published studies but which require further evaluation before recommendation or are recommended despite incomplete data as diagnostic or prognostic markers
　　Volume of cancer in needle biopsy specimens (recommended)
　　Volume of cancer in radical prostatectomy specimens (recommended)
　　Histological subtype of cancer
　　DNA ploidy

Category 3
Factors which have some scientific evidence to support their adoption as diagnostic or prognostic agents but are not currently recommended
　　Prostate-specific membrane antigen
　　Other serum tests (PSM, hK2, etc.)
　　Perineural invasion
　　Vascular/lymphatic invasion
　　Microvessel density (shows promise, but insufficient data)
　　Stromal factors, including TGF-β, integrins, etc.
　　Proliferation markers and apoptosis
　　Nuclear morphometry and karyometric analysis
　　Androgen receptors
　　Neuroendocrine markers
　　Genetic markers (show promise, but insufficient data)
　　All other factors which do not appear in Categories 1 or 2

---

variety of normal and neoplastic tissues. *In vivo*, studies have reported a complete lack of VEGF in benign prostate hyperplasia (BPH) and epithelial cells or, conversely, two isoforms (VEGF$_{165}$, VEGF$_{189}$) of the protein in stromal cells of BPH [58]. Numerous studies have described VEGF expression in organ-confined cancer, in cancer cell lines derived from metastases and in xenografts of prostate cancer [59]. Exogenous VEGF appears to promote the growth of xenograft tumours [60], and androgen deprivation inhibits VEGF expression. Taken together, these observations suggest that cancer cells express VEGF for angiogenesis of developing cancer, thereby circumventing oxygen diffusion as a rate limiting step in the growth of prostate cancer.

Conclusion

Histopathological assessment of prostate tissues taken at transrectal biopsy, transurethral resection or during a radical surgical procedure is the cornerstone of prostate cancer diagnosis. Despite publication of powerful new data with respect to prostate proteomics and genomics, detailed morphology remains the 'gold standard' of tissue analysis with respect to cancer diagnosis and prognosis. Fundamental to morphology is standardization of approach, without which surgical pathologists, urologists and the patients they serve all remain in isolation. Consensus agreement on those morphological features which define malignant neoplasia (Table 9.5) is not only an essential foundation for predicting individual patient prognosis, but also provides a powerful body of experience from which to gain further understanding of the biology of prostate cancer. This chapter has summarized the salient components of that consensus, as currently accepted. It is likely that many of the powerful analytical techniques currently under development will become deployed to assist the assessment of prostate cancer tissues and to accurately predict individual cancer behaviour or response to therapy. Surprisingly, although they are biologically fascinating, no such techniques have been shown to be as powerful, as effective or as reliable as experienced and skilled assessment of the histomorphological criteria outlined in this chapter.

References

1   Foster CS, Bostwick DG. Grading prostate cancer. In: Deshmukh N, Foster CS, eds. *Pathology of the Prostate*. London: WB Saunders, 1998: 191–227.
2   Cintra ML, Billis A. Histologic grading of prostatic adenocarcinoma: intraobserver reproducibility of the Mostofi, Gleason and Bocking grading systems. *Int Urol Nephrol* 1991; **23**: 449–54.
3   Di-Loreto C, Fitzpatrick B, Underhill S *et al*. Correlation between visual clues, objective architectural features and interobserver agreement in prostate cancer. *Am J Clin Pathol* 1991; **96**: 70–5.

4   Thickman D, Speers WC, Philpott PJ, Shapiro H. Effect of the number of core biopsies of the prostate on predicting Gleason score of prostate cancer. *J Urol* 1996; **156**: 110–14.

5   Cookson MS, Fleshner NE, Soloway SM, Fair WR. Correlation between Gleason score of needle biopsy and radical prostatectomy specimen: accuracy and clinical implications. *J Urol* 1997; **157**: 559–62.

6   Steinberg DM, Sauvageot J, Piantadosi S, Epstein JI. Correlation of prostate needle biopsy and radical prostatectomy Gleason grade in academic and community settings. *Am J Surg Pathol* 1997; **21**: 566–76.

7   Gleason DF. Histologic grading of prostate cancer: a perspective. *Human Pathol* 1992; **23**: 273–9.

8   Bostwick DG, Myers RP, Oesterling JE. Staging of prostate cancer. *Semin Surg Oncol* 1994; **10**: 60–73.

9   Allsbrook WCJ, Mangold KA, Yang X, Epstein JI. The Gleason grading system. *J Urol Pathol* 1999; **10**: 141–57.

10 Mostofi FK, Sesterhenn IA, Sobin LH. *WHO International Histological Classification of Prostate Tumours*. Geneva: WHO, 1980.

11 Schroeder FH, Hop WC, Bloom JH, Mostofi FK. Grading of prostate carcinoma: multivariant analysis of prognostic parameters. *Prostate* 1985; **7**: 13–20.

12 Brawer MK, Peehl DM, Stamey TA, Bostwick DG. Keratin immunoreactivity in the benign and neoplastic human prostate. *Cancer Res* 1985; **45**: 3663–7.

13 McIntire TL, Franzina DA. The presence of benign prostate glands in perineural spaces. *J Urol* 1986; **135**: 507–9.

14 Ro JY, Ayala AG, Ordonez NG, Cartwright JJ, Mackay B. Intraluminal crystalloids in prostatic adenocarcinoma: immunohistochemical, electron microscopic, and X-ray microanalytic studies. *Cancer* 1986; **57**: 2397–407.

15 Ahlering TE, Lieskovsky G, Skinner DG. Salvage surgery plus androgen deprivation for radioresistant prostatic adenocarcinoma. *J Urol* 1992; **147**: 900–2.

16 Wheeler JA, Zagars GK, Ayala AG. Dedifferentiation of locally recurrent prostate cancer after radiation therapy. *Cancer* 1993; **71**: 3783–7.

17 Schenken JR, Burns EL, Kahle PJ. The effect of diethylstilboestrol dipropionate on carcinoma of the prostate gland. II. Cytologic changes following treatment. *J Urol* 1942; **48**: 99–112.

18 Murphy WM, Soloway MS, Barrows GH. Pathological changes associated with androgen deprivation therapy for prostate cancer. *Cancer* 1991; **68**: 821–8.

19 Stamey TA, Freiha FS, McNeal JE, Redwine EA, Whittemore AS, Schmid HP. Localized prostate cancer: relationship of tumor volume to clinical significance for treatment of prostate cancer. *Cancer* 1993; **71**: 933–8.

20 Cupp MR, Bostwick DG, Myers RP, Oesterling JE. The volume of prostate cancer in the biopsy specimen cannot reliably predict the quantity of cancer in the radical prostatectomy specific antigen on an individual basis. *J Urol* 1995; **153**: 1543–8.

21 Bostwick DG, Graham SDJ, Napalkov P *et al*. Staging of early prostate cancer: a proposed tumor volume-based prognostic index. *Urology* 1993; **41**: 403–11.

22 Blackwell KL, Bostwick DG, Myers RP, Zincke H, Oesterling JE. Combining prostate specific antigen with cancer and gland volume to predict more reliably pathological stage: the influence of prostate specific antigen cancer density. *J Urol* 1994; **151**: 1565–70.

23 Sakr W, Wheeler TM, Blute M *et al*. Staging and reporting of prostate cancer: sampling of the radical prostatectomy specimen. *Cancer* 1996; **78**: 366–8.

24 Ohori M, Wheeler TM, Kattan MW, Goto Y, Scardino PT. Prognostic significance of positive surgical margins in radical prostatectomy specimens. *J Urol* 1995; **154**: 1818–24.

25 Stamey TA, Villers AA, McNeal JE, Link PC, Freiha FS. Positive surgical margins at radical prostatectomy: importance of the apical dissection. *J Urol* 1990; **143**: 1166–73.

26 Voges GE, McNeal JE, Redwine EA, Freiha FS, Stamey TA. Morphological analysis of surgical margins with positive findings in prostatectomy for adenocarcinoma of the prostate. *Cancer* 1992; **69**: 520–6.

27 Montie JE. Significance and treatment of positive margins or seminal vesicle invasion after radical prostatectomy. *Urol Clin North Am* 1990; **17**: 803–11.

28 Schroder FH, Hermanek P, Denis L, Fair WR, Gospodarowicz MK, Pavone-Macaluso M. The TNM classification of prostate carcinoma. *Prostate* 1992; **4**: 129–38.

29 British Association of Urological Surgeons TNM Sub-Committee. The TNM classification of prostate cancer: a discussion of the 1992 classification. *Br J Urol* 1995; **76**: 279–85.

30 Henson DE, Hutter RVP, Farrow GM. Practice protocol for the examination of specimens removed from patients with carcinoma of the prostate gland. *Arch Pathol Lab Med* 1994; **118**: 779–83.

31 Rifkin MD, Zerhouni EA, Garsonis CA *et al*. Comparison of magnetic resonance imaging and ultrasonography in staging early prostate cancer: results of a multi-institutional cooperative trial. *N Engl J Med* 1990; **323**: 621–7.

32 Labrie F, Dupont A, Suburu R *et al*. Serum prostate-specific antigen as pre-screening test for prostate cancer. *J Urol* 1992; **147**: 846–51.

33 Bostwick DG, Foster CS, Algaba F *et al*. Prostate tissue factors. In: Murphy G, Khoury S, Partin A, Denis L, eds. *Second International Consultation on Prostate Cancer*. Health Publications Ltd, 1999: 161–201.

34 Egan AJM, Bostwick DG. Prediction of extraprostatic extension of prostate cancer based on needle biopsy findings: perineural invasion lacks independent significance. *Lab Invest* 1997; **76**: 421.

35 Salamao DR, Graham SD, Bostwick DG. Microvascular invasion in prostate cancer correlates with pathological stage. *Arch Pathol Lab Med* 1995; **119**: 1050–4.

36 Hutter RVP, Montie JE, Busch C *et al*. Current prognostic factors and their relevance to staging. *Cancer* 1996; **78**: 369–71.

37 Blom JH, Ten Kate FJ, Schroeder FH, van der Heul RO. Morphometrically estimated variation in nuclear size: a useful tool in grading prostatic cancer. *Urol Res* 1990; **18**: 93–9.

38 Montironi R, Scarpelli M, Sisti S *et al*. Quantitative analysis of prostatic intraepithelial neoplasia on tissue sections. *Ann Quant Cytol Histol* 1990; **12**: 366–72.

39 Sesterhenn IA, Becker RL, Avallone FA, Mostofi FK, Lin TE, Davis CJ. Image analysis of nucleoli and nucleolar organizer regions in prostatic hyperplasia, intraepithelial neoplasia, and prostatic carcinoma. *J Urogen Pathol* 1991; **1**: 61–74.

40 Helpap B, Riede C. Nucleolar and AgNOR-analysis of prostatic intraepithelial neoplasia (PIN), atypical adenomatous hyperplasia (AAH) and prostatic carcinoma. *Pathol Res Pract* 1995; **191**: 381–90.

41 Cher ML, Chew K, Rosenau W, Carroll PR. Cellular proliferation in prostatic adenocarcinoma as assessed by bromodeoxyuridine uptake and Ki-67 and PCNA expression. *Prostate* 1995; **26**: 87–93.

42 Vesalainen S, Lipponen P, Talja M, Syrjanen K. Mitotic activity and prognosis in prostatic adenocarcinoma. *Prostate* 1995; **26**: 80–6.

43 Lipponen P, Vesalainen S, Kasurinen J, Alpa-Opas M, Syrjanen K. A prognostic score for prostatic adenocarcinoma based on clinical, histological, biochemical and cytometric data from the primary tumor. *Anticancer Res* 1996; **16**: 2095–100.

44 Kyprianou N, Isaacs J. Expression of transforming growth factor b in the rat ventral prostate during castration-induced programmed cell death. *Mol Endocrinol* 1989; **3**: 1515–22.

45 Limas C, Frizelle SP. Proliferative activity in benign and neoplastic prostatic epithelium. *J Pathol* 1994; **174**: 201–8.

46 Brown C, Sauvageot J, Kahane H, Epstein JI. Cell proliferation and apoptosis in prostate cancer – correlation with pathological stage? *Modern Pathol* 1996; **9**: 205–9.

47 Coetzee LJ, Layfield LJ, Hars V, Paulson DF. Proliferative index determination in prostatic carcinoma tissue: is there any additional prognostic value greater than that of Gleason score, ploidy and pathological stage? *J Urol* 1997; **157**: 214–18.

48 Foster CS. Prostatic cancer – a consensus. In: Waxman J., Williams G., eds. *Urological Oncology*. London: Edward Arnold, 1991: 67–91.

49 Colombel M, Symmans G, Gil S *et al*. Detection of the apoptosis-suppressing oncoprotein bcl-2 in hormone-refractory human prostate cancer. *Am J Pathol* 1993; **143**: 390–400.

50 Tu H, Jacobs SC, Borkowski A, Kyprianou N. Incidence of apoptosis and cell proliferation in prostate cancer: relationship with TGF-beta-1 and bcl-2 expression. *Int J Cancer* 1996; **69**: 357–63.

51 Kyprianou N, Tu H, Jacobs SC. Apoptotic versus proliferative activities in human benign prostatic hyperplasia. *Human Pathol* 1996; **27**: 668–75.

52 Korsmeyer SJ. Bcl-2: an antidote to programmed cell death. *Cancer Surv* 1992; **15**: 105–18.

53 Aihara M, Scardino PT, Truong LD *et al*. The frequency of apoptosis correlates with the prognosis of Gleason Grade 3 adenocarcinoma of the prostate. *Cancer* 1995; **75**: 522–9.

54 Siegal JA, Yu E, Brawer MK. Topography of neovascularity in human prostatic carcinoma. *Cancer* 1995; **75**: 2545–51.

55 Bostwick DG, Wheeler TM, Blute M *et al*. Optimized microvessel density analysis improves prediction of cancer stage from prostate needle biopsies. *Urology* 1996; **48**: 47–57.

56 Silberman MA, Partin AW, Veltri RW, Epstein JI. Tumor angiogenesis correlates with progression after radial prostatectomy but not with pathological stage in Gleason sum 5–7 adenocarcinoma of the prostate. *Cancer* 1997; **79**: 772–9.

57 Gettman MT, Bergstralh EJ, Blute M, Zincke H, Bostwick DG. Prediction of patient outcome in pathological stage T2 adenocarcinoma of the prostate: lack of significance for microvessel density analysis. *Urology* 1998; **51**: 79–85.

58 Jackson MW, Bentel JM, Tilley WD. Vascular endothelial growth factor (VEGF) expression in prostate cancer and benign prostatic hyperplasia. *J Urol* 1997; **157**: 2323–38.

59 Joseph IBJK, Isaacs JT. Potentiation of the antiangiogenic ability of linomide by androgen ablation involves down-regulation of vascular endothelial growth factor in human androgen-responsive prostatic cancers. *Cancer Res* 1997; **57**: 104–57.

60 Gridley DS, Andres ML, Slater JM. Enhancement of prostate cancer xenograft growth with whole-body radiation and vascular endothelial growth factor. *Anticancer Res* 1997; **17**: 923–8.

10: Prostate Radiotherapy

C. R. Lewanski & S. Stewart

Introduction

Treatment of prostate cancer with radiation was first attempted early in the twentieth century [1,2]. External beam radiotherapy was not established as a definitive treatment until the 1950s, following the lead of Bagshaw at Stanford University, where the treatment of patients with localized prostate cancer using linear accelerator beams was initiated in 1956 [3]. However, radiotherapeutic resources were limited and these early patients were treated using relatively simple techniques. Furthermore, most of these early patients were treated before the introduction of prostate-specific antigen (PSA) assays and modern staging techniques, thus inevitably leading to flaws in patient selection. The arrival of modern megavoltage equipment led to a rapid increase in the use of external beam irradiation, offering, at last, a serious therapeutic alternative to radical prostatectomy. Nevertheless, despite advances in the diagnosis, staging and treatment of localized prostate cancer, the optimal management of patients with localized prostate cancer remains unresolved, largely as a result of the fact that no large, well designed randomized clinical trial with long-term follow-up comparing surgery with radiotherapy has ever been completed. Indeed, the recent failure of the Medical Research Council's PR06 trial (a randomized trial comparing prostatectomy, radiotherapy and surveillance) to accrue patients has reiterated the difficulty in addressing this issue today. Thus, the choice of treatment for any one patient cannot be made on the basis of definitive evidence for the superiority of any one modality of treatment over another. Hence additional factors such as treatment morbidity and patient preference have gained in importance.

Comparison of external beam radiotherapy and radical prostatectomy

Radiotherapy is the most commonly used therapeutic modality in the UK for the radical treatment of prostate cancer. Retrospective comparison of the many series of patients treated with either surgery or radiation is difficult because of differences in patient selection. The surgical patients are frequently younger, suffer from fewer co-morbidities and undergo pathological pelvic lymph node staging as compared to patients offered radiotherapy. Furthermore, surgical series often select only well or moderately differentiated tumours, whereas radiation series do not exclude poorly differentiated ones.

Finally, the size of tumours within a stage reflects generally smaller tumours in surgical series. The only randomized trial comparing radical prostatectomy with radiotherapy recorded a higher rate of progression-free survival at 5 years in the surgical arm [4]. However, this trial was strongly criticized since some patients did not receive the treatment to which they were randomly assigned and the results in the radiotherapy arm were worse than those reported in other series at the time. The National Cancer Institute and the Office of Medical Application of Research convened a Consensus Development Conference in 1987 on the management of localized prostate cancer and concluded that the 10-year survival rates with radical prostatectomy and radiation therapy were similar [5].

Treatment results with external beam radiotherapy

The 5-year disease-free survival (DFS) rates with external beam radiotherapy (EBRT) are 95–100% for stage T1a, 80–90% for stages T1b and c, and 50–70% for stage T2. The corresponding 10-year DFS rates are 95%, 65–80% and 40–50%, respectively [6] (see Table 10.1a). It is difficult, however, to compare data in studies involving patients recruited before the advent of the PSA era. Pretreatment PSA levels have consistently been shown to be the most significant independent predictor of biochemical failure, with Gleason score and tumour stage also associated with biochemical control in multivariate analysis [7] (see Table 10.2). Nevertheless, even when patients are stratified by pretreatment PSA, marked variations in biochemical cure exist between various series. This can be explained at least in part by differences in definition of biochemical control following EBRT. Fortunately, the American Society for Therapeutic Radiology and Oncology (ASTRO) recently convened a panel of prostate cancer experts and established a standard definition of biochemical failure after EBRT, namely as three consecutive rises in posttreatment PSA after achieving a nadir, with failure recorded as the time midway between the nadir and the first rising PSA [8].

What is clear from the data amassed to date is that long-term survival rates for patients with T1 and T2 stage tumours treated by EBRT are close to that of an age-matched population cohort and for T1 and T2a tumours are essentially equal. Survival is less good for patients with T3 stage tumours (Table 10.1b) and poor for T4 tumours after EBRT alone. It would appear that other additional therapeutic modalities are required for these patients.

The importance of patient selection, in particular with respect to pretreatment PSA levels, is underscored by the observation that biochemical DFS at 4 years following EBRT is 65% in stage T1 and T2 patients if the pretreatment PSA is <15 ng/mL and only 7% if it is >15 ng/mL. Similarly, for T3 and T4 tumours the corresponding figures are 39% and 0% [9]. Thus a pretreatment PSA level >15 ng/mL is a powerful predictor of probable failure with conventional EBRT.

Table 10.1 Survival data for (a) stages T1 and T2 and (b) stage T3 carcinoma of the prostate with external beam radiotherapy

(a)

Reference	No. of patients		Overall survival (disease-free) (%)		
	T1	T2	5 years	10 years	15 years
26	308		85 (90)	65 (70)	40 (65)
		218	83 (87)	55 (65)	35 (50)
27	313		77 (87)	63 (86)	
28	48		85 (78)	70 (60)	
		252	82 (86)	65 (56)	
29	151		98	93	75
		346	94	68	41

(b)

Author and year	No. of patients	Overall survival (disease-free) (%)		
	T3	5 years	10 years	15 years
30	385	68 (70)	38 (50)	20 (35)
31	372	66 (77)	38 (63)	17 (50)
28	412	65 (58)	42 (38)	
32	551	72 (59)	47 (46)	27 (40)

Table 10.2 Rates of biochemical control (%) stratified by pretreatment PSA for external beam radiotherapy

Study centre and year	PSA level (ng/mL)			
	<4	4–10	10–20	>20
MD Anderson 1995 [33]	90	70	62	38
Massachusetts General Hospital 1994 [9]	82	44	30	8
University of Michigan 1995 [34]	90	85	56	20

Radiation therapy techniques

The margins of the target volume are chosen on the basis of the tumour extent palpable rectally and visualized on CT scanning. Prior to the advent of CT planning, prostate localization was achieved by means of a cystogram, with 10 mL of contrast introduced into the catheter balloon, which was then pulled down on to the bladder base. AP and lateral films were taken with barium in the rectum. The target volume was then reconstructed on to a transverse outline taken through the centre of the volume. As a rule, the anterior margin of the target volume passes through the mid-pubic symphysis and the posterior margin encompasses the anterior third of the rectum. Patients are treated daily in the supine position with a full bladder to remove small bowel and the bladder dome from the intended target volume. Three or four field arrangements are often utilized using at least 6 MV photons (Fig. 10.1). Day to day reproducibility of treatment is critical if a homogeneous dose is to be delivered to the target volume. Patient movement can be reduced by using ankle stocks or soft immobilization devices supporting the lower legs. More recently the

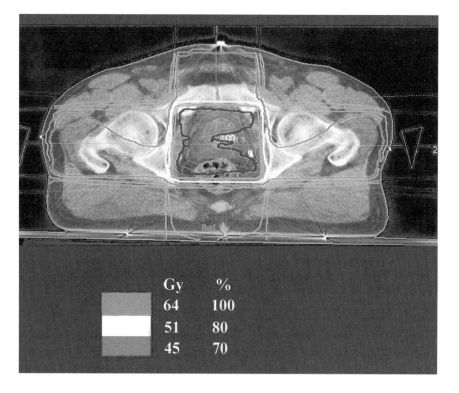

Gy	%
64	100
51	80
45	70

Figure 10.1 CT planning scan illustrating irradiation of the prostate gland with three 10 MV photon fields. (Shown in colour, Plate 6, facing p. 178.)

wider use of CT planning systems has permitted more accurate localization of the prostate, seminal vesicles and critical adjacent organs such as rectum and bladder.

The logical extension of accurate localization of the prostate by CT scanning is to use three-dimensional computer reconstruction of the prostate and seminal vesicles by integrating the treatment planning CT scan with a three-dimensional planning computer. One can then achieve a beam configuration for the prostate that conforms precisely to the shape of the organ at each individual CT slice, rather than forcing all prostates to fit into rectangular boxes. In 1987, the University of Michigan became the first US centre to treat patients with so-called three-dimensional conformal radiotherapy (3DCRT). Three key hypotheses underpin the rationale for 3DCRT. First, that more accurate prostate targeting could improve local control without the need to increase radiation dose. Second, a decrease in acute and late toxicities could be achievable from a reduction in the volume of normal tissue irradiated. Third, if the second hypothesis held true, then 3DCRT would allow dose escalation and potentially higher local control rates.

It is important, however, to ensure an adequate margin around the prostate during planning to take account of both patient movement between fractions and organ movement resulting from respiratory, bladder and bowel movement. One study observed movement of the prostate to be 1–5 mm in lateral directions, 5 mm on average in the craniocaudal axis and 5–7 mm in the antero-posterior direction [10]. Seminal vesicle motion may be even greater (10–20 mm), reflecting filling of the bladder and rectum. Thus, gross tumour volume (GTV) is grown by a margin of 5–10 mm to encompass sites of microscopic spread (to create a clinical target volume or CTV) and by a further 5–10 mm to allow for organ and patient movement (to create a planning target volume or PTV) (see Fig. 10.2).

The target volume

Should pelvic lymph nodes be routinely irradiated?

Few randomized studies have been designed to address this issue. The observation that patients die from distant metastases rather than pelvic node relapse, coupled with the fact that few patients with pelvic lymph node metastases can be cured of their disease, has limited interest in this area. Indeed there is a feeling that nearly all node positive patients with cancer of the prostate will develop distant metastatic disease if followed for sufficiently long periods of time. An early prospective randomized trial of extended field irradiation for prostate cancer giving 55 Gy to the whole pelvis had to be modified as a result of excessive small bowel toxicity [11]. This exemplifies the difficulty in

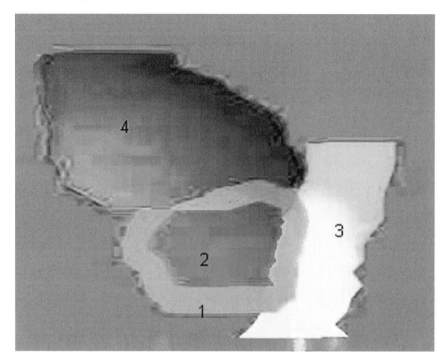

Figure 10.2 Three-dimensional computer reconstruction of conformal prostate radiotherapy showing (1) planning target volume, (2) clinical target volume, (3) rectum and (4) bladder. (Shown in colour, Plate 7, facing p. 178.)

administering sufficiently high doses of radiation in the pelvis to eradicate disease without incurring acute and late normal tissue toxicity. A more recent Radiation Therapy Oncology Group (RTOG) study randomized patients after negative surgical staging or lymphangiography to receive either 65 Gy to the prostate and paraprostatic tissues or 45 Gy to the whole pelvis and a 20 Gy boost to the prostate itself. In 445 evaluable patients, there was no significant difference in terms of local control, metastases or overall survival after a median follow-up of 7 years [12]. Although some non-randomized reports do show an advantage to pelvic nodal irradiation [13], until prospective randomized studies can demonstrate a proven efficacy to this, its use cannot be routinely recommended.

Indications for seminal vesicle irradiation

Several authors have attempted to define subgroups of patients in whom irradiation of the seminal vesicles could be avoided. The seminal vesicles are located high in the pelvis and posterior to the bladder, thus their exclusion can significantly reduce the volumes of rectum and bladder irradiated (44% and 9% respectively). Patients with pretreatment PSA levels of 0–4, 4–10 and

>10 ng/mL have seminal vesicle involvement rates of 3%, 8% and 33%, respectively [14]. The authors propose excluding the seminal vesicles in all patients with PSA levels of less than 4 ng/mL and in patients with PSA levels of 4–10 ng/mL and a Gleason score of 6 or less. A nonogram currently in use in the Medical Research Council (MRC) RT01 study suggests irradiation of the seminal vesicles if the patient has clinical stage T2b or T3a disease (high risk) or stage T1b/c or T2a disease with [PSA + (Gleason score – 6) × 10] >15 (moderate risk).

Radiation dose

Conventional EBRT doses deliver to the prostate 64 Gy in 32 fractions treating weekdays over 6.5 weeks. The observation that local recurrence within the radiation field occurs in up to 20% of T1b, 24% of T2 and 40% of T3 tumours within 10 years of treatment has confirmed suspicions that current radiation doses are inadequate, especially in larger tumours. Data from the Patterns of Care Study Outcome Survey in the US showed that 7-year actuarial local control rates for T3 tumours increased from 64% to 76% when the tumour dose increased from 60–65 Gy to >70 Gy [15]. However, the survey also demonstrated significantly increased complication rates with conventional treatment techniques when doses >70 Gy were used. The advent of 3DCRT has offered a renewed opportunity to perform dose escalation studies [16,17]. The Memorial Sloan–Kettering Cancer Center increased the tumour target dose from 64.8 Gy to 81 Gy in increments of 5.4 Gy.

Using the achievement of a PSA nadir of <1 ng/mL, after a median follow-up of 3 years, a clear dose-dependent response rate was observed. Ninety per cent of patients receiving 75.6 Gy or 81 Gy responded, compared with 76% receiving 70.2 Gy and 56% receiving 64.8 Gy. Severe toxicity rates were comparable with the lower doses of conventional EBRT [16]. Similarly, the Fox Chase Cancer Center observed improved biochemical control rates at 3 years for patients with pretreatment PSA levels >10 ng/mL when doses were escalated from 70 Gy stepwise to 80 Gy. No improvement in outcome was seen when the pretreatment PSA was <10 ng/mL [17]. The current MRC RT01 trial randomizes T1b–T3a N0 M0 patients with PSA levels <50 ng/mL to either standard dose (64 Gy/32 fractions) conformal EBRT or higher dose (74 Gy/37 fractions) irradiation.

Radiation morbidity

Radiation side-effects can be defined as acute or late. Late side-effects, defined as those that develop or persist more than 3 months after completion of treatment, are generally more dose limiting, since they are usually irreversible and may progress in severity. The development of such sequelae depends largely on the volume of normal tissue irradiated and the dose to which these tissues are subject. Acute side-effects of prostate radiotherapy include gastrointestinal symptoms such as diarrhoea, tenesmus and rectal bleeding resulting from a radiation proctitis, and genito-urinary symptoms such as dysuria, frequency and nocturia, coupled with a higher incidence of urinary tract infections from a radiation cystitis. Erythema and dry or moist skin desquamation may develop in the perineum. One or more of these features will develop in most patients undergoing prostate radiotherapy.

The overall incidence of late urinary or recto-sigmoid sequelae is approximately 3–5% for severe sequelae and 7–10% for moderate ones [18]. Urethral strictures, which are more common in patients irradiated after a transurethral resection of the prostate (TURP), bladder fistulas, haemorrhagic cystitis and stress incontinence as well as chronic proctitis presenting as rectal bleeding or diarrhoea are the major late toxicities. As expected, late toxicities increase with radiation dose; Hanks [19] showed the major complication rate to be 3.5% with doses <70 Gy and 7% with doses >70 Gy. Impotence is observed in 40–60% of patients after EBRT and is judged to be secondary to a radiation-induced endarteritis of the internal pudendal and penile arteries, which run lateral to the prostate. Conclusive proof that 3DCRT reduced late sequelae, in particular the chronic proctitis, compared with conventional EBRT came from a randomized study of 225 patients irradiated to a dose of 64 Gy [20]. It is now an accepted aim of radical radiotherapy to the prostate that it be accompanied by an incidence of severe late normal tissue damage of no more than 5% at 2 years [21].

Neoadjuvant and adjuvant hormones with radiation therapy

The poor results observed with T2b–T4 tumours and standard radiation treatment have stimulated interest in novel strategies in an attempt to improve treatment outcomes. One such strategy has involved combining androgen blockade prior to radiation therapy. Advantages of such an approach centre on down-sizing the prostatic tumour prior to irradiation, thus potentially reducing acute and long-term sequelae of treatment. Theoretically, this tumour shrinkage should result in improved blood flow with a concomitant decrease in tumour cell hypoxia, thereby increasing radiosensitivity. Additionally, the number of tumour clones that need to be eradicated may be reduced by androgen ablation. A total of six prospective randomized trials have been completed comparing radiotherapy alone or in combination with some form of hormonal manipulation. All six studies have shown improvements in some measure of local/regional control or DFS, but only two studies have shown an improvement in overall survival [22].

Two studies have compared the use of neoadjuvant hormone therapy and radiation with radiation alone. The RTOG study by Pilepich *et al.* [23] randomized 471 patients with bulky T2b–T4 tumours to receive either EBRT alone or total androgen blockade with goserelin and flutamide for 2 months before and during radiotherapy. With a median follow-up of 4.5 years, progression-free survival and local control rates were significantly improved in patients receiving the combined modality. No improvement in overall survival was noted. Laverdiere *et al.* [24] randomized 120 patients with T2b–T3 tumours to either radiotherapy alone or radiotherapy with 3 months of prior total androgen blockade, the hormonal therapy being continued during irradiation and for 6 months after completion. The prostate was biopsied 2 years later, revealing a positive biopsy rate of 68.8% in those treated with radiotherapy alone compared with only 5.6% in those treated with combination therapy. Whether this will translate into a meaningful benefit for the patient is as yet unknown. One large adjuvant hormonal study randomized 415 patients with T1–T4 tumours to either radiotherapy alone or radiotherapy and adjuvant goserelin commencing on the first day of radiotherapy and continued for 3 years. With a median follow-up of almost 4 years, overall survival in the combined group significantly exceeded that of the radiotherapy only group (79% vs. 62%, $P = 0.001$) [25].

The results from these studies are clearly encouraging, but a major criticism of them has been that they do not include a treatment arm of hormonal therapy alone. This is currently being addressed in a National Cancer Institute of Canada Clinical Trials Group/Canadian Uro-Oncology Group study. Furthermore, the optimal timing and duration of hormonal therapy has yet to be resolved, since none of the prospective studies have used consistent androgen deprivation schedules.

Prostate brachytherapy

Prostate brachytherapy is a form of radiation treatment where radioactive sources are directly implanted into the gland either temporarily or permanently. It offers the potential to deliver doses to the prostate some 2–3 times higher than conventional external beam radiation, with relative sparing of surrounding normal tissues by virtue of the short range of this type of radiation.

Early brachytherapy using radium inserted via a urethral catheter unfortunately exhibited high serious complication rates of 15–20% [2], which ultimately led to a decline in its use. The technique was superseded by the development of surgical techniques and subsequently megavoltage external beam irradiation. Some interest was restored after the publication in 1972 of a technique for retropubic implantation of iodine-125 (^{125}I) radionuclides [33]. However, the procedure required the freehand placement of iodine seeds with surgical exposure of the gland at laparotomy, and subsequent follow-up revealed a high rate of local failure [34].

The 1980s heralded several significant technological advances that have led to a renaissance of this technique. Most prominent amongst these has been the development of transperineal implantation using transrectal ultrasound and template guidance [35]. This allows the radiotherapist to reconstruct the gland three-dimensionally prior to implantation and, using sophisticated computerized dosimetry software, to ensure accurate radio-active seed placement. The availability of advanced radiation treatment planning computers capable of rapidly assessing radioactive seed numbers, activity and location has enabled a resumption of the technique to proceed with greater confidence.

Prostate brachytherapy can be accomplished by radioactive sources either left permanently in the tumour or inserted for a short period of time only. Although a number of radioactive sources exist, most experience has been gained with ^{125}I as a permanent implant. It has the advantage of being a low energy gamma emitter, enabling production of a dose confined to the prostate with easy protection of medical personnel. Its only potential drawback is its relatively low dose-rate, which may be inadequate in rapidly growing tumours [36]. The use of palladium-103 (^{103}Pd), with a higher dose-rate, may be more appropriate in such cases.

Both ^{125}I and ^{103}Pd are manufactured as seeds about the size of a grain of rice, enclosed within a titanium capsule. Transperineal seed implantation is usually performed as a single outpatient or overnight procedure under spinal or general anaesthesia. Between 80 and 100 seeds are implanted through a perineal template and directed to their destination within the gland under transrectal ultrasound guidance. The aim is to provide a homogeneous dose distribution to the prostate with a normal tissue margin of about 5 mm. The dose is prescribed to the edge of the target volume and is known as the matched peripheral dose (MPD), typically being 160 Gy for ^{125}I and 120 Gy for Pd-103. These doses are deemed radiobiologically equivalent as a result of palladium's higher dose-rate delivery. Since the MPD delineates the dose at the periphery of the gland, doses to the central parts of the prostate can be considerably higher (up to 200–240 Gy for ^{125}I). Post-implantation evaluation of seed distribution using CT-based dosimetry is useful (Fig. 10.3), since the oedema associated with radioactive implants can increase the prostate volume by a factor of 1.33–1.96 (mean 1.52), resolving exponentially with a half-life of approximately 9 days [37].

There have been no published randomized prospective trials comparing prostate brachytherapy with either radical prostatectomy or external beam radiation. Since modern prostate brachytherapy techniques are still relatively new, mature survival data are relatively scarce. The only modern brachy-therapy series at present to have mature follow-up data is from the Seattle

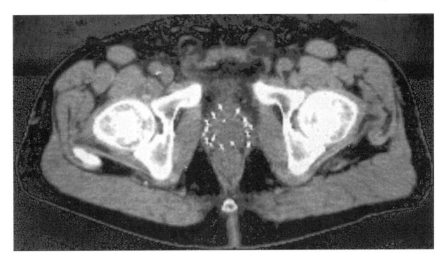

Figure 10.3 Post-brachytherapy implant CT scan illustrating multiple palladium-103 seeds within the prostate gland. (Shown in colour, Plate 8, facing p. 178.)

group [38]. In this series 64% of 152 patients received an I-125 implant alone (160 Gy MPD), with the remaining 36% receiving 45 Gy of external beam radiation to the pelvis followed in addition by a 120 Gy I-125 implant 2 weeks later, this latter group being judged to have a higher risk of extra-prostatic extension. Overall survival was 65% with a median follow-up of 10 years. Sixty-four per cent remained clinically and biochemically free of disease, with no significant difference between the two groups of patients, comparable with disease-free rates following radical prostatectomy. In common with other series, a period of 42 months following implantation was required to reach a PSA nadir.

The main technical limitation of prostate brachytherapy as sole therapy is the inability to treat effectively extra-capsular disease. Recently the American Brachytherapy Society has published selection criteria recommendations for permanent prostate brachytherapy [39] (see Table 10.3). D'Amico *et al.* [40], in a retrospective cohort study, showed that intermediate risk (stage T2b or Gleason score 7 or PSA >10 ng/mL) and high risk (stage T2c or above, or Gleason score >8 or PSA >20 ng/mL) patients fared worse when treated with brachytherapy alone than with radical prostatectomy or EBRT. Low risk patients (stage T1c, Gleason score 2–6, and PSA <10 ng/mL) showed no significant differences when treated with any of the three modalities.

In common with EBRT, brachytherapy shows a clear relationship between pretreatment PSA levels and achievement of biochemical control (see Table 10.4). Some form of early toxicity is experienced by most patients within 12 months of implantation and is characterized by symptoms of urgency, frequency, some degree of outflow obstruction and occasionally proctitis manifesting as tenesmus and diarrhoea. Most of these symptoms are mild and settle

Table 10.3 American Brachytherapy Society recommendations for transperineal permanent brachytherapy of prostate cancer (American Brachytherapy Society [39])

Indications	
Brachytherapy as monotherapy	*Brachytherapy as a boost to EBRT*
Stage T1 to T2a	Stage T2b or T2c
Gleason grade 2–6	Gleason grade 8–10
PSA < 10 ng/mL	PSA > 20 ng/mL
Relative contra-indications	**Contra-indications**
Previous TURP	Life expectancy < 5 years
Gland size > 60 cm³	Large or poorly healed TURP defect
High AUA score	Distant metastases
Positive seminal vesicles	Unacceptable operative risks
Severe diabetes	
Prominent median lobe	
History of multiple pelvic surgeries	
Previous pelvic irradiation	

Table 10.4 Rates of biochemical control (%) stratified by pretreatment PSA levels for prostate brachytherapy

Reference	Follow-up (years)	PSA level (ng/mL)							
		<4	<10	4–10	10–20	>10	20–30	>20	>30
38	10	—	70	—	—	60	—	—	—
40	5	—	85	—	30	—	—	10	—
49	5	94	—	70	47	—	38	—	33

Table 10.5 Incidence of some late complications of prostate brachytherapy (Ragde *et al.* [41])

Complication	Incidence (%)
Urinary incontinence	5.1 (overall)
Prior TURP	12.5
No prior TURP	0
Total incontinence requiring urinary diversion	1.7
Mild stress incontinence requiring no treatment	3.4
Severe vesico-urethral strictures requiring urinary diversion	2.5
Short bulbomembranous urethral strictures requiring one or more dilatations only	12

within a 5- to 10-month period. Some late complications are listed in Table 10.5. A striking feature is the observation that chronic urinary incontinence appears limited to patients undergoing a prior TURP. This reflects the high doses received by the central portion of the gland (which includes the bladder neck and urethra) with brachytherapy, which appear to be well tolerated by the intact gland and less so where the gland has been resected. A similar picture emerges with post-implant TURP [42], thus supporting the view that patients having previously undergone surgery or potentially requiring surgery to the prostate might be better served by other treatment modalities.

Overall most patients report an excellent quality of life post implantation (79%), with a minimal interruption of their social and economic function [43]. Potency rates vary from one series to another. The Seattle cohort observed a 30% incidence of complete impotence and an additional 30% incidence of partial erectile dysfunction [41], but others have reported that potency may be maintained in over 80% of patients following implantation [44]. A particular risk associated with prostate brachytherapy is the embolization of radioactive seeds to the lung. Although this can occur in up to 11% of patients, it is usually asymptomatic and can be reduced dramatically by the use of seeds embedded in a vicryl suture for the peripheral portions of the gland [45].

In summary, patients with T1–T2a cancers with PSA levels of <10 ng/mL and Gleason scores of 2–6 are good candidates for implantation with either ^{125}I or ^{103}Pd as monotherapy. Patients with T2b or T2c tumours or PSA levels >20 ng/mL or Gleason scores of 8–10 are probably better served by a combination of EBRT and implantation. However, the ultimate role of brachytherapy amongst the therapeutic options for prostate cancer awaits definition by randomized clinical trials.

The management of PSA failure after radical radiotherapy for localized prostate cancer

PSA levels decline over a period of many months following EBRT, and this is dissimilar to the changes following radical surgery. PSA progression can herald local recurrence alone, or the development of distant metastases, or both. There is some evidence to suggest that a rapid PSA doubling time (PSADT) of <6–8 months predicts for metastatic rather than local failure [46]. Longer PSADTs are typically associated with local relapse. If staging investigations confirm isolated local recurrence, then salvage prostatectomy should be considered if candidates who initially had T1 or T2 tumours have biopsy-proven recurrences more than 1 year after irradiation. The PSA should be <10–20 ng/mL with patients not receiving prior hormone therapy. Salvage prostatectomy is technically a more difficult operation following irradiation of the gland, due to the presence of radiation fibrosis. Operating times and hospital stays are longer and the morbidity of the procedure greater. Nerve-sparing procedures are generally impossible and so impotence is almost inevitable. There is little experience with salvage brachytherapy at present and so its use in this scenario must be considered experimental.

Role of salvage radiotherapy for PSA failures after radical prostatectomy

Patients who might be candidates for salvage radiotherapy after radical prostatectomy fall into three groups. The first group consists of patients with adverse histological features such as positive resection margins, seminal vesicle involvement or T3 disease, but undetectable PSA levels postoperatively. The second group consists of patients who had initially undetectable PSA levels postoperatively, subsequently rising 6 months or more following surgery. The third group consists of patients who have persistently detectable PSA levels after surgery. Hudson has reported a statistically significant difference in biochemical DFS among these three groups in a cohort of 106 patients given salvage/adjuvant radiotherapy [47]. Those who had a persistently detectable PSA level after surgery (group 3) had a biochemical failure rate of 82% with a follow-up in excess of 5 years. Those whose levels initially fell to normal after surgery and then rose subsequently (group 2) fared somewhat better with a 64% biochemical failure rate, but the adjuvantly treated group (group 1) fared best, with only a 25% failure rate. This would appear to indicate that postoperative radiotherapy is not helpful in patients with a persistently elevated PSA level following surgery, but may offer some advantage in the adjuvant setting.

Palliative radiation therapy

Metastases are limited to bone in 80–85% of patients with prostate cancer and these are effectively treated by single or fractionated radiation doses such as 8 Gy or 20 Gy in five fractions, respectively. Where lesions are widespread, treatment with hemi-body irradiation may be offered. Alternatively, strontium-89 administered intravenously offers similarly effective pain relief [48]. Strontium-89 is preferentially taken up and retained by sites of increased bone turnover. Retention at metastatic sites has been documented over 90 days after injection, despite a biological half-life of 14 days, implying targeted delivery of radiation to metastases. Strontium-89 emits β-particles with a range in tissues of 8 mm. It is possible that its emission characteristics may delay the progression of asymptomatic bony metastases in comparison with conventional hemi-body radiation field. The major toxicity of strontium-89 is haematological, with transient falls of 30–40% in platelets and leucocytes. Strontium-89 is also rather more expensive than a course of palliative radiotherapy.

New developments in prostate radiotherapy

The latest development in radiation treatment exploits varying the intensity of a radiation beam across a treatment field. This is known as intensity modulated radiation therapy (IMRT) and enables highly accurate shaping of dose distributions with complex geometries. For example, where the target is thickest the beam intensity is at its greatest, and where the target is thinnest the intensity is at its lowest. Thus the total dose delivered closely matches the shape of the target volume in three dimensions and avoids normal tissues. Hence, in contrast to 3DCRT, IMRT beams can produce concave dose patterns with exceptionally sharp dose fall-off. Although still in the experimental stages, this technology offers a further advance in the radiation treatment of prostate cancer.

Conclusion

There have been changes in radiotherapy techniques in the last two decades that have led to real improvements in patient management. New methods of radiation delivery have led to the opportunity of increasing local dosages without increasing toxicity.

References

1   Young HM. Technique of radium treatment of cancer of the prostate and seminal vesicles. *Surg Gynecol Obstet* 1992; **34**: 93–8.
2   Denning CL. Results in 100 cases of cancer of prostate and seminal vesicles treated by radium. *Surg Gynecol Obstet* 1992; **34**: 99–118.
3   Ray G, Cassady J, Bagshaw M. Definitive radiation of carcinoma of the prostate: a report on 15 years of experience. *Radiology* 1973; **106**: 407–18.
4   Paulson DF. Randomised series of treatment with surgery versus radiation for prostate adenocarcinoma. *Monogr Natl Cancer Inst* 1998; **7**: 127–31.
5   National Institutes of Health. *Consensus Development Conference Statement*. Washington, DC: US Government Printing Office, 1987: 6.
6   Leibel S, Expert Panel on Radiation Oncology. ACR appropriateness criteria. *Int J Radiat Oncol Biol Phys* 1999; **43**: 125–68.
7   Zagars G, Pollack A, Von Eschenbach A. Prognostic factors in clinically localised prostate cancer – analysis of 938 patients irradiated in the PSA era. *Cancer* 1997; **79**: 1370–80.
8   American Society for Therapeutic Radiology and Oncology (ASTRO) Consensus Panel. Consensus Statements on Radiation Therapy of Prostate Cancer: Guidelines for PSA following radiation therapy. *Int J Radiat Oncol Biol Phys* 1997; **37**: 1035–41.
9   Zeitman A, Coen J, Shipley W *et al*. Radical radiation therapy in the management of prostate adenocarcinoma: the initial PSA value as a predictor of treatment outcome. *J Urol* 1994; **151**: 640–5.
10 Crook JM, Raymond Y, Saihani D *et al*. Prostate motion during standard radiotherapy as assessed by fiducial markers. *Radiother Oncol* 1995; **37**: 35–42.

11   Pistenna DA, Bagshaw MA, Freiha FS *et al*. Extended field radiation therapy for prostatic adenocarcinoma: status report of a limited prospective trial. In: Johnson DE, Samuels ML, eds. *Cancer of the Genitourinary Tract*. New York: Raven, 1979: 229–47.

12   Asbell SO, Krall JM, Pilepich M *et al*. Elective pelvic irradiation in stage A2, B carcinoma of the prostate: analysis of RTOG 77-06. *Int J Radiat Oncol Biol Phys* 1988; **15**: 1307–16.

13   McGowan DE. The value of extended field radiation therapy in carcinoma of the prostate. *Int J Radiat Oncol Biol Phys* 1981; **7**: 1333–9.

14   Katcher J, Kupelian PA, Zippe C *et al*. Indications for excluding the seminal vesicles when treating clinically localised prostatic adenocarcinoma with radiotherapy alone. *Int J Radiat Oncol Biol Phys* 1997; **37**: 871–6.

15   Hanks G, Martz K, Diamond J. The effect of dose on local control of prostate cancer. *Int J Radiat Oncol Biol Phys* 1988; **15**: 1299–305.

16   Zelefsky M, Leibel S, Gaudin P *et al*. Dose escalation with three dimensional conformal radiation therapy affects the outcome in prostate cancer. *Int J Radiat Oncol Biol Phys* 1998; **41**: 491–500.

17   Hanks G, Schultheiss T, Hanlon A *et al*. Optimisation of conformal radiation treatment of prostate cancer: Report of a dose escalation study. *Int J Radiat Oncol Biol Phys* 1997; **37**: 543–50.

18   Shipley W, Zietman A, Hanks G *et al*. Treatment related sequelae following external beam radiation for prostate cancer: a review with an update in patients with stages T1 and T2 tumours. *J Urol* 1994; **152**: 1799–805.

19   Hanks G. External beam radiation therapy for clinically localised prostate cancer: Patterns of Care Studies in the United States. *Monogr Natl Cancer Inst* 1988; **7**: 75–84.

20   Dearnaley D, Khoo V, Norman A *et al*. Comparison of radiation side-effects of conformal and conventional radiotherapy in prostate cancer: a randomised trial. *Lancet* 1999; **353**: 267–72.

21   COIN. Guidelines on the management of prostate cancer. *Clin Oncol* 1999; **11**: S55–S88.

22   Vicini F, Kini V, Spencer W *et al*. The role of androgen deprivation in the definitive management of clinically localised prostate cancer treated with radiation therapy. *Int J Radiat Oncol Biol Phys* 1999; **43**: 707–13.

23   Pilepich M, Krall J, Al-Sarraf M *et al*. Androgen deprivation with radiation therapy compared with radiation therapy alone for locally advanced prostatic carcinoma: a randomised trial of the Radiation Therapy Oncology Group. *Urology* 1995; **45**: 616–23.

24   Laverdiere J, Gomez J, Cusan L *et al*. Beneficial effect of combination hormonal therapy administered prior and following external beam radiation therapy in localised prostate cancer. *Int J Radiat Oncol Biol Phys* 1997; **37**: 247–52.

25   Bolla M, Gonzalez D, Warde P *et al*. Improved survival in patients with locally advanced prostate cancer treated with radiotherapy and goserelin. *New Engl J Med* 1997; **337**: 295–300.

26   Bagshaw M, Cox R, Ramback J. Radiation therapy for localised prostate cancer: justification by long-term follow-up. *Urol Clin North Am* 1990; **17**: 787–802.

27   Hanks G, Krall J, Martz K *et al*. The outcome of treatment of 313 patients with T1 prostate cancer treated with external beam irradiation. *Int J Radiat Oncol Biol Phys* 1988; **14**: 243–8.

28   Perez C, Lee H, Georgiou A *et al*. Technical and tumour related factors affecting outcome of definitive irradiation for localised carcinoma of the prostate. *Int J Radiat Oncol Biol Phys* 1993; **26**: 565–81.

29   Hahn P, Baral E, Cheang M *et al*. Long-term outcome of radical radiation therapy for prostate carcinoma: 1967–1987. *Int J Radiat Oncol Biol Phys* 1996; **34**: 41–7.

30   Bagshaw M, Cox R, Ray G. Status of radiation therapy of prostate cancer at Stanford University. *Monogr Natl Cancer Inst* 1988; **7**: 47–60.

31 Del Regato J, Trailings A, Pittman D. Twenty years follow-up of patients with inoperable cancer of the prostate (stage C) treated by radiotherapy: Report of a National Co-operative Study. *Int J Radiat Oncol Biol Phys* 1993; **26**: 197–201.

32 Zagars GK, Von Eschenbach AC, Johnson DE *et al*. Stage C adenocarcinoma of the prostate: an analysis of 551 patients treated with external beam irradiation. *Cancer* 1987; **60**: 1489–99.

33 Whitmore WF, Hilaris B, Grabstald H. Retropubic implantation of iodine-125 in the treatment of prostatic cancer. *J Urol* 1972; **108**: 918–20.

34 Zelefsky MJ, Whitmore WF. Long-term results of retropubic permanent 125 iodine implantation of the prostate for clinically localised prostatic cancer. *J Urol* 1997; **158**: 23–9.

35 Holm HH, Juul N, Pedersen JF *et al*. Transperineal iodine-125 seed implantation in prostate cancer guided by trans-rectal ultrasonography. *J Urol* 1983; **130**: 283–6.

36 Freeman ML, Goldhaggen P, Sierra E *et al*. Studies with encapsulated iodine-125 sources. *Int J Radiat Oncol Biol Phys* 1982; **8**: 1347–53.

37 Waterman FM, Yuen N, Corn BW *et al*. Edema associated with I-125 or Pd-103 prostate brachytherapy and its impact on post-implant dosimetry: an analysis based on serial CT acquisition. *Int J Radiat Oncol Biol Phys* 1998; **41**: 1069–77.

38 Ragde H, Elgamal AA, Snow PB *et al*. Ten-year disease-free survival after transperineal sonography-guided I-125 brachytherapy with or without 45 Gy external beam irradiation in the treatment of patients with clinically localised, low to high Gleason grade prostate carcinoma. *Cancer* 1998; **83**: 989–1001.

39 Nag S, Beyer D, Friedland J *et al*. American Brachytherapy Society recommendations for trans-perineal permanent brachytherapy of prostate cancer. *Int J Radiat Oncol Biol Phys* 1999; **44**: 789–99.

40 D'Amico AV, Whittington R, Malkowicz SB *et al*. Biochemical outcome after radical prostatectomy, external beam radiation therapy, or interstitial radiation therapy for clinically localized prostate cancer. *JAMA* 1998; **280**: 969–74.

41 Ragde H, Blasko JC, Grimm PD *et al*. Interstitial I-125 radiation without adjuvant therapy in the treatment of clinically localized prostate carcinoma. *Cancer* 1997; **80**: 442–53.

42 Hu K, Wallner K. Urinary incontinence in patients who have a TURP/TUIP following prostate brachytherapy. *Int J Radiat Oncol Biol Phys* 1998; **40**: 783–6.

43 Artebery VE, Frazier A, Dalmia P *et al*. Quality of life after permanent prostate implants. *Semin Surg Oncol* 1997; **13**: 461–4.

44 Stock RG, Stone NN, Iannuzzi C. Sexual potency following interactive ultrasound guided brachytherapy for prostate cancer. *Int J Radiat Oncol Biol Phys* 1996; **35**: 267–72.

45 Tapen EM, Blasko JC, Grimm PD *et al*. Reduction of radioactive seed embolization to the lung following prostate brachytherapy. *Int J Radiat Oncol Biol Phys* 1998; **42**: 1063–7.

46 Zagars G, Pollack A. Kinetics of serum PSA after external beam radiation for clinically localised prostate cancer. *Radiother Oncol* 1997; **44**: 213–21.

47 American Society for Therapeutic Radiology and Oncology (ASTRO) Consensus Panel. Consensus Statements on Radiation Therapy of Prostate Cancer: Guidelines for prostate re-biopsy after radiation and for radiation therapy with rising PSA levels after radical prostatectomy. *J Clin Oncol* 1999; **17**: 1155–63.

48 Quilty P, Kirk D, Bolger J *et al*. A comparison of the palliative effects of strontium-89 and external beam radiotherapy in metastatic prostate cancer. *Radiother Oncol* 1994; **31**: 33–40.

49 Beyer DC, Priestley JB. Biochemical disease free survival following 125-I prostate implantation. *Int J Radiat Oncol Biol Phys* 1997; **37**: 559–63.

11: Prostate Cancer: Immediate vs. Deferred Treatment

D. Kirk

Introduction

Androgen deprivation continues to be the main treatment for advanced prostate cancer [1]. Although some response is seen in most patients, it will be temporary and relapse will occur, usually within two years in patients with metastases. While radiotherapy and other palliative measures may then be helpful in relieving symptoms, relapse after hormone therapy is usually fatal within a matter of months [2]. Ever since the introduction of hormone treatment for prostate cancer, there has been discussion as to its timing [3]. The issue depends on a balance between the benefits of treatment on the one hand and its side-effects and toxicity on the other.

The debate has been accentuated by recent improvements in diagnostic techniques, which have created new categories of 'advanced disease'. Examples are lymph node involvement found at radical prostatectomy, and prostate specific antigen (PSA) detected relapse after definitive treatment for localized disease [4]. These clinical situations would not have been unearthed in the days before radical surgery and the use of PSA testing, and such patients, if given hormone treatment, are destined to receive it, and be exposed to its side-effects, for many years. Ultimately it is to be hoped that the causes of hormone refractory disease can be understood and prevented, and that methods of delivering androgen deprivation while avoiding its side-effects will be developed. Meanwhile it remains essential to identify those men who will benefit from this treatment and to start treatment at the most appropriate time. This chapter addresses this important issue.

Why defer treatment?

Although there are clear indications for hormone treatment—metastatic prostate cancer presenting with bone pain or other symptoms, ureteric obstruction, retention of urine in an elderly man—many men with advanced disease are asymptomatic. It is here that the possibility of deferring treatment arises. Although it might be expected that treatment at diagnosis would prolong survival, even this has been disputed [5]. It is possible that treatment could be delayed until symptoms occur and this might be followed by a further asymptomatic period. Survival may be similar in both patient groups [6].

Immediate or deferred treatment: the swinging pendulum

The idea of deferring treatment was considered in the 1940s [3], and has been a recurring theme ever since. Over-optimism about the results of treatment, based on the use of historical controls [3], left unquestioned for several years the effectiveness of hormone treatment in prolonging survival. Then the Veterans Administration Cooperative Research Group (VACURG) studies [6] seemed to indicate that deferring treatment until progression occurred might not affect survival.

Thus, in the early 1980s, there was a balance of opinion. On the one hand, there were the potential advantages of deferring treatment, with any side-effects resulting from treatment occurring for a shorter period of time, and the possibility that many patients might not need treatment as they would die first from an unrelated cause.

However, a number of potential harmful effects could arise from delaying treatment [7] (Table 11.1). In addition, it is a good oncological principle that treatment while tumour bulk is smaller should be more effective.

The development of new methods of hormone manipulation, such as LHRH analogues, seemed to reduce the disadvantages of hormone treatment, thus favouring early treatment [8]. At the same time, these new treatments are expensive, and added an economic component to the argument in favour of deferred treatment. Recently, the long-term toxicity of chronic androgen deprivation has been recognized, with particular concern about osteoporosis [9].

Table 11.1 Potential hazards of delaying treatment in advanced prostate cancer

Deferring treatment may reduce survival
Prostate cancer may become less hormone sensitive as it progresses
Local progression in the absence of treatment increases the number of patients requiring TURP
  for recurrent outflow obstruction and those who develop ureteric obstruction
Catastrophic events such as spinal cord compression and pathological fractures may occur in
  untreated patients
The absence of specific symptoms might mask a general malaise associated with uncontrolled
  cancer
Patients managed by deferred treatment may die from prostate cancer without receiving
  hormone therapy

The need for clinical trials

It was recognized that for many reasons, not least the selected group of patients studied (mainly elderly veterans of World War I), the results of the VACURG studies were inconclusive and more studies were required. The study sponsored by the British Medical Research Council (MRCPR03) [10], which finished recruitment in 1993, was but one of these. Further studies by the European Organization for Research and Treatment of Cancer (EORTC) on somewhat different groups of patients are under way [11], but may not be in a position to report results for some time. The outcome of studies of adjuvant hormone treatment in patients receiving radiotherapy have been reported from the EORTC [12] and Radiation Therapy Oncology Group (RTOG) [13]. These are in effect trials of immediate vs. deferred hormone treatment. As data are accumulated from these studies, a picture is developing. It does not define the relative value of immediate or deferred treatment, but has focused the issues, both in terms of advising patients of the options, and in directing future research.

Progression in prostate cancer

Once prostate cancer has been diagnosed, and is beyond curative treatment, its future impact on the patient can develop in a number of ways (Table 11.2). Immediate treatment is instituted in the hope of delaying or preventing them. Deferred treatment accepts that some of them will occur, and will become an indication to start treatment, which it is hoped will reverse them.

Table 11.2 Development of advanced prostate cancer

Disease progression
Local
  Bladder outflow obstruction
  Ureteric obstruction
Metastatic disease
  Progression from M0 disease
  Progression of metastases
    Symptoms
    Complications—Spinal cord compression
              —Pathological fracture
Extraskeletal metastases

Death
  Prostate cancer
  Other causes

Impact of hormone treatment on disease outcome

The results of MRCPR03 have been presented elsewhere [14], and widely discussed [10]. In summary, disease specific survival and to a lesser extent overall survival were increased in those treated immediately (Fig. 11.1). However, on subgroup analysis improved survival occurred only in those with M0 disease at diagnosis. Distant progression in those with M0 disease occurred more rapidly, and metastatic pain occurred sooner if treatment was deferred. This is to be expected, and was used in many cases as an indication to start deferred treatment. However, local progression is an important problem in advanced prostate cancer. In the MRC study, 82 of the patients receiving immediate treatment have required a transurethral resection of the prostate (TURP) for outlet obstruction. However, within the group whose treatment was deferred, 141 required a TURP. In addition, ureteric obstruction occurred more rapidly and more frequently with deferred treatment (43 vs. 58, immediate vs. deferred). However, response of this complication to treatment makes it reversible in previously untreated patients, while ureteric obstruction in those already treated is usually a pre-terminal event. Other events—spinal cord compression, pathological fracture and extraskeletal distant metastases—were all more common in patients whose treatment was deferred. It is important to note that of 23 patients who developed spinal cord compression in the deferred treatment arm of the study, 18 had already had treatment initiated for another reason, and in 17 patients, treatment had been started more than 6 months previously. It can be seen that in the MRCPR03 study spinal cord compression was not an insidious event occurring without warning in untreated

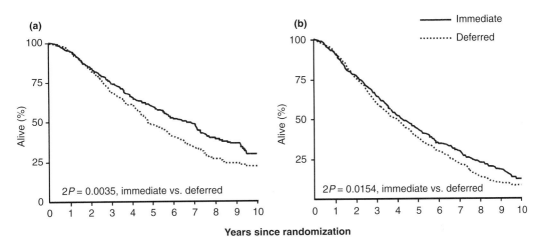

Figure 11.1 MRCPR03 trial of immediate vs. deferred treatment. Disease specific and overall death rates compared by randomization group: (a) time to death from prostate cancer (all patients); (b) time to death from any cause (all patients).

patients, nor, as has been suggested [10], did it arise from clinical neglect of the trial patients. The observation that this complication was preceded by other disease-related events suggests that during deferred treatment the inevitable disease progression which occurs is not reversed when treatment is started — this may also account for the higher incidence of extraskeletal metastases.

It should also be noted that only 7 of the 33 cases of paraplegia occurred in M0 patients — this seems to be a danger mainly to those with metastases at presentation. This is an argument in favour of treatment in those with metastatic disease. It may also explain the absence of cases of paraplegia in the EORTC studies commented on by Schröder [11] in his critique of MRCPR03 — the difference is in the study population not in the trial conduct.

Patients who die without treatment

Comment must be made on the 82 patients in the MRCPR03 study who died without treatment [15]. Fifty-six of these were thought to have died from causes other than prostate cancer. This perhaps is the ultimate success of deferred treatment, as these are patients for whom treatment proved to be unnecessary. However, there were also 26 patients who, on first collection of data, possibly died from prostate cancer without treatment. This should not have been a great surprise, as a report on deferred treatment from Newcastle in 1986 recorded 17% of patients dying in this way [16]. The data on these 26 patients have been reviewed. In 15, death did appear to be from prostate cancer. However, it occurred mainly in elderly patients, and reflected the problems of managing cancer in the elderly. For example, three patients refused treatment when it was advised, and in two post-mortem examination after death with non-specific symptoms demonstrated previously unsuspected metastases. In the remaining 11 of these 26, although the certified cause of death was prostate cancer, on detailed review this seems unlikely. Some certainly died from cancer but so atypical of prostate cancer, with little evidence of recent progression of the prostatic tumour, that a second, but undiagnosed, malignancy was probably to blame. Conflicting pathology producing similar problems to prostate cancer (e.g. Parkinson's disease affecting bladder function) also caused fatal complications attributed to prostate cancer on the death certificate.

It should be noted that there was a clustering of most of these deaths in the early part of the study. This was before PSA testing was widely available. It is clear that PSA allows earlier identification of progression and better discrimination between prostate cancer and other causes of death. This probably explains why it is reported that this problem has not been encountered in studies commenced more recently [10].

The author has dwelled on this issue for two reasons. First, it is important in interpreting data from trials to realize that accurate identification of the cause of death, particularly in the elderly, can be difficult. Data collection on an annual basis, as in MRCPR03, while having a number of advantages, might cause difficulty when a death has occurred in the early part of the period. A carefully defined death reporting procedure is needed when cause of death is a critical endpoint, and overall survival, the fact and date of death itself being without dispute, must be considered the most accurate measure.

The second reason is its relevance to the trial survival data. At any one time, the difference in numbers surviving between the trial arms is small. It has been suggested that this difference is simply due to the patients who died without treatment and that the survival difference would not have been seen if these deaths had been avoided by more careful follow-up [10]. This argument is unsustainable for a number of reasons. By the time the data had been published, most of these patients had died several years before. Thus even if their deaths had been postponed by hormone treatment, they would still have died by the time the data were analysed. However, this argument has a deeper flaw. All men with advanced prostate cancer treated with hormones will die from the disease unless another condition occurs first. Before too long, the mortality in both arms of the study will approach 100%. The important parameter is duration of survival as measured by survival curves. We have addressed this issue by considering the effects on these curves assuming the worst (and unlikely) case of all 26 patients having died from prostate cancer. To have abolished the disease specific survival difference would have required treatment of these patients to have prolonged survival by an average of 6.5 years (Fig. 11.2), and this is clearly unlikely.

Is the case for immediate treatment proved?

Confirmation of definite advantages from immediate treatment is reflected in the improved survival seen in the EORTC study of adjuvant treatment with radiotherapy [12], although in the study of the RTOG this was noted only in those with high grade disease [13]. The reported data from both these studies are still somewhat immature. Hormone treatment will also reduce the risk of complications from local progression. The increased risk of spinal cord compression seems to transcend the start of deferred treatment, warning that disease progression occurring during the period without treatment may not be reversed when treatment is started. There is also the risk that, for whatever reason, the appropriate time of starting treatment may be missed.

On the other hand, are there problems with immediate treatment? The immediate side-effects—impotence, hot flushes, etc.—have been long recognized. However, just as studies have started to show that clear benefits may result from immediate treatment, so has the possibility emerged that serious

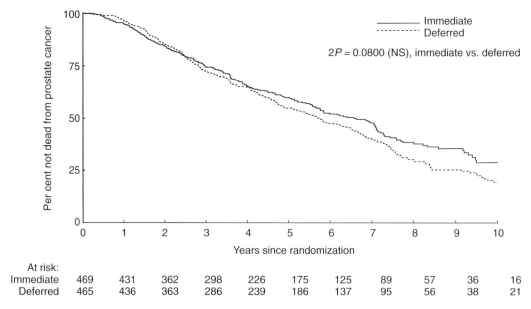

Figure 11.2 MRCPR03 trial of immediate vs. deferred treatment. Hypothetical survival curves, immediate vs. deferred, assuming all 26 patients who died or may have died from prostate cancer survived 6.5 years longer. Shorter survival leaves a significant survival difference.

harmful effects may result from androgen treatment. Some of these are specific to particular therapies: cardiovascular complications of oestrogens, liver toxicity of anti-androgens. However, testosterone deficiency, including androgen deprivation from orchiectomy or LHRH analogues, long considered 'safe' options, is now recognized to cause weight increase, loss of muscle mass and loss of energy [17]. Anaemia may be a particular problem in patients treated with combined androgen blockade [18]. Recently, osteoporosis has been described as a significant problem after androgen deprivation, analogous to that in post-menopausal women [9].

Is there a more serious possibility? The difference between disease specific and overall survival has been noted, and may be explained by the background influence of coincidental deaths (Fig. 11.1). However, it was recognized in the VACURG studies that oestrogens in high dosage cause increased cardiovascular mortality [6]. Could other methods of androgen deprivation cause death? Does hormone treatment affect overall survival, or does it merely reduce cancer deaths at the expense of a compensating increase in mortality from other causes?

Table 11.3 MRCPR03: Deaths from causes other than prostate cancer

Cause of death	Immediate treatment	Deferred treatment
Cardiovascular disease	77	91
Cancer	27	15
Respiratory disease	22	9
Other	21	14
Total	147 (37%)	129 (31%)

Table 11.4 MRCPR03: Deaths from cancer other than prostate cancer

Type of cancer	Immediate treatment	Deferred treatment
Bronchus	5	5
Colorectal	7	3
Stomach	5	1
Oesophagus	3	1
Bladder	2	1
Kidney	2	—
Pancreas	—	2
Other	3	2
Total	27	15*

*Eleven had already received hormone treatment; six died from cancer other than prostate before treatment started.

Is hormone treatment dangerous?

Are there disadvantages to treatment? If there are, are we in a position to be able to identify the fatal complication of androgen deprivation? If there is one, it should be identified in MRCPR03 since those treated immediately were exposed to hormone treatment for longer, and demonstrate an excess of deaths from whatever is the condition [19]. Cardiovascular disease seems the most plausible culprit. In fact, more deaths from cardiovascular disease occurred in the deferred arm (Table 11.3). The clearest risk factor for cardiovascular death was age (Fig. 11.3). Looking at all the causes of non-prostate cancer death, the clearest increase is in the incidence (Table 11.4) and rate (Fig. 11.4) of death from other types of cancer in immediately treated patients. These, it must be admitted, were usually cancers which are rapidly fatal, consistent with the hypothesis that immediate treatment allowed time for them to occur by delaying prostate cancer death. However, the possibility of hormone treatment

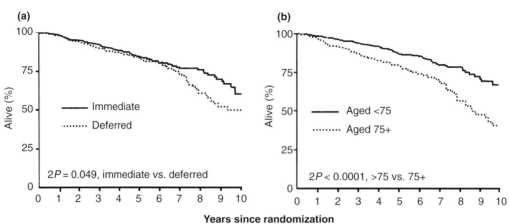

Figure 11.3 MRCPR03 trial of immediate vs. deferred treatment. Survival curves for cardiovascular deaths: (a) immediate vs. deferred; (b) age greater or less than 75.

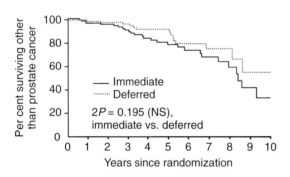

Figure 11.4 MRCPR03 trial of immediate vs. deferred treatment. Survival curves for deaths from cancer other than prostate cancer.

in some way accelerating the later stages of cancer expression remains an intriguing one.

Practical management of prostate cancer

Thus, the decision to start hormone treatment continues to involve a careful analysis of the relative advantages and disadvantages of treatment, and the symptoms caused by prostate cancer. The debate, started over 50 years ago, continues. Where are we in 2001?

Metastatic disease

It is probably advisable to consider treatment in the majority of men with metastatic disease. Clearly, where metastases are symptomatic, treatment is mandatory. Deferring treatment will only delay its need for a few months.

In MRCPR03 it was in men with M1 disease at presentation that the risk of spinal cord compression and pathological fractures was greatest. Men with metastatic disease will not usually survive long enough to allow long-term ill-effects from androgen deprivation to be experienced. In the short term, an improvement in non-specific well being from reduction in tumour load may well outweigh any side-effects. In MRCPR03, the increased need for TURP was as common in patients with M1 as in those with M0 disease, and a possible source of troublesome morbidity in the terminal stages of disease, with 10% of patients needing a TURP in the last year of their life [20].

Where deferred treatment is considered, perhaps at the request of the patient, clear criteria can be identified as to suitability. The patient with a large metastasis in the spine, the patient with bone destruction threatening pathological fracture, the patient who is anaemic or suffers from other, more subtle causes of ill health, or who has a large aggressive primary tumour—especially if the tumour is poorly differentiated—should probably be advised to start treatment immediately. When treatment is deferred, it should be with the full co-operation and understanding of the patient and his general practitioner. In this situation, the patient must be regularly reviewed in the Clinic with close monitoring of his symptoms, so that treatment can be initiated as soon as significant progression occurs. It follows that where the patient is unable or unwilling to comply with close follow-up, deferred treatment is unsuitable.

Localized disease

How does this debate affect the management of localized disease? The use of adjuvant treatment in confined disease, as tamoxifen is used in breast cancer [21], is currently the subject of a large international study. It will presumably delay the clinical appearance of progression in those for whom definitive treatment has not eradicated the disease. Whether this will improve the outcome compared with treatment delayed until that progression has occurred, or indeed increase those who have been truly cured by definitive treatment, is to be shown. So, how should men with early prostate cancer and involved lymph nodes or positive margins at surgery, or in PSA-detected relapse, be managed? Anecdotal reports have shown that radiotherapy and/or hormonal treatment is effective in reducing the PSA. However, there is a risk in managing prostate cancer in the modern era that the patient's PSA is treated rather than his disease. Suffice to say that currently there is a lack of trial evidence to support early treatment in these circumstances—a fall in PSA will occur, but how much impact this has on later development of the disease remains to be determined. One randomized study of early vs. deferred treatment of patients with positive lymph nodes has been presented [22]. Although showing a statistically significant advantage for early treatment, in terms of both progression and survival, the overall numbers were too small (46 early vs. 52 deferred), with six deaths in the early group vs. 18 in the deferred group, for the result to have statistical power and may have resulted from an uneven balance between the groups. A larger study from the EORTC is awaited.

Essentially, in these patients the balance between advantage and disadvantage is clear. With adjuvant treatment, many patients will have been cured by definitive treatment, thus being unable to benefit from hormone treatment. In others, including those with detectable PSA after treatment, the prognosis is such that clinical progression and death may be years away, possibly after they have died from another disease. On the other hand, treatment will be taken for years and thus the risks of toxicity are greater compared with those treated for advanced disease. It is certainly inappropriate to extrapolate from trials in advanced disease (such as MRCPR03) to earlier disease.

Locally advanced disease

A number of strategies can be considered for those patients with locally advanced T3/T4 cancer. Deferred treatment is considered on the basis that many of these patients will be incurable, but have slowly progressive disease which may not threaten life or health for some years. Data from MRCPR03 would support this approach in elderly patients. This is because 30% of men with M0 disease who were over 80 died from other causes before requiring treatment. However, the main recruitment into MRCPR03 took place prior to the full impact of PSA testing and transrectal ultrasound (TRUS) biopsy. Most patients were diagnosed following a TURP, and even then substantial numbers required further TURP for local progression, a risk substantially reduced in those treated immediately. Nowadays, the diagnosis is more likely to result from a needle biopsy. Patients presenting with symptoms of outflow obstruction will require treatment, while others might progress to obstruction in its absence. For the symptomatic man, a TURP will palliate the symptoms, but without further treatment may be only a temporary expedient.

Although early T3 tumours can be managed by surgery [23], in most centres radiotherapy, hormone treatment, or a combination would be considered. Radiotherapy, usually now preceded by neoadjuvant treatment [24], is logical for localized disease, for which systemic treatment is perhaps inappropriate. However, there is clear evidence that hormone treatment is effective in controlling localized disease. An earlier MRC study (PR02) demonstrated no difference between radiotherapy or hormone treatment in terms of TURP rates during follow-up, although numbers were small and radiotherapy techniques have moved on [25]. Adjuvant hormone treatment has been shown to improve survival compared with radiotherapy alone [11]. Is this the result of the combination, or would survival have been as good if patients had received only hormone treatment? Studies exploring this possibility by comparing hormone therapy alone with combined treatment are under way in both Canada and the UK.

Conclusion

We still have a dilemma with hormone treatment. Not treating cancer is a difficult concept for patients and many doctors. Treatment has possible benefits, benefits which recent trial data have made firmer. Yet treatment is also a source of side-effects and potential toxicity. Hormone treatment is only temporarily beneficial—hormone refractory relapse is inevitable. Future clinical research must address a number of issues, which include quality of life and treatment related toxicity. Meanwhile, in the laboratory, efforts must be directed towards understanding the mechanisms for the development of hormone refractory relapse. Prevention of androgen insensitivity would change hormone therapy from a palliative to a curative treatment. If hormone treatments could be improved so that there is benefit without toxicity, the therapeutic balance would be swayed towards immediate treatment.

Meanwhile, those of us who manage men with prostate cancer have to use treatments that are currently available. Imperfect though they are, current methods of hormone treatment are effective to an extent that is not available for many other types of cancer. We must recognize that this is a disease which varies in its impact from individual to individual. One notable aspect of participating in MRCPR03 was the importance of the effect of information on the patient. Having received a balanced account of the arguments for and against immediate treatment, and despite knowing that the trial was based on uncertainty, many men were clear which approach they wanted for themselves. Although this adversely affected trial recruitment, it tells us a lot about men's attitude to treatment of prostate cancer. Our patients deserve this level of information. They need to share our uncertainties, and ultimately our role is to help them make a decision as to which method of management is right for them. We then need to be aware of the risks associated with the course of action chosen, and alert to the possible problems which might occur. The urologists or oncologists who decide that there is an answer to the question 'immediate or deferred treatment?' have come to the wrong conclusion and their patients will suffer from their certainty.

References

1   Jacobi GH. Hormonal treatment of metastatic carcinoma of the prostate. In: Fitzpatrick JM, Krane RJ, eds. *The Prostate*. Edinburgh: Churchill Livingstone, 1989: 389–99.

2   Beynon LL, Chisholm GD. The stable state is not an objective response in hormone-escaped carcinoma of the prostate. *Br J Urol* 1984; **56**: 702–70.

3   Nesbit RM, Baum WC. Endocrine control of prostatic cancer: clinical survey of 1818 cases. *JAMA* 1950; **143**: 1317–20.

4   Kirby RS. Avoidance and management of rising prostate-specific antigen after radical prostatectomy. In: Belldegrun A, Kirby RS, Newling DWW, eds. *New Perspectives in Prostate Cancer*, 2nd edn. Oxford: Isis Medical, 2000: 147–55.

5   Lepor H, Ross A, Walsh PC. The influence of hormonal therapy on survival of men with advanced prostatic cancer. *J Urol* 1982; **128**: 335–40.

6   Byar DP. The Veterans Administration Cooperative Research Group's studies of cancer of the prostate. *Cancer* 1973; **32**: 1126–30.

7   Kirk D. Deferred treatment for advanced prostatic cancer. In: Waxman J, Williams G, eds. *Urological Oncology*. Sevenoaks: Edward Arnold, 1991: 117–25.

8   Kozlowski JM, Ellis WJ, Grayhack JT. Advanced prostatic carcinoma: early versus late endocrine therapy. *Urol Clin North Am* 1991; **15**: 15–24.

9   Daniell HW. Osteoporosis after orchiectomy for prostate cancer. *J Urol* 1997; **157**: 439–44.

10 Kirk D. Trials and tribulations in prostatic cancer. *Br J Urol* 1987; **59**: 375–9.

11 Schröder FH. Endocrine treatment of prostate cancer—recent developments and the future. Part 1: maximal androgen blockade. Early vs delayed endocrine treatment and side effects. *BJU Int* 1999; **83** [European Urology Update Series]: 161–70.

12 Bolla M, Gonzalez D, Ward P *et al*. Improved survival in patients with locally advanced prostate cancer treated with radiotherapy and goserelin. *New Engl J Med* 1997; **337**: 295–300.

13 Pilepich MV, Caplin R, Byhardt RW *et al*. Phase III trial of androgen suppression using goserelin in unfavourable-prognosis carcinoma of the prostate treated with definitive radiotherapy: report of Radiation Therapy Oncology Group Protocol 85-31. *J Clin Oncol* 1997; **15**: 1013–21.

14 Medical Research Council Prostate Cancer Working Party Investigators Group. Immediate versus deferred treatment for advanced prostatic cancer: initial results of the Medical Research Council Trial. *Br J Urol* 1997; **79**: 235–46.

15 Kirk D, Medical Research Council Prostate Cancer Working Party Investigators Group. MRC immediate versus deferred treatment study: patients dying without treatment. *Br J Urol* 1998; **81** (Suppl. 4): 31 (Abstract).

16 Carr TW, Handley RC, Travis D, Powell PH, Hall RR. Deferred treatment of prostate cancer. *Br J Urol* 1988; **62**: 249–53.

17 Morley JE, Kaiser FE, Hajjar R, Perr HM III. Testosterone and frailty. *Clin Geriat Med* 1997; **13**: 655–95.

18 Strum SB, Mcdermed JE, Scholz MC, Johnson H, Tisman G. Anaemia associated with androgen deprivation in patients receiving combined hormone blockade. *Br J Urol* 1997; **79**: 933–41.

19 Kirk D, Medical Research Council Prostate Cancer Working Party Investigators Group. Does hormonal treatment for prostate cancer cause excess deaths: data from the MRC immediate versus deferred hormone treatment study. *BJU Int* 1999; **83** (Suppl. 4): 9 (Abstract).

20 Kirk D, Medical Research Council Prostate Cancer Working Party Investigators Group. MRC immediate versus deferred treatment study: how important is local progression in advanced prostate cancer. *Br J Urol* 1998; **81** (Suppl. 4): 30 (Abstract).

21 Early Breast Cancer Trialists Collaborative Group. Systemic treatment by hormonal, cytotoxic or immune therapy. *Lancet* 1992; **339**: 1–15.

22 Messing E, Manola J, Sarosdy M, Wilding G, Crawford D, Trump D. Immediate hormonal

therapy compared with observation after radical prostatectomy and pelvic lymphadenectomy in men with node positive protate cancer. *N Eng J Med* 1999; **341**: 1781–8.

23 Zinke H, Utz DC, Benson RC, Patterson DE. Bilateral lymphadenectomy and radical retropubic prostatectomy for stage C prostate cancer. *Urology* 1984; **24**: 532–9.

24 Dearnaley DP. Combined modality treatment with radiotherapy and hormonal treatment in localised prostate cancer. In: Belldegrun A, Kirby RS, Newling DWW, eds. *New Perspectives in Prostate Cancer*, 2nd edn. Oxford: Isis Medical, 2000: 169–80.

25 Fellows GJ, Clark PB, Beynon LL *et al.* Treatment of advanced localised prostatic cancer by orchiectomy, radiotherapy, or combined treatment. (A Medical Research Council study.) *Br J Urol* 1992; **70**: 304–9.

12: Hormone Therapy of Prostate Cancer

R. Agarwal & J. Waxman

Introduction

The history of the treatment of prostatic cancer dates back over 100 years, to when patients with prostatic 'conditions' were first castrated. Hormonal therapy has been widely used only since 1941, following the demonstration by Huggins & Hodges [1] of the androgen dependence of prostate cancer and the therapeutic effects of orchiectomy and oestrogen administration. The next historical development was in 1945 when the benefits of adrenalectomy in patients with prostate cancer were demonstrated [2]. The next major development occurred in the 1970s when the anti-androgens cyproterone acetate and flutamide were synthesized. The gonadotrophin releasing hormone analogues (GnRH-A) buserelin, goserelin and leuporelin were developed in the late 1970s and 1980s, and more recently the selective 5α-reductase inhibitor finasteride and the anti-androgen bicalutamide have become available. Research is continuing into novel methods of androgen deprivation including the use of GnRH agonists and GnRH receptor antibodies and vaccines [3].

The significant advances that have been made over the last century have established hormone therapy as the principal treatment modality for advanced disease. Within this area of hormonal therapy there remain significant unresolved controversies. These include the role of specific hormonal therapies as single agents or in combination, and the place of newer agents within the treatment algorithm. The most significant issue in prostatic cancer remains our failure to cure advanced disease: at present all treatment is palliative to improve outcome while minimizing the toxicity of treatment.

The rationale for hormonal therapy in prostate cancer

The normal development of prostatic tissue is dependent on testosterone, and to a minor extent on growth hormone and prolactin. Approximately 95% of plasma testosterone in men is produced by testicular Leydig cells under the influence of luteinizing hormone (LH), which is secreted in a pulsatile manner by the anterior pituitary. At puberty, the secretion of GnRH by the hypothalamus into the hypophyseal circulation results in the synthesis and release into the systemic circulation of LH and consequently a rise in serum testosterone levels. The prostate gland enlarges under the influence of testosterone and this influence is responsible for its normal development as well as benign prostatic hyperplasia and prostate cancer in older men. Testosterone's effects on the prostate are mediated by its interaction with the androgen receptor after conversion to 5-hydroxytestosterone (5-HT) by intracellular 5α-reductase. The androgen receptor/5-HT complex translocates to the nucleus and via binding to specific androgen response elements on chromosomal DNA regulates gene expression involved in growth, proliferation and inhibition of apoptosis [4].

There are other sources of circulating androgens. The adrenal glands produce approximately 5% of the total plasma testosterone in non-castrate men. However, adrenal androgen synthesis is not regulated by LH, and may instead reflect overall glucocorticoid synthesis, which is controlled by adrenocorticotrophin-releasing hormone (ACTH). There are also dietary androgens, which vary considerably between vegetarians and omnivores.

Serum androgen levels are regulated via a negative feedback loop involving the hypothalamic–pituitary axis. Androgen, progesterone and oestrogen receptors are present in the hypothalamus and anterior pituitary, which when activated by their cognate ligands inhibit GnRH and LH release, respectively, thereby suppressing testicular androgen synthesis [4].

Initially in prostate cancer cells the androgen dependent mitogenic and anti-apoptotic signalling pathways are maintained, and are necessary for the survival and proliferation of these malignant cells. Indeed the Nobel Prize was awarded to Huggins & Hodges [1] for this important discovery and the demonstration of the regression of prostate cancer following androgen deprivation via orchiectomy.

A number of strategies for androgen deprivation have been developed based on an understanding of normal androgen physiology. This has resulted in the use of oestrogens and progestagens to inhibit GnRH synthesis, and the development of the GnRH 'super' agonists, 5α-reductase inhibitors, and androgen receptor antagonists [3].

However, despite their initial sensitivity to androgen deprivation when patients relapse, prostate cancer cells become relatively androgen independent, though they may remain sensitive to hormonal manipulations for a further period of time before eventually becoming hormone independent [5]. The exact mechanism underlying this progression from androgen independent to hormone independent disease has become clear over the past decade. This area has been reviewed by Oh and Kantoff [6], who highlight the development of p53 mutations, overexpression of bcl-2 and the importance of cytokine receptors such as for the IGF and her2/neu receptors in providing alternate growth and proliferation signals to prostate cancer cells thereby preventing apoptosis in response to androgen deprivation. Alternatively, amplification and mutation of the androgen receptor (AR) can also lead to apparent androgen independence. Taplin *et al.* [7] and Zhao *et al.* [8] have shown how mutations of the AR can result in increased affinity for and activation of the AR by anti-androgens, oestrogens, progestagens and glucocorticoids.

Hormonal therapies

Orchiectomy

Orchiectomy has remained the gold standard against which pharmacological treatments have been assessed. It is argued that orchiectomy is cheap and safe [9]. However, the argument that orchiectomy is cheap is not altogether accurate. This is because the procedure is frequently performed as an inpatient operation. The argument is also irrelevant because patient choice is the real issue and patient preference is for medical therapy [10]. Simply put, it is bad enough to have cancer, but to be castrated for it results in a rapid and permanent fall in testosterone levels within hours of surgery. There is one situation where orchiectomy is the treatment of first choice and this is in patients presenting with cord compression, where a rapid reduction in testosterone levels is required.

Castration, whether medical or surgical, can result in loss of libido, impotence, fatigue, depression, hot flushes, osteoporosis and gynaecomastia [11]. Prophylactic irradiation of the breasts has been shown to reduce the incidence of gynaecomastia to a degree, but frequently breast tissue grows around the irradiated breast bud. Hot flushes may be controlled with clonidine, progestational agents or venlafaxine [11].

Oestrogens

The most commonly used oestrogen in prostate cancer has been diethylstilboesterol (DES). It was initially used at a dose of 5 mg/day to inhibit hypothalamic and pituitary release of GnRH and LH, respectively, and has been shown to reduce testosterone levels to castrate levels in 2–3 weeks [12]. However, its use has declined following studies by the Veterans Administration Cooperative Urological Research Group (VACURG) showing a significant increase in cardiovascular morbidity and thromboembolic events in patients treated with DES [11]. Subsequent studies using 1 mg/day of DES have shown similar efficacy to 5 mg/day DES, with fewer but still significant cardiac and thromboembolic side-effects [12,13]. This cardiovascular toxicity remains a problem even when aspirin is given [14].

DES-diphosphate (fosfesterol), a derivative of DES, has been developed in a bid to minimize systemic toxicity and enhance the therapeutic index [15]. The theoretical basis for this reduction in toxicity is that conjugated DES-diphosphate is inactive until dephosphorylated, and so it was initially assumed that the high concentration of phosphatases in prostatic tissue would result in high local concentration of DES with minimal systemic exposure. Subsequent studies have failed to demonstrate a differential distribution of DES after fosfesterol between prostatic and non-prostatic tissue compared with the administration of DES itself. Other oestrogens that have been used in the treatment of prostate cancer are ethinyl oestradiol and chlortrianisene, which have inferior therapeutic and side-effect profiles to DES [16].

The cardiotoxicity and increase in thromboembolic events with the use of the oral oestrogens have prevented their widespread use in spite of their low cost and potentially beneficial effects on bone and lipid metabolism. However, recent studies have shown that the above toxicities of oral oestrogen are mediated by its first pass metabolism in the liver which results in an increase in synthesis of procoagulant factors such as factor VIII [17]. This has led to a resurgence in interest in the use of oestrogens in prostatic carcinoma. The parenteral administration of oestrogens such as polyoestradiol phosphate (PEP) avoids first pass metabolism and would be expected to result in diminished cardiovascular and thromboembolism related toxicity [18]. Randomized trials of PEP as an alternative to medical or surgical castration are under way in Sweden. It should be noted that oestrogens also affect platelet function and cause fluid retention, both of which contribute to cardiovascular toxicity [18].

Estramustine, a conjugate of an oestrogen with a nitrogen mustard (a DNA alkylating agent), was synthesized in an attempt to exploit the expression of oestrogen receptors in prostatic tissue [19]. In this case oestrogen was to serve as a targeting mechanism, to enable the specific release of the nitrogen mustard within the prostate. However, the conjugate cannot be degraded intracellularly, preventing the release of the nitrogen mustard moiety. Despite this, estramustine does appear to have a minor degree of anti-tumour activity in prostate cancer, which seems to be via a novel mechanism of interference with microtubule assembly and disassembly [19]. Estramustine is therefore not regarded as a form of hormonal therapy generally.

Progestational agents

The most commonly used agents in this class are medroxyprogesterone acetate, megesterol acetate and cyproterone acetate (CPA). All three act via the suppression of GnRH and LH release via hypothalamo-pituitary progesterone receptors, resulting in a reduction in testicular androgen synthesis [20]. In addition, they are also androgen receptor antagonists. In comparisons of the three agents, CPA, which is complex in its effects, is superior to the other two in terms of efficacy in first line therapy of metastatic prostate cancer [21]. Indeed, monotherapy with CPA 250 mg/day is equivalent in terms of overall survival to DES 3 mg/day in patients with locally advanced or metastatic disease [21]. CPA has been used extensively in the treatment of prostate cancer in combination with orchiectomy or a GnRH analogue. However, because of the hepato-toxicity associated with chronic CPA administration, it is no longer recommended for complete androgen blockade, or as monotherapy. Instead, CPA has gradually been replaced by the pure anti-androgens in combined androgen blockade therapy. Currently CPA is indicated for transient use to prevent 'tumour flare' associated with the GnRH analogues. CPA, like other forms of androgen deprivation, may cause a loss of libido, impotence, fatigue, depression and gynaecomastia [21].

Medroxyprogesterone acetate (MPA) has been shown in both the EORTC-30761 and VACURG trials to be inferior at both 30 mg/day and 200 mg/day (after parenteral loading) to both cyproterone acetate and diethylstilboesterol in patients who have not previously received any form of hormonal therapy [12,21]. However, MPA has also been shown to be useful in controlling hot flushes caused by medical or surgical castration.

Megesterol acetate, like CPA, also results in a reduction in plasma androgens to just above castrate levels [22]. However, over a period of 2–6 months testosterone levels gradually return to normal. Megesterol acetate has therefore been used in combination with DES 0.1 mg/day in the first line therapy of prostate cancer, with equivalent progression-free survival to orchiectomy [23]. In patients who have relapsed after castration, single agent megesterol acetate is associated with response rates of only 0–9% [6]. At a dose of 40 mg/day, however, it is successful in controlling hot flushes in over 70% of men who have been castrated [6].

All the progestogens have cardiovascular toxicity due either to direct effects on platelet function or to fluid retention because of their steroidal properties [21].

GnRH analogues

The deca-peptide sequence of GnRH was elucidated and the first GnRH analogues (GnRH-A) developed in the early 1970s [3]. Leuporelin and goserelin were derived from GnRH through the substitution of amino acids at the C-terminus and at position 6. This served to increase the affinity of the synthetic peptide for the GnRH receptor and leads to a relative resistance to enzymatic degradation by pituitary amarylidases. Other drugs licensed for use in prostate cancer in this class include buserelin and triptorelin.

When GnRH-A are administered they initially bind to hypothalamic GnRH receptors with the release of LH and follicle-stimulating hormone [3]. These peptides are not released from their binding sites and receptor down-regulation occurs with suppression of LH release and testicular androgen synthesis. Over a period of 3–4 weeks castrate levels of plasma androgens are achieved. Leuporelin and goserelin are both administered as subcutaneous injections, which are available as monthly or 3-monthly depot preparations. Six-monthly and yearly depot preparations are in development [3].

The side-effects of GnRH-A are identical to those of surgical orchiectomy: hot flushes, impotence, loss of libido, mood disturbance, anaemia and osteo-porosis [11]. A minor degree of gynaecomastia is reported. In addition, the initial stimulation of LH and testosterone release may be associated with progression of prostate cancer, known as 'tumour flare' [24]. These agents are therefore contra-indicated in patients with signs of spinal cord compression or ureteric obstruction. Tumour flare can also be associated with increased bone pain from metastases in up to 40% of patients [24]. In these circumstances the use of an anti-androgen commenced at least 3 days prior to the GnRH-A and continued for a further 3–4 weeks is recommended.

GnRH-A, as monotherapy, is equivalent to orchiectomy and DES in patients with metastatic prostatic carcinoma with respect to response rate and survival [9]. Although GnRH-As do not have the thromboembolic or cardiac side-effects of DES, they are significantly more expensive [9]. In a survey of patients who were given a choice between orchiectomy and long-term GnRH-A therapy, results were significantly in favour of medical castration [10].

GnRH antagonists are now entering clinical trial [3]. These agents have a very long development history. The initial agonists caused immune responses because the conformational change rendered them significantly structurally different from the parent peptide. Newer antagonists do not cause as significant an immune response because the structural changes are less major than in previous compounds.

The recent development of GnRH receptor antibodies and anti-GnRH receptor vaccines, which are currently in clinical trials, may enable long-term medical castration without the need for monthly or 3-monthly injections [3].

Anti-androgens

A series of non-steroidal pure competitive androgen receptor antagonists

(AR-A), flutamide, nilutamide and bicalutamide, have been developed over the past 25 years [3]. Flutamide and bicalutamide are the only two androgen receptor antagonists currently licensed in the United Kingdom.

AR-As work by competitively binding to and inhibiting the transcriptional activity of the androgen receptor in prostatic tissue. Malignant cells deprived of the growth and proliferation signals of testosterone will then undergo apoptosis. The inhibition of the pituitary and hypothalamic androgen receptors, however, results in increased LH release and testicular androgen synthesis. This, coupled with only partial antagonism of the androgen receptor, is probably responsible for their inferiority as monotherapy compared with medical or surgical castration at standard doses [9]. In addition trials of high-dose bicalutamide (150 mg/day) have shown inferior response rates in patients with metastatic disease [25]. In patients with locally advanced disease only response and survival appeared equivalent; however, the trials were of insufficient power to prove equivalence [25]. Indeed this conclusion is supported by a meta-analysis on AR-As vs. castration conducted by the Agency for Health Care Policy and Research (AHCPR), which showed a trend in favour of castration over AR-A monotherapy [9].

Flutamide, nilutamide and bicalutamide may all cause loss of libido, impotence, lethargy, mood alteration, gynaecomastia and breast tenderness [11,20]. In comparative trials with orchiectomy or GnRH-As, AR-As cause less sexual dysfunction, fewer hot flushes and less muscle wasting, but are associated with an increase in breast tenderness and gynaecomastia [25]. In addition, flutamide causes diarrhoea in approximately 10% of patients, and may occasionally be associated with fatal hepato-toxicity [26]. By contrast, nilutamide has been associated with an increased risk of interstitial pneumonitis and night blindness [27]. Bicalutamide has the highest affinity for the AR and the longest half-life of the AR-As, enabling once daily dosing. It is also associated with a lower incidence of diarrhoea than flutamide [28].

Adrenal androgen inhibitors

In the late 1940s, following the widespread use of castration, the importance of adrenal androgens was recognized, and the therapeutic benefits of bilateral adrenalectomy demonstrated by Huggins and Scott, in patients with disease relapse following orchiectomy [2]. A response rate of between 20% and 60% has been reported in various series [6]. However, the surgical morbidity associated with the procedure has prompted the use of adrenal enzyme synthesis inhibitors such as aminoglutethimide and ketoconazole to achieve a medical adrenalectomy.

Ketoconazole is an imidazole antifungal agent, which inhibits both adrenal and testicular hydroxylases and the P450 cytochrome system involved in the synthesis of androgens [6]. At a dose of 1200 mg/day a rapid reduction in plasma testosterone to castrate levels occurs within 24 h. However, long-term use of ketoconazole results in significant gastrointestinal toxicity, and testosterone suppression is transient. It may be of marginal use in patients with spinal cord compression, where rapid reduction in testosterone is required without inducing the 'flare' associated with GnRH analogues, until castration can be performed. Ketoconazole has also been used in patients who have relapsed following castration, at a lower dose of 600 mg/day, with an objective response rate of about 30%.

Aminoglutethimide inhibits adrenal and testicular hydroxylases and aromatase and thereby the synthesis of androgens [6]. However, aminoglutethimide is associated with significant nausea and vomiting, skin rashes, and thyroid dysfunction and may precipitate adrenal insufficiency. The effects of aminoglutethimide are transient. Aminoglutethimide is administered with replacement doses of hydrocortisone, and it is the steroids that are significant. Plowman *et al.* [29] showed that the inhibition of adrenal steroidogenesis achieved with hydrocortisone alone was equivalent to that achieved with combination therapy, without the associated toxicity of aminoglutethimide. Indeed, Tannock *et al.* [30] have very elegantly demonstrated the efficacy of low dose prednisolone in the palliation of androgen independent disease. In this study a symptomatic response rate of 30% was seen.

Overall response rates of 15–20% are seen in patients with relapsed disease after castration with adrenal androgen inhibition, with a median survival of up to 15–20 months in responders [6].

5α-Reductase inhibitors

Finasteride, a specific 5α-reductase inhibitor, prevents the conversion of testosterone to dihydroxytestosterone (DHT), which has a hundred-fold greater affinity for AR compared with testosterone [31]. DHT is normally the principal activator of the AR in prostatic tissue, and the use of finasteride in benign prostatic hyperplasia has been shown to result in a clinically significant reduction in prostatic tissue volume. Its efficacy in prostatic carcinoma is limited due to a compensatory increase in plasma testosterone via feedback to the hypothalamic axis, and as a single agent only a 20–25% reduction in prostate-specific antigen (PSA) is seen with doses of 10 mg/day [31]. This has stimulated studies of finasteride in combination with anti-androgens such as flutamide or GnRH-As [32,33]. Randomized controlled trials of the benefits of combination therapy with finasteride relative to castration alone are being performed.

Therapeutic strategies

Hormonal therapy only

With the utility of androgen deprivation in metastatic prostate cancer established, questions regarding the optimal strategy of androgen deprivation, duration of therapy and its efficacy in earlier stages of disease have emerged.

COMBINED ANDROGEN BLOCKADE

Orchiectomy, DES and GnRH-A as monotherapies have been shown to be equivalent in terms of disease control and survival [9]. However, in all three cases adrenal androgen synthesis remains unaffected, which may contribute to the continued growth of prostate cancer cells. This has led to the development of combined androgen blockade (CAB) or maximum androgen blockade (MAB), in which medical or surgical castration is combined with long-term administration of an anti-androgen. Several large well-conducted studies comparing the relative efficacy of CAB and monotherapy have been conducted over 15 years, with apparently conflicting results. In a recent individual patient meta-analysis of 27 randomized controlled trials by the Prostate Cancer Trialists' Collaborative Group, CAB with a non-steroidal androgen was found to provide a statistically significant 3% (95% confidence interval 0.4–5.4%) survival advantage at 5 years relative to castration alone [34]. By contrast, CAB with CPA appeared to result in a poorer outcome, with a 5-year survival of 15.4% vs. 18.1% for castration alone [34]. The clinical utility of the survival advantage with non-steroidal anti-androgens has been questioned in view of the greater toxicity of CAB due to an increased incidence of gastrointestinal side-effects and emotional fluctuation. In addition the cost of CAB, especially in combination with a GnRH, is substantially greater than of castration alone. In a recent cost-effectiveness analysis conducted by the AHCPR the cost-effectiveness threshold for CAB with a GnRH-A was estimated to be US$ 100 000 per quality adjusted life year [9]. However, despite these reservations CAB does offer a survival advantage for the patient, and a pragmatic strategy of initiating CAB with withdrawal of the anti-androgen in patients with side-effects may provide an optimization of both quality of life and survival in such patients.

INTERMITTENT ANDROGEN BLOCKADE

The significant toxicity associated with medical or surgical castration has led to the strategy of intermittent androgen blockade [35,36]. Patients treated with intermittent therapy initially undergo CAB with serial monitoring of PSA until it either plateaus or becomes undetectable. After a further defined period of CAB, androgen deprivation is discontinued and the serum PSA monitored. CAB is reinstituted when the PSA reaches a predefined level or a patient becomes symptomatic, and the cycle is repeated. This approach is supported by experimental evidence from prostate cancer cell lines in which a longer period of androgen dependence has been demonstrated with intermittent therapy compared with continuous androgen deprivation [37].

In clinical trials the success of repeated cycles of androgen deprivation has been demonstrated with treatment cycles of 70–75 weeks, an overall mean percentage time off therapy of 40–45%, and a median of 8 weeks from discontinuation of CAB to recovery of serum testosterone to normal levels [35]. However, no data demonstrating a significant benefit are currently available from the ongoing randomized controlled trials comparing intermittent therapy with continuous CAB.

SEQUENTIAL ANDROGEN DEPRIVATION

Sequential androgen deprivation is the logical opposite of CAB and is based on the use of finasteride with or without an anti-androgen initially, followed by the addition of or substitution with a GnRH-A at disease progression. This strategy has the advantage of initially preserving potency and deferral of the toxicities of castration. However, controlled trials demonstrating this benefit are required.

EARLY VS. DEFERRED THERAPY

Several trials have been performed to try to address the issue of whether androgen deprivation therapy should be instituted at diagnosis or deferred until symptoms develop in patients with prostate cancer. The rationale for deferring treatment is based on the potentially long interval from presentation to the development of symptoms in patients with prostate cancer, especially those with small volume and low grade tumours, who may die without ever becoming symptomatic. These patients, if treated 'early', would be subjected to several years of potentially harmful androgen deprivation without apparent benefit. However, delayed treatment risks the development of complications such as spinal cord or ureteric compression and also the development of androgen independent malignant cell clones.

In the first trial conducted by VACURG a significant survival advantage of adjuvant DES 1 mg/day after prostatectomy compared with prostatectomy only at presentation was demonstrated [12]. However, because of a 41% nonprostate cancer related mortality in that trial it was felt that a large number of patients treated early would not benefit from androgen deprivation.

In 1997 the first results of a randomized trial of early vs. delayed hormonal therapy in prostate cancer performed by the Medical Research Council (MRC) reported an overall survival advantage for immediate therapy with orchiectomy or GnRH-A over deferred treatment, in patients with locally advanced or metastatic prostate cancer [38]. In addition, patients with known metastatic disease in the deferred treatment arm required hormonal therapy at a median of 9 months for symptomatic progression. Moreover, the deferral of hormonal therapy was associated with a significantly increased rate of complications such as spinal cord and ureteric compression and early death in this group of patients with metastatic disease [38]. Based on these results patients who are ineligible for curative therapy such as prostatectomy, external beam radiotherapy or brachytherapy should be considered for early androgen deprivation.

However, two additional trials of early vs. deferred hormonal therapy, EORTC 30846 and 30891, are ongoing, and interim analyses of these have not yet demonstrated a significant survival advantage for early therapy [39].

CHEMOPREVENTION

The increasing incidence of prostate cancer over the last two decades and the efficacy and good toxicity profile of finasteride have led to a trial of cancer chemoprevention organized by the National Institutes of Health, USA, in which 18 000 men over the age of 55 have been randomized to finasteride or placebo [40]. Results from the trial are not expected for several years. Concern has been raised on the use of finasteride in view of its limited efficacy in prostate cancer, but in the treatment of an asymptomatic population the use of agents with significant side-effects, such as AR-As and GnRH-As, is not justified.

Neoadjuvant and adjuvant hormonal therapy

RADICAL PROSTATECTOMY

The concept of neoadjuvant hormonal therapy prior to radical prostatectomy has recently gained favour, as neoadjuvant hormonal therapy has the potential of downstaging tumours, which may facilitate radical prostatectomy and enable complete tumour excision. Several randomized trials assessing its value are under way in which patients are treated with either a GnRH-A or CAB for approximately 3 months prior to radical prostatectomy. Preliminary results from all trials so far have consistently demonstrated a reduction in the proportion of radical prostatectomies with positive margins and also complete pathological responses of approximately 6% [41,42]. Although this is encouraging, longer follow-up will be required before the impact on overall survival of neoadjuvant hormonal therapy with radical prostatectomy can be judged.

The issue of adjuvant hormonal therapy after radical prostatectomy was first addressed in the VACURG trial of radical prostatectomy in combination with DES at a dose of 0.1 mg, 1 mg or 5 mg per day or placebo for stage I or II prostate cancer [12]. This trial showed a benefit in favour of adjuvant hormonal therapy at a dose of 1 mg, but not 0.1 or 5 mg. It may be argued that the cardiotoxicity of DES and tumour under-staging may have diluted any benefit of hormonal therapy at higher doses of DES.

Similarly, Messing *et al.* [43] have demonstrated an advantage in both progression-free and overall survival for immediate orchiectomy (medical or surgical) in patients who have radical prostatectomy and are found to have node-positive cancers.

The issue of if and when to institute hormonal therapy after PSA relapse in patients who have undergone radical prostatectomy has so far not been addressed in any randomized trial. The results of the MRC trial of early vs. deferred treatment are not applicable, as patients in this group may remain asymptomatic and free of metastases for a median of 8 years and appear to have a median survival of 5 years from the development of metastatic disease [44]. Specific trials designed to answer this question are therefore required.

RADIOTHERAPY

The high incidence of positive prostate biopsies after radiotherapy and an overall 80% relapse rate at 10 years following radiotherapy have resulted in several trials over the past three decades exploring the potential benefits of adjuvant hormonal therapy and/or neoadjuvant hormonal therapy [45]. Neoadjuvant hormonal therapy, by reducing tumour volume, may facilitate radiotherapy and minimize morbidity. This benefit has indeed been confirmed for patients with large tumours due to undergo radiotherapy where prior to neoadjuvant hormonal therapy greater than a third of rectal mucosa would have had to be irradiated [46]. Following neoadjuvant hormonal therapy the smaller radiotherapy fields necessary result in a lower incidence of proctitis in these patients [46].

In addition, all trials of neoadjuvant hormonal therapy and/or adjuvant hormonal therapy with radiotherapy have demonstrated an improvement in local tumour control and progression-free survival with varying periods of hormonal therapy [9,42]. Although only two trials so far have shown a survival advantage for adjuvant hormonal therapy or neoadjuvant hormonal therapy, this may simply be a reflection of the shorter period of follow-up relative to tumour stage in some of the negative studies [9,42,47,48]. A qualitative systematic review of randomized controlled trials of adjuvant hormonal therapy or neoadjuvant hormonal therapy with radiotherapy concluded that insufficient information was available to support the value of combined hormonal therapy and radiotherapy in improving cancer specific and overall survival [49]. However, quantitative meta-analysis, performed by both the Radiation Therapy Oncology Group (RTOG) and AHCPR, confirmed a survival advantage for adjuvant hormonal therapy with radiotherapy [9,50]. The hazard ratio for 5-year overall survival in the AHCPR meta-analysis was 0.63 (95% confidence interval 0.48–0.83) in favour of adjuvant hormonal therapy [9].

ADJUVANT CHEMOTHERAPY

Adjuvant chemotherapy has been given in an attempt to improve upon remission rates and duration [51]. Treatment is tempered by the performance status, age and marrow reserve of the patients with prostate cancer. The studies in this area are few, and have used toxic agents. We have shown that adjuvant treatment with mitoxantrone has doubled survival in patients with localized prostate cancer but not metastatic disease. This demonstration, in a small randomized study, may be of significance and requires confirmation in larger randomized trials, which are currently under way in the USA.

Hormonal therapy of relapsed disease

Tumour relapse in patients initially treated by radical prostatectomy or radiotherapy alone may be treated with hormonal therapy with an overall response rate of 80% and a median duration of response of 18 months [6]. Patients whose tumours relapse after castration, however, have a poor prognosis, with an expected median survival of 8 months [6].

In patients relapsing after CAB, withdrawal of the anti-androgen is associated with a tumour response in 10–40% of cases with a median survival of 7 months, as AR-As may paradoxically simulate the androgen receptor in these tumours [52]. In patients who have received CAB and had flutamide withdrawn, treatment with 150–200 mg/day of bicalutamide may result in a significant improvement in symptoms and a PSA response [52]. Megesterol acetate following AR-A withdrawal also produces PSA responses of 12–14%, though objective response is rare. Adrenal androgen inhibition with aminoglutethimide, ketoconazole and/or low-dose corticosteroids produces objective response rates of 10–20% in this setting [6,52]. High-dose tamoxifen has also been shown to produce objective responses of 0–9% in small case series [6]. Progression following third line endocrine therapy is inevitably hormone independent, and in this setting mitoxantrone, in particular, and a number of other chemotherapeutic agents have been shown to have some efficacy [3,53].

Conclusion

Significant advances have been made in the understanding of the hormonal control of prostate cancer, yielding novel therapies. A number of questions regarding optimal hormone therapy are presently being tested in clinical trials. These are likely to extend the role of hormonal therapy beyond that of palliation of locally advanced or metastatic disease. We look to the future with hope for the development of curative treatments of this malignant condition.

References

1   Huggins C, Hodges CV. Studies on prostate cancer 1: the effect of castration, of oestrogen and of androgen injection on serum phosphatases in metastatic carcinoma of the prostate. *Cancer Res* 1941; **1**: 293–7.
2   Huggins C, Scott WW. Bilateral adrenalectomy in prostatic cancer: clinical features and urinary excretion of 17-ketosteroids and oestrogens. *Ann Surg* 1945; **122**: 1031–41.
3   Fitzpatrick JM. New developments in the pharmacological management of prostate cancer. *BJU Int* 2000; **85**: 31–7.
4   Osterling J, Fuks Z, Lee CT, Scher HI. Cancer of the prostate. In: Devita JV Jr, Hellman S, Rosenberg SA, eds. *Cancer: Principles and Practice of Oncology*, 5th edn. New York: Lippincott-Raven, 1997: 1322–86.
5   Crawford ED, Rosenblum M, Ziada AM, Lange PH. Overview: hormone refractory prostate cancer. *Urology* 1999; **54**: 1–7.
6   Oh WK, Kantoff PW. Management of hormone refractory prostate cancer: current standards and future prospects. *J Urol* 1998; **160**: 1220–9.
7   Taplin ME, Bubley GJ, Shuster TD *et al.* Mutation of the androgen-receptor gene in metastatic androgen independent prostate cancer. *N Engl J Med* 1995; **332**: 1393–8.
8   Zhao XY, Malloy PJ, Krishnan AV *et al.* Glucocorticoids can promote androgen-independent growth of prostate cancer cells through a mutated androgen receptor. *Nature Med* 2000; **6**: 703–6.
9   Agency for Health Care Policy and Research. *Relative effectiveness and cost-effectiveness of methods of androgen suppression in the treatment of advanced prostatic cancer.* Summary Evidence Report/Technology Assessment No. 4. Rockville, MD: Agency for Health Care Policy and Research, 1999.
10 Chon JK, Jacobs SC, Naslund MJ. The cost value of medical versus surgical hormonal therapy for metastatic prostate cancer. *J Urol* 2000; **164**: 735–7.
11 Schröder FH. Endocrine treatment of prostate cancer—recent developments and the future. Part 1: maximal androgen blockade, early vs. delayed endocrine treatment and side-effects. *BJU Int* 1999; **83**: 161–70.
12 Byar DP, Corle DK. Hormone therapy for prostate cancer: results of the Veterans' Administration Cooperative Urological Research Group studies. *Monogr Natl Cancer Inst* 1998; **7**: 165–70.
13 Robinson MRC, Smith PJ, Richards B, Newling DWW, de Pauw M, Sylvester R. The final analysis of the EORTC genito-urinary tract cancer co-operative group phase III clinical trial (protocol 30805) comparing orchidectomy plus Cyproterone acetate and low dose

234   *Chapter 12*

Stilboestrol in the management of metastatic carcinoma of the prostate. *Eur Urol* 1995; **28**: 272–83.

14 Bishop MC. Experience with low-dose oestrogen in the treatment of advanced prostate cancer: a personal view. *Br J Urol* 1996; **78**: 921–8.

15 Ferro MA, Gillatt D, Symes MO, Smith PJ. High-dose intravenous estrogen therapy in advanced prostatic carcinoma: use of PSA to monitor response. *Urology* 1989; **34**: 134–8.

16 Crawford ED. Hormonal therapy of prostatic carcinoma: defining the challenge. *Cancer* 1990; **66** (Suppl.): 1035–8.

17 Henriksson P, Blombäck M, Bratt G, Edhag O, Eriksson A. Activators and inhibitors of coagulation and fibrinolysis in patients with prostatic cancer treated with estrogen or orchidectomy. *Thromb Res* 1986; **44**: 783–91.

18 Henriksson P, Carlström K, Pousette A *et al*. Time for revival of estrogens in the treatment of advanced prostatic carcinoma? Pharmacokinetics, and endocrine and clinical effects of a parenteral estrogen regimen. *Prostate* 1999; **40**: 76–82.

19 Hudes GR, Greenberg R, Krigel RL *et al*. Phase II study of estramustine and vinblastine, two microtubule inhibitors, in hormone-refractory prostate cancer. *J Clin Oncol* 1992; **10**: 1754–61.

20 Mahler C, Verhelst J, Denis L. Clinical pharmacokinetics of the antiandrogens and their efficacy in prostate cancer. *Clin Pharmacokinet* 1998; **34**: 405–17.

21 Pavone-Macaluso M, de Voogt HJ, Viggiano G *et al*. Comparison of diethylstilbestrol, cyproterone acetate and medroxyprogesterone acetate in the treatment of advanced prostatic cancer: final analysis of a randomised phase III trial of the European Organisation for Research on Treatment of Cancer Urological Group. *J Urol* 1986; **136**: 624–31.

22 Geller J. Megesterol acetate plus low-dose oestrogen in the management of advanced prostatic carcinoma. *Urol Clin North Am* 1991; **18**: 83–91.

23 Johnson DE, Babaian RJ, Swanson DA, von Eshenback AC, Wishnow KI, Tenney D. Medical castration using megestrol acetate and minidose estrogen. *Urology* 1988; **31**: 371–4.

24 Waxman J, Man A, Hendry WF *et al*. Importance of early tumour exacerbation in patients treated with long acting analogues of gonadotrophin releasing hormone for advanced prostatic cancer. *Br Med J* 1985; **291**: 1387.

25 Boccardo F, Rubagotti A, Barichello M *et al*. Bicalutamide monotherapy versus flutamide plus goserelin in prostate cancer patients: results of an Italian Prostate Cancer Project Study. *J Clin Oncol* 1999; **17**: 2027–38.

26 Geller J. Overview of enzyme inhibitors and anti-androgens in prostate cancer. *J Androl* 1991; **12**: 364.

27 Janknegt RA, Abbou CC, Bartoletti R *et al*. Orchiectomy and nilutamide or placebo as treatment of metastatic prostate cancer in a multi-institutional double-blind randomised trial. *J Urol* 1993; **149**: 77.

28 Schellhammer P, Sharifi R, Block N *et al*. A controlled trial of bicalutamide versus flutamide, each in combination with luteinizing hormone-releasing hormone analogue therapy, in patients with advanced prostate cancer. *Urology* 1995; **45**: 745–52.

29 Plowman PN, Perry LA, Chard T. Androgen suppression by hydrocortisone without aminoglutethimide in orchiectomised men with prostatic cancer. *Br J Urol* 1987; **59**: 252–7.

30 Tannock I, Gospodarowicz M, Meakin W, Panzarella T, Steward L, Rider W. Treatment of metastatic prostatic cancer with low-dose prednisone: evaluation of pain and quality of life as pragmatic indices of response. *J Clin Oncol* 1989; **7**: 590–7.

31 Presti JC Jr, Fair WR, Andriole G *et al*. Multicenter, randomized, double-blind, placebo controlled study to investigate the effect of finasteride (MK906) on stage D prostate cancer. *J Urol* 1992; **148**: 1201–4.

32 Fleshner NE, Fair WR. Anti-androgenic effects of combination finasteride plus flutamide in patients with prostatic carcinoma. *Br J Urol* 1996; **78**: 907–10.

33 Kirby R, Robertson C, Turkes A *et al*. Finasteride in association with either flutamide or goserelin as combination hormonal therapy in patients with stage M1 carcinoma of the prostate gland. *Prostate* 1999; **40**: 105–14.

34 Prostate Cancer Trialists' Collaborative Group. Maximum androgen blockade in advanced prostate cancer: an overview of the randomised trials. *Lancet* 2000; **355**: 1491–8.

35 Goldenberg SL, Bruchovsky N, Gleave ME, Sullivan LD, Akakura K. Intermittent androgen suppression in the treatment of prostate cancer: a preliminary report. *Urology* 1995; **45**: 839–45.

36 Strum SB, Scholz MC, McDermed JE. Intermittent androgen deprivation in prostate cancer patients: factors predictive of prolonged time off therapy. *Oncologist* 2000; **5**: 45–52.

37 Gleave M, Bruchovsky N, Bowden M, Goldenberg SL, Sullivan LD. Intermittent androgen suppression prolongs time to androgen-independent progression in the LNCaP prostate tumor model. *J Urol* 1994; **151**: 457a.

38 The Medical Research Council Prostate Cancer Working Party Investigators Group. Immediate versus deferred treatment for advanced prostatic cancer: initial results of the Medical Research Council Trial. *Br J Urol* 1997; **79**: 226–34.

39 Eisenberger MA, Walsh PC. Early androgen deprivation for prostate cancer? *N Engl J Med* 1999; **341**: 1837–8.

40 Thompson IM, Coltman CA Jr, Crowley J. Chemoprevention of prostate cancer: the Prostate Cancer Prevention Trial. *Prostate* 1997; **33**: 217–21.

41 Vaillancourt L, Ttu B, Fradet Y *et al*. Effect of neoadjuvant endocrine therapy (combined androgen blockade) on normal prostate and prostatic carcinoma. *Am J Surg Pathol* 1996; **20**: 86–93.

42 Lee HHK, Warde P, Jewett MAS. Neoadjuvant hormonal therapy in carcinoma of the prostate. *BJU Int* 1999; **83**: 438–48.

43 Messing EM, Manola J, Sarosdy M, Wilding G, Crawford ED, Trump D. Immediate hormonal therapy compared with observation after radical prostatectomy and pelvic lymphadenectomy in men with node-positive prostate cancer. *N Engl J Med* 1999; **341**: 1781–8.

44 Gerber GS, Thisted RA, Scardino PT *et al*. Results of radical prostatectomy in men with clinically localised prostate cancer. *JAMA* 1996; **276**: 615–19.

45 Zietman AL, Prince EA, Nakfoor BM, Shipley WU. Neoadjuvant androgen suppression with radiation in the management of locally advanced adenocarcinoma of the prostate: experimental and clinical results. *Urology* 1997; **49** (Suppl. 3A): 74–83.

46 Zelefsky MJ, Harrison A. Neoadjuvant androgen ablation prior to radiotherapy for prostate cancer: reducing the potential morbidity of therapy. *Urology* 1997; **49** (Suppl. 3A): 38–45.

47 Bola M, Gonzalez D, Warde P *et al*. Improved survival in patients with locally advanced prostate cancer treated with radiotherapy and goserelin. *N Engl J Med* 1997; **337**: 295–300.

48 Granfors T, Modig H, Damber J-E, Tomic R. Combined orchiectomy and external radiotherapy versus radiotherapy alone for nonmetastatic prostate cancer with or without pelvic lymph node involvement: a prospective randomised study. *J Urol* 1998; **159**: 2000–34.

49 Vicini FA, Kini VR, Spencer W, Diokno A, Martinez AA. The role of androgen deprivation in the definitive management of clinically localised prostate cancer treated with radiation therapy. *Int J Radiat Oncol Biol Phys* 1999; **43**: 707–13.

50 Roach M, Lu J, Pilepich MV *et al*. Predicting long-term survival, and the need for hormonal

therapy: a meta-analysis of RTOG prostate cancer trials. *Int J Radiat Oncol Biol Phys* 2000; **47**: 617–27.

51   Pettaway CA, Pisters LL, Troncoso P *et al.* Neoadjuvant chemotherapy and hormonal therapy followed by radical prostatectomy: feasibility and preliminary results. *J Clin Oncol* 2000; **18**: 1050–7.

52   Kantoff PW, Small E, George DJ. Management of hormone-refractory prostate cancer. *Am Soc Clin Oncol* 1999; **18**: 1092.

53   Tannock IF, Osoba D, Stockler MR *et al.* Chemotherapy with mitoxantrone plus prednisone or prednisone alone for symptomatic hormone-resistant prostate cancer: a Canadian randomised trial with palliative end points. *J Clin Oncol* 1996; **14**: 1756–64.

13: Chemotherapy in Hormone Refractory Prostate Cancer

J. J. Knox & M. J. Moore

Introduction

Prostate cancer is the second leading cause of cancer mortality in men, accounting for an estimated 45 000 deaths annually in the USA and Canada. Hormonal therapy is the mainstay of treatment for disseminated prostate cancer, with clinical improvement seen in approximately 75% of patients treated with androgen ablation. However, all such patients will eventually become resistant to hormonal therapy. Hormone refractory prostate cancer (HRPC) is a more difficult problem, with no clear consensus about the optimal management strategy. Older studies of systemic chemotherapy demonstrated few responses and no survival benefit, leading many reviewers to conclude that it has little role in the standard management of these patients. Ongoing research includes the critical re-examination of older treatments as well as evaluating new agents and combinations. There may be cause for optimism. First these newer combinations are demonstrating greater activity against this disease in phase I/II studies than previously reported. In addition, the measurements of outcome used are more likely to translate into patient benefit. Recognition of the cost and overall burden that HRPC places on patients and society has contributed to an ongoing effort to develop newer agents that may soon change the natural history of this disease.

HRPC is characterized by a median survival of approximately 1 year with a system complex of pain from bony metastases, decreasing functional status, fatigue and bone marrow failure. Once symptoms develop most patients are significantly disabled by their disease. These patients are intolerant of aggressive cytotoxic therapies because of their age, poor performance status and limited marrow reserve. Intensive investigational therapies, studied in selected patients at a tertiary care centre, are often not suitable for the majority of those with HRPC seen in routine practice.

Definition of hormone refractory prostate cancer (HRPC)

A stringent description of HRPC would require disease progression in the presence of optimal hormonal management with castrate levels of testosterone, along with the lack of response to anti-androgen withdrawal or any other hormonal therapies. Disease progression may be demonstrated by a sequential elevation in prostate-specific antigen (PSA) levels, new or worsening metastatic lesions, or increasing symptoms related to tumour growth. In the past most patients would be identified on the basis of symptomatic progression. Recently, more asymptomatic patients are being identified on the basis of a rising PSA. The criteria used to define HRPC and the proportion of patients who are symptomatic will influence outcome in clinical studies. An apparent increase in median survival from approximately 6–9 months in older studies of chemotherapy to 10–13 months in more recent ones is probably more a reflection of differences in the population treated than of any improvements in therapy.

Supportive treatments

A number of simple measures other than chemotherapy have demonstrated benefit in HRPC. External beam radiation therapy is effective in controlling pain from bony metastases, with complete resolution of pain in approximately 40% of cases. Radioisotopes such as strontium-89 accumulate in osteoblastic metastasis and can relieve bony pain. In randomized trials there was a lower usage of analgesia and a reduced incidence of pain at new sites associated with the use of strontium-89 [1]. The main toxicity was haematological, with a 33% incidence of grade 3 thrombocytopenia.

   Low doses of corticosteroids will lead to improvements in pain and reduction in PSA in approximately 20% of patients. This improvement lasts for a median of 4 months; whether it is related to a suppression of adrenal androgens or to a non-hormonally mediated mechanism is not clear [2]. Corticosteroids have been used as the control arm in several phase III studies in HRPC. A response to the withdrawal of flutamide or other anti-androgens has been reported in 20–40% of patients on long-term treatment [3]. The mechanism may be a stimulation of an aberrant androgen receptor. Both the use of corticosteroids and an anti-androgen withdrawal response can confound interpretation of other approaches such as chemotherapy if they are instituted coincident with the start of such treatment. Most new studies of chemotherapy require an interval of not less than 4 weeks following stopping anti-androgens to control for the withdrawal response. Finally, the role of bisphosphonates in delaying the progress of bony metastases in HRPC is currently under investigation by a National Cancer Institute of Canada (NCI) randomized phase III trial completing accrual in the year 2001.

Evaluation of the response and benefits of therapy

There are some unique aspects to prostate cancer that make response to therapy difficult to assess. The most prevalent metastatic site is bone (80–90%) which is non-measurable, and thus changes are difficult to interpret. Therefore the restriction of phase II trials to the less common patients with bidimensionally measurable soft tissue and visceral lesions may not reflect the activity of the treatment in the group as a whole. Controversy exists over the use of disease stabilization as an indicator of response, since this category may be a manifestation of slow tumour growth rather than an effect of therapy. As most patients with prostate cancer have non-measurable disease, changes in serum PSA have been used as a surrogate measure of activity of treatment [4]. Reductions in PSA may represent evidence of anti-tumour activity of the treatment, although PSA may be produced by only a small component of the tumour and there have been reports of patients with falling PSA values in the setting of disease progression.

There has also been little consistency in reporting of PSA, which makes comparisons between studies difficult. The Prostate-Specific Antigen Working Group have recently published guidelines on the reporting of a PSA response [5]. They define a PSA response as a decline from pretreatment baseline of at least 50% confirmed at least 4 weeks later without clinical or radiographic evidence of progression. It is agreed that PSA changes do not meet the criteria for surrogacy in that they cannot substitute for a true endpoint of clinical benefit. However, standardization of the PSA response is necessary to help decide what agents should be investigated further in phase III trials.

Measures of patient benefit are survival, quality of life and symptom scales. Many phase III trials in HRPC have reported overall survival as a study endpoint, but few in the past have included quality of life assessments in their analyses. The comparison of survival between responders and non-responders is an invalid measure of treatment benefit [6]. Irrespective of treatment, patients with indolent disease will survive longer than those with rapid progression [7]. Changes in measurable disease are also often used as surrogates for patient benefit, on the assumption that if there is less cancer the patient will feel better. This is not necessarily valid as any benefits from a reduction in the extent of cancer may be neutralized by the toxicity of treatment. Conversely, patients may feel better without the criteria for a partial response being met.

Older studies of chemotherapy

The role of cytotoxic chemotherapy in the management of HRPC has been frequently reviewed [5,8,9]. Systemic chemotherapy, whether administered as single agents or in multidrug combinations, has not been shown to prolong survival in HRPC. Response rates of single agents vary depending on the criteria employed. For example, in two early National Prostate Cancer Project

(NPCP) trials, protocols 100 and 300, overall response rate (complete re-sponse plus partial response) for single-agent cyclophosphamide was 0% and 7%, respectively [10]. When patients with stable disease were included, the rate increased to 26% and 46%, respectively. By the same token, most of the other drugs evaluated in the treatment of HRPC, such as platinum com-pounds, anthracyclines, 5-fluorouracil, methotrexate, mitomycin C and the vinca alkaloids, produce objective overall response rates of only about 10% when given alone [9]. In two important NPCP trials carried out in the 1970s, single-agent chemotherapy was compared with standard treatment without chemotherapy [10]. The higher rate of response/stable disease on the chemo-therapy arms did not translate into any survival advantages when compared with the control arms.

No definite survival benefit has thus far been demonstrated in randomized trials comparing single vs. combination agents in HRPC, although the latter may produce higher objective response rates (and higher toxicity). This is not surprising since no cytotoxic drug has shown remarkable single-agent activity and so a dramatic effect is unlikely to occur from combination of relatively in-active drugs, unless there is clinical synergy. In a Southwest Oncology Group study, patients were randomized to receive either doxorubicin plus cyclophos-phamide in combination or hydroxyurea alone [11]. Twenty-six per cent of the patients on the combination arm and 13% on the single-agent arm had symptomatic improvements ($P = 0.048$). Among the 43 patients with measur-able disease, 32% and 4% responded to the combination and single agent, re-spectively ($P = 0.06$). No significant survival difference was observed in the 137 evaluable patients allocated to the two treatment arms. Another regimen that had been tested by several groups in phase II trials consisted of 5-fluorouracil, doxorubicin and mitomycin C (FAM) [12–14]. Although re-sponse rates as high as 48% have been reported with this combination, its use was associated with significant toxicity. Balance must be sought between the amelioration of disease-related symptoms if a treatment is successful, and the side-effects created by the treatment. It is only recently that palliative endpoints such as quality of life analyses, pain indices and analgesic scores have been formally evaluated in the clinical trials of HRPC [15].

Mitoxantrone plus prednisone

Mitoxantrone is a semi-synthetic anthracenedione with some structural simi-larities to doxorubicin (Fig. 13.1). Early studies with mitoxantrone in HRPC showed that it had modest activity using conventional response criteria but was well tolerated, with improvements in disease-related symptoms, particu-larly bone pain [16,17]. Canadian studies of mitoxantrone and low-dose prednisone broke from the usual response criteria with the approach that the

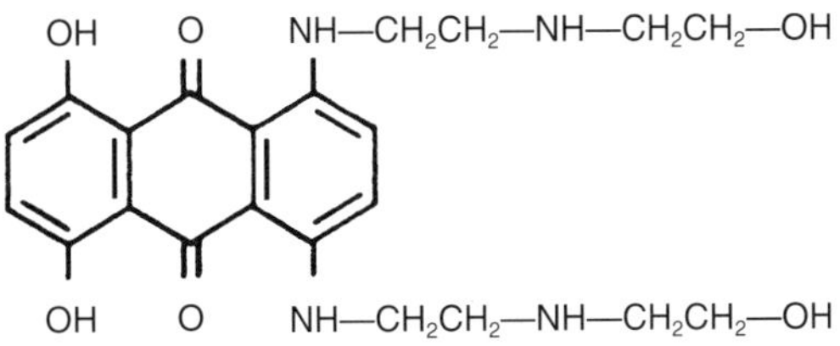

Figure 13.1 The chemical structure of mitoxantrone.

best way to measure disease palliation is to assess directly the effects of therapy on disease-related symptoms and quality of life [15,18]. As the most common symptom is pain secondary to bone metastases and most patients require narcotic analgesia, this is achieved through pain assessment, analgesic diaries and quality of life assessments done by the patient.

A multicentre phase II study of mitoxantrone plus prednisone using palliative response criteria was performed [15]. The methods of assessment used in this trial included the 'core' European Organization for Research and Treatment of Cancer (EORTC) quality of life questionnaire, a quality of life module for prostate cancer, a 6-point scale for pain assessment (PPI) and a record of analgesic intake. The primary endpoint in this trial was a 'palliative response' defined as a decrease in PPI by two or more integers with no increase in analgesic usage *or* a decrease in analgesic usage from baseline by $\geq 50\%$ without an increase in PPI. Response had to be maintained for two or more consecutive cycles.

In this study 9 of 25 evaluable men (36%) achieved a palliative response on the basis of PPI and analgesic scores. Response was maintained for an average of 4.7 courses (range 2–12). The quality of life analyses showed improvements in two dimensions (social functioning and emotional functioning) and two symptoms (pain and anorexia) from baseline. Toxicity was primarily myelosuppression, there was no serious non-haematological toxicity and no patient required hospitalizations for the treatment of febrile neutropenia.

A larger study randomizing patients between mitoxantrone plus prednisone and prednisone alone using the same palliative endpoints and quality of life analyses was then instituted. In this study by Tannock *et al.* [18], 161 patients in 11 Canadian institutions were randomized to receive mitoxantrone 12 mg/m^2 intravenously every 3 weeks plus prednisone 10 mg per day or to prednisone alone. Patients on prednisone could cross over to mitoxantrone on progression.

The results of this trial showed superior palliation from mitoxantrone plus prednisone, with an overall palliative response rate of 38% as defined by a stringent reduction in pain without an increase in analgesic medication, or by a $\geq 50\%$ reduction in analgesia without increase in pain. This compared with a palliative response rate of 21% in patients receiving prednisone alone

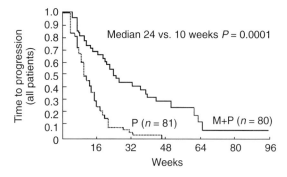

Figure 13.2 Time to symptomatic progression in patients randomized to receive prednisone alone (P) or mitoxantrone plus prednisone (M + P) (Tannock *et al.* [18]).

Table 13.1 Phase III trials of mitoxantrone plus steroids in hormone refractory prostate cancer

Reference	Therapy	No. of patients	PSA response* (%)	Pain improved (%)	Time to progression (months)	Overall survival (months)
18	Mitoxantrone + prednisone	80	44	38	6.0	12.1
	Prednisone alone	81	23	21	2.5	11.8
19	Mitoxantrone + hydrocortisone	119	38	Not reported	3.7	12.3
	Hydrocortisone alone	123	22	Not reported	2.2	12.6
20	Mitoxantrone + prednisone	56	48	N/A†	10.5	No difference
	Prednisone alone	63	24	N/A†	3.8	No difference

*Denotes ≥ 50% decline from baseline.
†All patients in this study were free of pain at baseline.

($P < 0.025$). In addition, the time to symptomatic progression in all patients was significantly greater for those receiving the chemotherapy (medians of 24 weeks vs. 10 weeks, $P < 0.0001$) (Fig. 13.2 and Table 13.1). The patients who met the criterion for palliative response also had improvements in most domains of quality of life, including highly significant improvements in overall well-being. Unfortunately, there was no significant difference in overall survival.

The trial also showed a PSA response rate (≥50% on two occasions >3 weeks apart) of 34% on mitoxantrone as compared with 23% on prednisone alone. Time to PSA progression was also delayed in patients receiving chemotherapy. Two additional phase III trials of mitoxantrone with steroids in patients with HRPC have been conducted (Table 13.1). The Cancer and Leukemia Group B (CALGB) randomized 242 patients (both symptomatic and asymptomatic) to either mitoxantrone plus hydrocortisone or to hydrocortisone alone. The results were similar to the Canadian study, with improved pain, PSA response and time to progression with chemotherapy but no impact upon overall survival [19]. The US Oncology Group conducted a similar trial in 124 asymptomatic patients and demonstrated improvements in PSA response (48 vs. 24%) and time to progression (10.5 vs. 3.8 months) without any impact on overall survival [20]. The lack of survival benefit in all these studies may be partially explained by a cross-over phenomenon in which the majority of patients received chemotherapy following progression on steroids.

Estramustine

Estramustine, composed of nornitrogen mustard and oestradiol joined via a carbamate ester linkage, produces some cytotoxic activity independent of its alkylating and hormonal constituents (Fig. 13.3) [21]. The anti-neoplastic effects of estramustine in HRPC patients are exerted through its non-covalent binding to microtubule-associated proteins (MAPs), resulting in depolymerization of formed microtubules and hence disruption of mitosis [21,22]. There is also *in vitro* and *in vivo* evidence that estramustine binds to the nuclear matrix and possibly induces cell death via disturbances in macromolecular synthesis [22].

Estramustine has been extensively tested in HRPC patients, and as a single agent its benefits are minimal [10,23–32]. The comparison of these studies, mainly from the pre-PSA era, is difficult due to the use of variable tumour response including the controversial category of stable disease as well as variable patient selection criteria [5]. In six randomized NPCP trials, only 6 of 217 HRPC patients (2.8%) achieved an objective response to single-agent estramustine [10,25–29]. No improvement in mean survival time was seen over patients who received no chemotherapy [10,25,30]. In addition, estramustine was not found to be superior to other single-agent regimens such as cisplatin, methotrexate, mitomycin C or vincristine. In two Scandinavian studies where estramustine was compared with low-dose epirubicin with or without medroxyprogesterone acetate, no difference in survival was recorded [31,32].

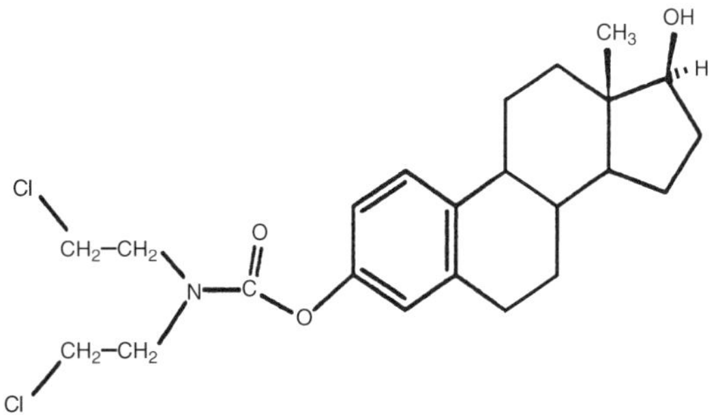

Figure 13.3 The chemical structure of estramustine.

Table 13.2 Phase II trials of estramustine combinations in hormone refractory prostate cancer

Reference	Therapy (including estramustine)	No. of patients	PSA response* (%)	OR†	Median survival (weeks)
22	Vinblastine (i.v.)	36	31	1/7	48
33		25	54	2/5	32
34		31	46	3/13	33
36	Etoposide (oral)	42	55	9/18	44
37		62	39	8/15	56
38		56	58	15/33	56
39	Vinorelbine	25	38	0/5	Not reported
40	Paclitaxel 96 h	34	53	4/9	68
41	Paclitaxel/etoposide	37	65	10/22	56
42	Docetaxel	27	62	0/3	Not reported
43	Docetaxel/hydrocortisone	40	69	9/40	?‡
44	Docetaxel short course	18	39	2/8	?

*Denotes ≥ 50% decline from baseline.
†Objective response rate (partial and complete responses of measurable disease).
‡Not yet reached.

However, one of these studies employed pain and performance scores as end-points, and found that epirubicin plus medroxyprogesterone acetate offered the best palliation. Although it did not utilize validated quality of life instruments, this study is one of few that addressed the issue of symptomatic benefit in patients.

The more recent trials of estramustine use in HRPC involve its combination with other chemotherapeutic agents, especially those which provide synergistic cytotoxicity *in vitro* (Table 13.2). The current emphasis is to determine which combinations and what schedules are worthy of evaluation in phase III trials. The initial trials evaluated the combined regimen of estramustine and vinblastine, two recognized microtubule inhibitors with distinct yet complementary molecular targets [22,33,34] (Table 13.2). The PSA response rate, defined as the percentage of patients with greater than 50% decrease in PSA for a minimum of three biweekly or monthly measurements, ranged from 31% to 54%. In these studies, partial responses were noted in 1/7 (14%), 2/5 (40%) and 3/13 (23%) of patients with bidimensionally measurable non-osseous disease. This regimen was then compared with vinblastine alone in a randomized trial of the Hoosier Oncology Group. This study by Hudes *et al.* [35] showed that the combination was superior for time to progression (3.7 months vs. 2.2 months, $P < 0.001$) and for a significant PSA response (25.2% vs. 3.2%, $P < 0.001$). Overall survival was the primary endpoint; however, the study was underpowered to detect modest improvements and failed to do so. Quality of life measures were included, but compliance with these measures was too poor to draw any meaningful conclusions. Toxicity included considerable nausea in the combined arm while the expected granulo-cytopenia was surprisingly worse in the vinblastine alone arm.

Given the results of this trial estramustine/vinblastine has not been adopted routinely for HRPC, and studies continue to find a more active and less toxic treatment. It is also notable that the PSA response rate for this regimen in a multicentre randomized trial was much lower than that originally reported. This study, as well as the subsequent phase III suramin trial, demonstrates that promising results in a phase II study need confirmation in larger studies before such therapies are routinely adopted. Subsequent phase III trials of estramustine combinations will need meaningful quality of life measures as well as the power to detect potentially modest but important improvements in survival.

A series of phase II studies have examined estramustine in combination with oral etoposide [36–38] (Table 13.2). Both objective and PSA responses were approximately 50%. Considerable nausea was seen despite attempts to test progressively lower doses of estramustine. Owing to concerns about the toxicity of this combination, these regimens have not been tested in phase III studies.

A number of other studies have combined estramustine with other plant alkaloids such as vinorelbine, paclitaxel and docetaxel [39–44] (Table 13.2). In phase II trials these also appear to be active combinations, with PSA responses in the 40–60% range and objective responses about 25%. The combination of intermittent estramustine and docetaxel [43] is attractive, based on its convenient schedule and low side-effect profile. It is this combination which has been advanced to a phase III trial where it is being compared with the current standard of mitoxantrone and prednisone and should address the question of superiority.

This study, being undertaken by the Southwest Oncology Group (SWOG 9916), is comparing estramustine, docetaxel and dexamethasone with mitoxantrone and prednisone as first or second line therapy for HRPC [45]. Each arm will accrue about 300 patients with a power to detect a 33% increase in median survival. Other endpoints include time to progression, PSA response, toxicity and quality of life. The quality of life measures are intended to duplicate the standard set by Tannock and colleagues in the previous randomized trial of mitoxantrone.

There is also some question regarding the actual contribution made by estramustine in combinations for treating HRPC. Docetaxel as a single agent shows activity in this disease comparable to the combination. A phase II trial showed PSA responses of 46%, and 7 of 35 evaluable patients had partial responses (20%) [46]. Docetaxel plus prednisone in two dosing schedules is being compared with mitoxantrone plus prednisone in a large international study planned to open in the year 2001. Endpoints will be survival (powered to detect a 33% improvement), palliation and quality of life.

Suramin

Suramin is a polysulphonated naphthylurea originally synthesized 80 years ago and used as a treatment for a variety of parasitic diseases. In the 1980s suramin was noted to have inhibitory effects on the binding of a variety of autocrine growth factors, including platelet-derived growth factor (PDGF), fibroblast-derived growth factor (FGF) and transforming growth factor-β (TGF-β). It was also noted to have cytotoxic activity against human prostatic cell lines *in vitro*. Subsequently it has been shown to have a wider range of effects including inhibition of binding of other growth factors, inhibition of DNA polymerase, protein kinase C and topoisomerase II, and inhibition of angiogenesis [47]. Which of this plethora of effects is responsible for the cytotoxic activity remains unclear.

The original clinical trial of suramin done at the NCI did demonstrate some evidence of activity against HRPC [48]. However, it also demonstrated an impressive range of side-effects, the most troublesome of which was a Guillain Barre type sensory-motor polyneuropathy which appeared to be related to variable plasma concentrations of suramin. Subsequent studies of suramin all included extensive plasma pharmacokinetic monitoring to establish a safe schedule. Differences of opinion existed about the relative merits of suramin in HRPC. The most promising data were from a study by Eisenberger *et al.* [49] which demonstrated objective responses in 6 of 12 patients with measurable disease, a reduction in PSA by 50% in (24/31) 77% and by 75% in (17/31) 55%. The duration of response was notable, with several lasting longer than 1 year. However, suramin is known to inhibit PSA release and 9 of the 24 patients with a PSA decrease of >50% had evidence of disease progression during therapy. In addition, treatment was discontinued in 28 of 35 (80%) because of dose-limiting toxicity that was primarily a syndrome of fatigue, malaise and lethargy. Suramin suppresses adrenocortical function and is therefore given in conjunction with hydrocortisone. The concomitant use of corticosteroids and that of anti-androgen withdrawal have made it difficult to establish the true responses attributed to suramin. In another study patients received suramin only after documented progression following anti-androgen withdrawal and the use of corticosteroids [50]. In this case minimal activity was seen, with no responses in patients with measurable disease, and only 5 of 28 (18%) having a reduction of PSA of >50%.

The question of suramin's activity and benefit in prostate cancer is addressed in ongoing and recently reported large phase III trials. A large double-blind, multicentre trial completed in the USA and Canada randomized symptomatic patients with HRPC between suramin given by a fixed intravenous injection schedule over 11 weeks plus hydrocortisone and hydrocortisone alone [51]. The primary endpoint was patient-derived measures of palliation using pain scales and opioid use while controlling for confounders such as anti-androgen withdrawal, steroid use and placebo. A total of 458 patients were randomized. A pain response was achieved in a higher proportion of patients receiving suramin than placebo (43% vs. 28%, $P = 0.001$) and duration of response was greater for suramin responders (median 240 vs. 69 days, $P = 0.0027$). No survival advantage was seen, although the cross-over design may prevent such a determination. Measurable disease response was documented in <4% of the suramin-treated patients (3/76 vs. 0/80). PSA responses were reported as 33% vs. 16% ($P = 0.01$) favouring the suramin arm.

Interpretation of a PSA response with suramin is complex; this phase III response rate is considerably less than the more than 70% PSA response reported in some phase II studies [49]. Validated quality of life measures were quite similar in both arms despite somewhat worse toxicity and more adverse events in the suramin arm. Toxicities were primarily mild to moderate in intensity and similar in both arms except for increased incidence of rash with suramin (57% vs. 13%). Neurological, renal, hepatic and coagulation complications were rare. Overall, this trial demonstrates that this particular suramin regimen provides a modest pain palliation, but with no overall impact on quality of life. A subsequent randomized study of three different dose levels of suramin was done by the CALGB [52]. This showed PSA response rates of less than 20% on all three arms, with considerable toxicity. Owing to the poor activity seen in randomized trials, as well as the toxicity and inconvenience, suramin will not enter into significant clinical use.

Novel targets for therapy

In recent years there has been a tremendous increase in the development of biological targets for cancer therapy. Given the relative insensitivity of prostate cancer to cytotoxic agents, this area holds much potential. Various types of gene therapy and immune therapy based on antigen-presenting cells are under evaluation in laboratory models and early phase trials. Similarly, anti-angiogenesis therapies, differentiation therapies, pro-apoptotic therapies, cell signalling inhibitors and matrix metalloproteinase inhibitors are under early investigation in a number of tumour sites including HRPC. While the clinical impact of all these approaches has been minimal to date, the appropriate clinical settings and combinations in which to use these agents remain an area of active research.

The anti-apoptotic protein product of Bcl-2 is overexpressed in androgen-independent human cancer specimens [53]. Agents such as antisense oligonucleotides, small molecules or specific enzymes designed to specifically inactivate Bcl-2 are currently in preclinical studies. Another area of study involves the role of p53 mutations in allowing the metastatic, hormone refractory phenotype. Overcoming this block to apoptosis may be achieved through a number of pathways currently being worked out in preclinical studies. There is also evidence that hormonal regulation of prostate cancer cells is linked to changes in epidermal growth factor receptors. Erb2(Her-2/neu) is one member of this family of receptors that may be disregulated in HRPC. The Her-2/neu antibody, herceptin, is marketed for use in metastatic breast cancer either alone or in combination with chemotherapy. Whether this agent would also be therapeutic in prostate cancer remains a question of investigation.

Chemotherapy in earlier stage prostate cancer

The clinical use of chemotherapy in prostate cancer is currently restricted to patients with hormone refractory disease. However, there is an increased interest in studying the benefits of chemotherapy earlier in the course of the illness. This has been stimulated by results in other tumours such as breast and colorectal cancer where the benefits of chemotherapy have been greatest when used as adjuvant therapy in the setting of clinically localized disease. To date the only data available are from older studies where the chemotherapy used may not have been optimal, the follow-up was short and the sample size did not provide sufficient power to detect modest differences in outcome. There is an older study of adjuvant cyclophosphamide for locally advanced prostate cancer carried out by the NPCP which showed no survival benefit [54]. The anti-tumour activity of a regimen like mitoxantrone plus prednisone has a comparable level of activity against HRPC as does 5-FU plus leucovorin against advanced colorectal cancer. When used in the adjuvant setting following removal of a primary colon tumour 5-FU plus leucovorin will reduce relapse rates by about 30% and improve overall survival.

Recently, two very large phase III studies examining the role of chemotherapy in earlier stage prostate cancer have been opened. The Southwest Oncology Group will randomize 1360 patients with defined high risk characteristics following radical prostatectomy to either androgen therapy for 2 years or androgen therapy plus six cycles of mitoxantrone plus prednisone. The Radiation Therapy Oncology Group will randomize 1440 patients to receive either radiotherapy plus hormones or the same regimen plus four cycles of estramustine, paclitaxel and oral etoposide. Both studies have sufficient power to detect a 15–20% improvement in median or 5-year survival, although it will be at least 10 years until results are sufficiently mature to answer this question.

Conclusion

It is reasonable to conclude that there is a role for chemotherapy in the management of hormone refractory prostate cancer. Studies have demonstrated that mitoxantrone plus prednisone is a useful palliative therapy that provides improvements in pain and quality of life for approximately 40% of those treated. Other promising regimens such as the estramustine combinations or docetaxel are currently undergoing further testing in randomized trials. It will be important to see if they can show superiority to mitoxantrone and prednisone and be the first chemotherapy treatments to impact on survival in HRPC. There is a general increase in investigation into understanding the mechanisms of hormonal resistance and in developing more novel strategies to prevent or treat this problem. These should eventually translate into better systemic therapies for the treatment of this difficult problem.

References

1 Porter AD, McEwan AJB, Powe JE *et al*. Results of a randomized phase III trial to evaluate the efficacy of strontium[89] adjuvant to external beam irradiation in the management of endocrine resistant metastatic prostate cancer. *Int J Radiation Oncol Biol Phys* 1993; **25**: 805–13.

2 Tannock IF, Gospodarowicz M, Meakin W *et al*. Treatment of metastatic prostate cancer with low dose prednisone: evaluation of pain and quality of life as pragmatic indices of response. *J Clin Oncol* 1989; **7**: 590–7.

3 Scher HI, Kelly WK. Flutamide withdrawal syndrome: its impact on clinical trials in hormone resistant prostate cancer. *J Clin Oncol* 1993; **11**: 1566–72.

4 Kelly WK, Scher HI, Mazumdar M *et al*. Prostate-specific antigen as a measure of disease outcome in metastatic hormone-refractory prostate cancer. *J Clin Oncol* 1993; **11**: 607–15.

5 Bubley GJ, Carducci M, Dahut W *et al*. Eligibility and response guidelines for phase II clinical trials in androgen-independent prostate cancer: recommendations from the Prostate-Specific Antigen Working Group. *J Clin Oncol* 1999; **17**: 3461–7.

6 Anderson JR, Cain KC, Gelber RD. Analysis of survival by tumour response. *J Clin Oncol* 1983; **1**: 710–19.

7 Tannock IF. Is there evidence that chemotherapy is of benefit to patients with carcinoma of the prostate? *J Clin Oncol* 1985; **3**: 1013–21.

8 Eisenberger MA, Simon R, O'Dwyer PJ *et al*. A reevaluation of nonhormonal cytotoxic chemotherapy in the treatment of prostatic carcinoma. *J Clin Oncol* 1985; **3**: 827–41.

9 Kreis W. Current chemotherapy and future directions in research for the treatment of advanced hormone-refractory prostate cancer. *Cancer Invest* 1995; **13**: 296–312.

10 Schmidt JD, Scott WW, Gibbons R *et al*. Chemotherapy programs of the national prostate cancer project (NPCP). *Cancer* 1980; **45**: 1937–46.

11 Stephens RL, Vaughn C, Lane M *et al*. Adriamycin and cyclophosphamide versus hydroxyurea in advanced prostate cancer. *Cancer* 1984; **53**: 406–10.

12 Logothetis CJ, Samuels ML, von Eschenbach AC *et al.* Doxorubicin, mitomycin-C, and 5-fluorouracil (DMF) in the treatment of metastatic hormonal refractory adenocarcinoma of the prostate, with a note on the staging of metastatic prostate cancer. *J Clin Oncol* 1983; **1**: 368–79.

13 Blumenstein B, Crawford ED, Saiers JH *et al.* Doxorubicin, mitomycin C and 5-fluorouracil in the treatment of hormone refractory adenocarcinoma of the prostate: a SWOG study. *J Urol* 1993; **150**: 411–13.

14 Laurie JA, Hahn RG, Therneau TM *et al.* Chemotherapy for hormonally refractory advanced prostate carcinoma. *Cancer* 1992; **69**: 1440–4.

15 Moore MJ, Osoba D, Murphy K *et al.* Use of palliative end points to evaluate the effects of mitoxantrone and low-dose prednisone in patients with hormonally resistant prostate cancer. *J Clin Oncol* 1994; **12**: 689–94.

16 Osborne CK, Drelichman A, Von Hoff D *et al.* Mitoxantrone: modest activity in a phase II trial in advanced prostate cancer. *Cancer Treat Rep* 1983; **67**: 1133–5.

17 Raghavan D, Bishop J, Woods J *et al.* Mitoxantrone, a non-toxic, moderately active agent for hormone resistant prostate cancer. *Proc Am Soc Clin Oncol* 1986; **5**: 102.

18 Tannock IF, Osoba D, Stockler M *et al.* Chemotherapy with mitoxantrone plus prednisone or prednisone alone of symptomatic hormone-resistant prostate cancer: a Canadian randomized trial with palliative endpoints. *J Clin Oncol* 1996; **14**: 1756–64.

19 Kantoff PW, Halabi S, Conaway M *et al.* Hydrocortisone with or without mitoxantrone in hormone-refractory prostate cancer: results of the cancer and leukemia group B 9182 study. *J Clin Oncol* 1999; **17**: 2506–13.

20 Gregurich MA. Phase III study of mitoxantrone/low-dose prednisone vs low-dose prednisone alone in patients with asymptomatic hormone-refractory carcinoma of the prostate. *Proc Am Soc Clin Oncol* 2000; **19**: 336 (Abstract 1321).

21 Sheridan VR, Tew KD. Mechanism based chemotherapy for prostate cancer. *Cancer Surveys* 1991; **2**: 239–54.

22 Hudes GR, Greenberg R, Krigel RL *et al.* Phase II study of estramustine and vinblastine, two microtubule inhibitors, in hormone-refractory prostate cancer. *J Clin Oncol* 1992; **10**: 1754–61.

23 Pienta KJ, Redman B, Hussain M *et al.* Phase II evaluation of oral estramustine and oral etoposide in hormone-refractory adenocarcinoma of the prostate. *J Clin Oncol* 1994; **12**: 2005–12.

24 Loening SA, Beckley S, Brady MF *et al.* Comparison of estramustine phosphate, methotrexate and cis-platinum in patients with advanced, hormone refractory prostate cancer. *J Urol* 1983; **129**: 1001–6.

25 Murphy GP, Gibbons RP, Johnson DE *et al.* A comparison of estramustine phosphate and streptozotocin in patients with advanced prostatic carcinoma who have had extensive irradiation. *J Urol* 1977; **118**: 288–91.

26 Murphy GP, Gibbons RP, Johnson DE *et al.* The use of estramustine and prednimustine versus prednimustine alone in advanced metastatic prostatic cancer patients who have received prior irradiation. *J Urol* 1979; **121**: 763–5.

27 Soloway MS, DeKernion JB, Gibbons RP *et al.* Comparison of estramustine phosphate and vincristine alone or in combination for patients with advanced, hormone refractory, previously irradiated carcinoma of the prostate. *J Urol* 1981; **125**: 664–7.

28 Soloway MS, Beckley S, Brady MF *et al.* A comparison of estramustine phosphate versus cis-platinum alone versus estramustine phosphate plus cis-platinum in patients with advanced hormone refractory prostate cancer who had had extensive irradiation to the pelvis or lumbosacral area. *J Urol* 1983; **129**: 56–61.

29 DeKernion JN, Murphy GP, Priore R. Comparison of flutamide and emcyt in hormone-refractory metastatic prostatic cancer. *Urology* 1988; **31**: 312–17.

30 Newling DWW, Fossa SD, Tunn UW *et al*. Mitomycin C versus estramustine in the treatment of hormone resistant metastatic prostate cancer: the final analysis of the European Organization for Research and Treatment of Cancer, genitourinary group prospective randomized phase III study (30865). *J Urol* 1993; **150**: 1840–4.

31 Tveter KJ, Hagen S, Holme I *et al*. A randomized study on hormone-resistant prostatic cancer: estramustine phosphate versus low dose epirubicin with or without medroxyprogesterone acetate. *Scand J Urol Nephrol* 1990; **24**: 243–7.

32 Anderstrom C, Eddeland A, Folmerz P *et al*. Epirubicin and medroxyprogesterone acetate versus estramustine phosphate in hormone-resistant prostatic cancer: a prospective randomized study. *Eur Urol* 1995; **27**: 301–5.

33 Seidman AD, Scher HI, Petrylak D *et al*. Estramustine and vinblastine: use of prostatic specific antigen as a clinical trial end point for hormone refractory prostatic cancer. *J Urol* 1992; **147**: 931–4.

34 Amato RJ, Ellerhorst J, Bui C *et al*. Estramustine and vinblastine for patients with progressive androgen-independent adenocarcinoma of the prostate. *Urol Oncol* 1995; **1**: 168–72.

35 Hudes G, Einhorn L, Ross E *et al*. Vinblastine versus vinblastine plus oral estramustine phosphate for patients with hormone-refractory prostate cancer: a Hoosier Oncology Group and Fox Chase Network phase III trial. *J Clin Oncol* 1999; **17**: 3160–6.

36 Pienta KJ, Flaherty LE, Hussain M *et al*. Report of an extended phase II trial of oral estramustine and oral etoposide in the treatment of hormone refractory prostate cancer patients. *Proc Am Soc Clin Oncol* 1996; **15**: 261 (Abstract 681).

37 Pienta KJ, Redman BC, Bandekar R *et al*. A phase II trial of oral estramustine and oral etoposide in hormone refractory prostate cancer. *Urology* 1997; **50**: 401–7.

38 Dimopoulos MA, Panopoulos C, Bamia C *et al*. Oral estramustine and oral etoposide for hormone refractory prostate cancer. *Urology* 1997; **50**: 754–8.

39 Carles J, Domenech M, Gelabert-Mas A *et al*. Phase II study of estramustine and vinorelbine in hormone refractory prostate carcinoma patients. *Acta Oncol* 1998; **37**: 187–91.

40 Hudes GH, Nathan F, Khater C *et al*. Phase II trial of 96-hour paclitaxel plus oral estramustine phosphate in metastatic hormone refractory prostate cancer. *J Clin Oncol* 1997; **15**: 3156–63.

41 Smith DC, Esper P, Strawderman M *et al*. Phase II trial of oral estramustine, oral etoposide and IV paclitaxel in hormone refractory prostate cancer. *J Clin Oncol* 1999; **17**: 1664–71.

42 Petrylak DP, Macarthur R, O'Connor J *et al*. Phase I/II studies of docetaxel combined with estramustine in men with hormone refractory prostate cancer. *Semin Oncol* 1999; **26**: 28–33.

43 Savarese D, Taplin ME, Halabi S *et al*. A phase II study of docetaxel, estramustine and low-dose hydrocortisone in men with hormone refractory prostate cancer: preliminary results of cancer and leukemia group B trial 9780. *Semin Oncol* 1999; **26**: 39–44.

44 Sinibaldi VJ, Carducci M, Laufer M *et al*. Preliminary evaluation of a short course of estramustine phosphate and docetaxel in the treatment of hormone refractory prostate cancer. *Semin Oncol* 1999; **26**: 45–8.

45 Hussain M, Petrylak D, Fisher E *et al*. Docetaxel and estramustine versus mitoxantrone and prednisone for HRPC: scientific basis and design of Southwest Oncology Group study 9916. *Semin Oncol* 1999; **26**: 55–60.

46 Picus J, Schultz M. Docetaxel (Taxotere) as monotherapy in the treatment of HRPC: preliminary results. *Semin Oncol* 1999; **26**: 14–18.

47 Takano S, Gately S, Neville ME *et al*. Suramin, anticancer and angiosuppressive agent, inhibits endothelial cell binding of basic fibroblast growth factor, migration, proliferation and induction of urokinase-type plasminogen activator. *Cancer Res* 1994; **54**: 2654–60.

48   Myers C, Cooper M, Stein C *et al*. Suramin: a novel growth factor antagonist with activity in hormone refractory metastatic prostate cancer. *J Clin Oncol* 1992; **10**: 881–9.

49   Eisenberger MA, Reyno LM, Jodrell DI *et al*. Suramin, an active drug for prostate cancer: interim observations in a phase I trial. *J Natl Cancer Inst* 1993; **85**: 611–21.

50   Kelly WK, Curley T, Leibertz C *et al*. Prospective evaluation of hydrocortisone and suramin in patients with androgen-independent prostate cancer. *J Clin Oncol* 1995; **13**: 2208–13.

51   Small EJ, Meyer M, Marshall ME *et al*. Suramin therapy for patients with symptomatic hormone-refractory prostate cancer: results of a randomized phase III trial comparing suramin plus hydrocortisone to placebo plus hydrocortisone. *J Clin Oncol* 2000; **18**: 1440–54.

52   Small RH, Ansari G, Wilding DP *et al*. Results of CALGB 9480, a phase III trial of 3 different doses of suramin for the treatment of hormone refractory prostate cancer (HRPC). *Proc Am Soc Clin Oncol* 2000; **19**: 328 (Abstract 1291).

53   McDonnel TJ, Navone NM, Troncoso P *et al*. Expression of bcl-2 oncoprotein and p-53 protein accumulation in bone marrow metastases of androgen independent prostate cancer. *J Urol* 1997; **157**: 569–74.

54   Schmidt JD, Gibbons RP, Murphy GP *et al*. Adjuvant therapy for clinical localised prostate cancer treated with surgery or irradiation. *Eur Urol* 1996; **29**: 425–33.

14: Radical Prostatectomy

T. J. Christmas & A. P. Doherty

Introduction

An increase in public awareness of prostate cancer, coupled with screening for prostate cancer by digital rectal examination and measurement of serum prostate specific antigen (PSA) in at risk men over the last 10–15 years, have enabled urologists to identify more men with clinically localized prostate cancer. However, the benefits of screening for prostate cancer are not yet proven and early detection of clinically insignificant (Gleason 1 + 1 tumours) and low stage prostate cancer in elderly men, in whom the disease is most prevalent, would not be likely to reduce mortality from the disease. The death rate from prostate cancer remains high on both sides of the Atlantic although the treatment strategies have been very different. There is now increasing evidence that the large numbers of radical prostatectomies performed in the USA over the last 15 years are beginning to have an impact, and a stepwise reduction in the death rate from prostate cancer has become apparent over the last 5 years [1]. The same phenomenon should be occurring in European countries but data collection deficiencies may be hampering its demonstration.

It is important to carefully assess each individual patient with prostate cancer before deciding on the most appropriate therapy. Many men die with prostate cancer rather than from prostate cancer. Cure for prostate cancer by radical prostatectomy is feasible, but we have to identify the individuals for whom this procedure is appropriate and necessary.

Patient selection for radical prostatectomy

There is no international consensus on the criteria for selecting patients for radical prostatectomy, although this would be desirable. Conservative management of some men with well-differentiated adenocarcinoma of the prostate has been shown to be a safe policy providing that they are kept under surveillance [2]. In Scandinavia, where conservative therapy has been the norm for clinically localized prostate cancer, a study of the long-term survival after treatment with non-curative intent in 301 men with localized prostate cancer showed that 50% died of prostate cancer. Eighty-two per cent of those diagnosed at age 60 years or less died of prostate cancer whilst only about a quarter of men over 80 years suffered the same fate [3]. The background data provided by studies of conservative management of localized prostate cancer have aided the construction of guidelines for the selection of patients for radical prostatectomy. Inevitably there are some urologists who are proactive whilst others, particularly in the United Kingdom, have sustained a nihilistic policy and regard radical prostatectomy as an 'unnecessary operation with serious complications performed by surgeons purely for pecuniary gain' [4]. Some would argue that in the hands of such nihilists, who have advocated radiotherapy for various urological cancers when surgery is clearly the best option, surgical technical ineptitude has driven the decision making process. All patients should be offered the best and most appropriate treatment for their prostate cancer even if this necessitates transfer to another urologist capable of delivering the treatment.

At the Charing Cross Hospital we have adopted a protocol for selecting men for radical retropubic prostatectomy. A confirmed histological diagnosis of prostate cancer from biopsies of Gleason grade 2+2 or more is mandatory. The tumour should be clinically localized stage T1–2 staged by trans-rectal ultrasound, CT and/or MR scan. Evidence of metastatic disease within bone, lymph nodes or other sites is an absolute contraindication for surgery. The patient should have a life expectancy of 10 years or more and have no serious co-morbidity such as a history of significant myocardial ischaemia or stroke. There should be no other surgical contraindications. Jehovah's Witnesses who refuse blood transfusion are accepted for surgery. Written informed consent describes all possible surgical complications.

Radical retropubic prostatectomy

Surgical technique

We admit patients to hospital the afternoon before their surgery for preoperative investigations such as chest X-ray and electrocardiograph and to cross match two units of blood. On the morning of surgery the patient is given a suppository, fitted with thigh length anti-thrombo-embolism stockings and given a subcutaneous injection of 5000 units of heparin. Antibiotic prophylaxis with a third-generation cephalosporine is commenced at the time of anaesthetic induction.

After induction of general anaesthesia the patient is placed in a supine position and the operating table broken to hyperextend the patient at the level of the pelvic brim. An 18 French urethral catheter is inserted with 20 mL in the balloon. We prefer a midline incision extending from the pubis to the umbilicus. The rectus abdominis muscle is split and the pelvis entered without opening the peritoneal cavity. A self-retaining retractor facilitates excellent exposure to the pelvis.

The first step is to perform bilateral iliac lymphadenectomy. The group of lymph nodes that lie in the space bordered by the external iliac vein, obturator nerve and vessels, internal iliac artery and the obturator internus muscle are removed *en bloc* from each side and the lymphatic vessels sealed with ligaclips. If macroscopic examination of the lymph nodes raises the possibility of the presence of metastases then the nodes are sent for frozen section examination. Frozen section examination of the lymph nodes is often considered if the pre-operative PSA is greater than 25 ng/mL. If frozen section reveals metastases within the nodes then the surgical procedure is abandoned.

The next step in radical retropubic prostatectomy is to open the endopelvic fascia on both sides to release the prostate from its lateral connections to the musculature of the pelvic floor. The prostate is fixed to the pubis by two pubo-prostatic ligaments, and after division of these the dorsal venous complex of Santorini is exposed. A right-angled clamp is used to tunnel a space between the venous complex and the urethra and two ligatures are used to secure the venous complex before its division. Next, a surgical plane is created between the prostate apices and the distal striated urethral sphincter mechanism. The anterior wall of the urethra is incised to expose the urethral catheter, which is then clamped and divided. The catheter is used to retract the prostate in a cephalad direction. At the urethral resection margin the veru montanum should be apparent. Next the posterior urethra is divided at the level of the veru montanum to expose the underlying recto-urethralis muscle, which is usually divided to expose the anterior wall of the rectum. In most patients it is possible to preserve the neurovascular bundles that lie in the groove between prostate and rectum which have been shown to be important for erectile function [5]. Division of one or both of the neurovascular bundles may lead to erectile dysfunction [6]. Careful dissection of the lateral apices should reveal the neurovascular bundles, and they are preserved while the prostate is dissected from the rectum. The lateral pedicles are divided after application of ligaclips. As the prostate is retracted the ampullary parts of the vas deferens and the seminal vesicles are exposed.

The next stage of the operation is the bladder neck dissection. Most surgeons choose to preserve the circular muscle fibres of the bladder neck—the so-called bladder neck preservation technique—although this may not be practical in patients who have previously undergone trans-urethral resection of the prostate (TURP). There is good evidence that preservation of the bladder neck during radical prostatectomy improves continence and reduces the risk of strictures without compromising cancer cure [7]. The anterior bladder neck is divided just proximal to the prostate and a bladder neck spreader inserted. Then the posterior bladder neck is divided; at this point care should be taken to avoid damage to the ureteric orifices, which may be difficult after a prior TURP. Division of the entire bladder neck will expose the upper ampullary parts of the vasa and the seminal vesicles. The remaining lateral pedicles are clipped and divided to leave the prostate attached to just the vasa and seminal vesicles. The vasa are clipped and divided and the seminal vesicles dissected free. Care should be taken to avoid damage to the autonomic ganglia at the tip of the seminal vesicles since these give rise to the nervi erigentes. After removal of the prostate the pelvis should be washed out with water to destroy any free malignant cells that might have been released from the prostate.

The next step in the operation is to reconstruct the bladder neck. The techniques for this have been modified over the years to prevent postoperative complications. Eversion of the bladder mucosa at the bladder neck has been shown to reduce the risk of subsequent anastomotic stricture [8]. We use six 3-0 Monocryl sutures to evert the bladder mucosa. After mucosal eversion the bladder neck is reconstructed so that it is the same diameter as the urethra. There are several different techniques for bladder neck reconstruction but we favour a technique that plicates a triangle of detrusor muscle postero-laterally on each side. The 2-0 Monocryl continuous suture used for this aids haemostasis and re-enforces the detrusor muscle at the bladder neck. It is important to create a leak-proof anastomosis at the bladder neck since urinary leakage can lead to scarring and subsequent anastomotic stricture [8].

A new urethral catheter is inserted after lubrication with gel. We favour a 20-French Simplastic catheter with a whistle-tip since it is very unlikely to block with blood clots by virtue of its high internal to external diameter ratio. A suture is placed through the eye of the catheter to allow manoeuvre of the catheter in and out of the sphincter whilst constructing the anastomosis. Six 3-0 Monocryl sutures on 26-mm-diameter round-bodied needles are utilized for the anastomosis. These are initially placed and clipped but not tied. The posterior middle suture is first inserted and should be placed through the distal remnant of the recto-urethralis muscle, the striated sphincter and the veru montanum. Care must be applied when placing the two postero-lateral sutures to avoid incorporating the neuro-vascular bundles; however, a large bite including the striated sphincter and the pelvic floor muscles is recommended. After insertion of the three posterior anastomotic sutures the catheter is placed in the bladder and 20 mL of saline inserted into the balloon. The final three anterior sutures should be inserted through the sphincter and stump of the dorsal venous plexus. The bladder is then parachuted down onto the sphincter and all six sutures tied, starting with the back middle suture. All the knots should end up on the outside of the anastomosis.

The catheter is flushed to ensure free drainage and a Yeates drain placed in the pelvis. The wound is closed with 1 PDS, 2-0 Vicryl and skin staples.

Post-operative care

Most patients are able to tolerate normal oral intake within 48 h of surgery. We start to shorten the Yeates drain at 48 h and remove it on the fifth post-operative day. Antibiotics are continued for 72 h. We remove the urethral catheter at 7 days providing the drain site is dry. However, in many centres the catheter is left for 2 weeks. After catheter removal pelvic floor exercises are commenced. Heparin is discontinued on the eighth day when most patients are discharged home.

Perineal prostatectomy

A few surgeons prefer a perineal approach for radical prostatectomy. The patient is placed in an exaggerated lithotomy position and the prostate is approached through an inverted U incision just anterior to the anus. Although the postoperative recovery is quicker with the perineal approach than the retropubic approach there are no other advantages. Long-term results of perineal prostatectomy carried out by experts are undoubtedly excellent. Iselin and colleagues [9] have reported the results in 1242 men over a 20-year period. However, synchronous pelvic lymphadenectomy is not possible through the perineum, and doubts have been expressed regarding the ability to perform a truly radical operation through the perineum. Furthermore, in a retrospective study of 94 men who underwent radical prostatectomy via the retropubic ($n = 46$) or perineal ($n = 48$) routes, there was a significantly greater risk of capsular incisions, surgically induced positive margins and biochemical (PSA) failure in the perineal group, in spite of the fact that the risk factors in the two groups were comparable [10]. Radical perineal prostatectomy has remained popular in a few centres but should be reserved for men with small centrally placed tumours and a low PSA.

Laparoscopic radical prostatectomy

Minimally invasive surgical techniques have advanced rapidly over the last 10 years assisted by enormous improvements in the quality of the laparoscope, television cameras, training and experience. Doubts have been expressed regarding the application of this technology in the field of cancer surgery. In a recent meta-analysis of the results of videoscopic surgery for malignancy a total of 164 cases of port site recurrences were reported. The primary tumours were colon, gall bladder, lung, ovary and kidney. The aetiology of the port site recurrence appeared to be a result of the tumour manipulation, local trauma and high-pressure carbon dioxide insufflation [11]. In spite of concerns in other malignant diseases there has been increasing interest in laparoscopic radical prostatectomy. Initial reports on this procedure showed that it was very time consuming with an average operative time of 9.4 h [12] and was associated with major haemorrhage requiring conversion to open surgery. The most renowned pioneer in the field of laparoscopic radical prostatectomy is undoubtedly Professor Guy Vallancien from Paris. Between 1998 and 1999 120 men underwent laparoscopic radical prostatectomy by the Paris group and the mean operative time was only 4 h. Conversion to open surgery was necessary in seven (5.8%) and the mean intraoperative bleeding was 402 mL. Postoperative complications were similar to those of open retropubic radical prostatectomy but follow-up is very short-term [13]. Most prostate cancer patients are not concerned about the cosmetic aspects of abdominal scars, but are keen to be cured of prostate cancer, even if it requires a prolonged hospital stay. Laparoscopic radical prostatectomy is now technically feasible in specialist centres but we must await the long-term results before drawing any conclusions. Will port site recurrence develop later in these patients?

Radical prostatectomy results

Radical prostatectomy appears to offer the best chance of cure for men with prostate cancer. At the Charing Cross Hospital we have performed radical retropubic prostatectomy on 239 men of median age 61 years (range 41–72 years) with a median PSA of 10.7 ng/mL (range 1–65 ng/mL) between 1993 and 2000. Histopathological examination of the specimens revealed apparently positive surgical margins in 127 (53%) of the patients. However, it is now apparent in our own experience, and in other reported series that the presence of positive surgical margins, particularly at the apices of the prostate, is not independently associated with an increased risk of clinical or PSA disease progression and hence should be interpreted with caution [14]. The PSA level is the most precise measure of persistent disease and a steady rise implies recurrence. Super-sensitive PSA assay allows earlier detection of recurrence by up to 2.3 years sooner than conventional assays [15]. We have utilized a super-sensitive PSA assay in the follow-up of our patients. A PSA nadir of 0.05 ng/mL or less has been achieved in 66%. These results are similar to those reported from many centres in the USA, where follow-up is longer. Partin *et al.* [16] have reported a PSA non-progression rate of 83% at five years and 70% at 10 years in a series of 894 radical prostatectomy patients, however, this was not using the super-sensitive assay throughout.

Mortality in the Charing Cross hospital series has been remarkably low — only one of our patients (0.41%), a man with a preoperative PSA of 26 ng/mL and micrometastases in his pelvic lymph nodes, has died of prostate cancer 78 months after surgery. Four other men (2.8%) have died of unrelated conditions — two of myocardial infarction, one from pulmonary embolus and one of myeloid leukaemia. Four patients have clinical evidence of metastatic disease and are currently having hormonal therapy. Peri-operative mortality figures in large series from the USA are similar to our own experience.

Radical prostatectomy complications

All men are rendered infertile by radical prostatectomy and this should be detailed on the patient's consent form. The few men of this age group who wish to father children after their surgery can have sperm storage. Only two of our patients have made use of this facility over the last seven years.

The most commonly encountered complication of radical prostatectomy is erectile dysfunction. There is no doubt that nerve-sparing surgery reduces the risk of erectile dysfunction after radical prostatectomy. The best results, in terms of preservation of erectile function from this type of surgery, have been reported by the Johns Hopkins group, who have a 68% potency rate after radical prostatectomy in men who were potent preoperatively [17]. However, the results published by the Stanford group were not comparable—a potency rate of 13.3% for unilateral nerve-sparing and 31.9% for bilateral nerve-sparing radical prostatectomy [18]. At the Charing Cross hospital, where we are dealing with a very different patient population from the USA, in particular more elderly men with more advanced tumours, approximately 45% of men are troubled by erectile dysfunction, but the response to treatment is encouraging.

The second most common complication of radical prostatectomy is stricture at the anastomosis, and this usually occurs within the first three months after surgery. This complication is more likely to occur in patients who have not had mucosal eversion at the bladder neck or have had prolonged urinary leakage through the anastomosis. Also patients who have had prior TURP are at particular risk of anastomotic stricture. The incidence of anastomotic stricture in our series is 15/239 (6.2%). Other large series of radical prostatectomies have reported a similar incidence of bladder neck anastomotic stricture [19,20].

The incidence of incontinence of urine after radical prostatectomy has been exaggerated in our view and this has created unjustified concern about this potential complication in many patients. The incidence of incontinence after radical prostatectomy is variable. Although about 50–66% may leak immediately after catheter removal, by six months only 12% should leak, and by one year only 2% will have significant leakage [21]. In our own experience only 2% leak to the extent that they require use of a pad beyond three months after surgery.

The need for blood transfusion during or after radical prostatectomy is very low in experienced hands. We have transfused only two out of the last 50 cases. There are a number of other rare complications such as urethro-vesical anastomotic leakage, persistent lymphatic leakage and lymphocele, wound infection, deep venous thrombosis and pulmonary embolism. Two patients (0.8%), both with stage T3 tumours, have suffered a rectal injury. In both cases the rectum was repaired and covered with a patch of greater omentum without the need for a defunctioning colostomy.

Treatment of complications

Fortunately, most patients with erectile dysfunction following radical prostatectomy respond well to standard treatments, especially if the impotence is primarily neurogenic. Intra-cavernosal injections, intraurethral pellet insertion, oral sildenafil citrate (Viagra) and vacuum devices are the most popular modalities. The insertion of penile prostheses is an option in selected patients who have failed to respond to more conservative treatments. A variety of agents can be used for intracavernosal injection therapy. They can be broadly divided into phosphodiesterase inhibitors such as papaverine, alpha-adrenergic receptor blockers such as phenoxybenzamine and prostaglandin E1 (PGE1) agents such as alprostadil. There is some evidence that early treatment, starting one month after radical prostatectomy, with intracavernosal alprostadil injection results in an improved potency rate [22]. The mechanism of action is thought to be that the PGE1 maintains cavernous oxygenation and avoids hypoxia-induced damage to erectile tissue, which can subsequently impair erectile function. Intra-cavernosal injection of alprostadil will produce an erectile response in 75% or more of men who suffer from erectile dysfunction following prostate surgery.

Trans-urethral alprostadil therapy with the medicated urethral system for erection (MUSE) is well tolerated with few side-effects. In a study of 384 radical prostatectomy patients with erectile dysfunction 70.3% of men were able to achieve an erection sufficient for sexual intercourse with MUSE therapy [23]. Similar excellent results have been reported with the oral agent sildenafil citrate. In a study of 15 men with erectile dysfunction following bilateral nerve-sparing radical prostatectomy 80% had a positive response to oral sildenafil citrate. Those in whom the erectile nerves had been sacrificed had a poor response [24].

In the future, other treatments for erectile dysfunction in prostate cancer may become available. One possibility is intraoperative reconstruction of damaged cavernous nerves using a sural or genito-femoral nerve interposition graft. This technique has been successfully used in rats to restore erectile function following surgical damage to the neurovascular bundle [25] and more recently has been tried in humans [26]. Inhibitors of lipid peroxidation, which is probably an important mediator of cavernous nerve dysfunction following crushing injury, are also being investigated in the rat to determine whether prophylactic administration of these agents might have a role in preventing operative neural damage [27].

Anastomotic strictures, which are usually located proximal to the distal sphincter mechanism, can be successfully treated by bladder neck incision or resection without leading to incontinence [19]. In our series only one of the 15 (6.7%) patients treated this way has had a recurrence of his stricture.

In all but 2% of cases of urinary incontinence after radical prostatectomy there will be spontaneous resolution of the problem without therapy. The advice of a continence nurse is helpful in the early postoperative period. Pelvic floor exercises and pelvic floor interferential therapy will help to speed up the process of recovery of continence. Men with irritative symptoms and detrusor instability may benefit from treatment with anticholinergic drugs such as oxybutynin or tolterodine. The few men who are suffering from stress incontinence at three months can be considered for injection therapy. This is administered under general anaesthetic via the urethral or trans-vesical route. Injecting collagen or macroplastique can tighten the bladder neck and sphincter areas, and quite good results have been reported with this treatment [28,29].

Conclusion

The benefits of radical prostatectomy in men with clinically localized prostate cancer are exemplified by the large number of patients, many of whom research the subject extensively, who choose this treatment rather than alternative therapies such as external-beam radiotherapy and brachytherapy. In our view, radical prostatectomy offers men the best chance of cure from prostate cancer according to the currently available data. The trade off for cure has historically been the side-effects of surgery, especially erectile dysfunction. However, modifications of surgical technique and recent developments in the therapy of erectile dysfunction have made this a less important issue.

Radical prostatectomy is an excellent treatment for prostate cancer but should only be recommended in patients who fulfil established selection criteria. Sadly, this operation has been performed inappropriately and ineffectively by some surgeons, with disastrous consequences. There is strong evidence that the success of radical prostatectomy depends upon the experience and training of the surgeon in terms of both cancer cure and reduction of postoperative side-effects. Patients contemplating surgical therapy for their prostate cancer should be advised to seek an experienced surgeon. Close follow-up after surgery is mandatory since about 20% relapse biochemically. Providing that there is no spread of prostate cancer away from the close environs of the prostate the prognosis after radical prostatectomy is very good.

References

1 Greenlee RT, Murray T, Bolden S, Wingo PA. Cancer statistics 2000. *CA Cancer J Clin* 2000; **50**: 7–33.
2 Chodak GW, Thisted RA, Gerber GS *et al.* Results of conservative management of clinically localized prostate cancer. *N Engl J Med* 1994; **330**: 242–8.
3 Aus G, Hugosson J, Norlen L. Long-term survival and mortality in prostate cancer treated with noncurative intent. *J Urol* 1995; **154**: 460–5.
4 MRCS STEP course. *Urology Section.* London: Royal College of Surgeons of England, 1995.
5 Walsh PC, Donker PJ. Impotence following radical prostatectomy: insight into etiology and prevention. *J Urol* 1982; **128**: 492–7.
6 Walsh PC, Epstein JI, Lowe F. Potency following radical prostatectomy with wide unilateral excision of the neurovascular bundle. *J Urol* 1987; **138**: 823–7.
7 Shelfo SW, Obek C, Soloway MS. Update on bladder neck preservation during radical retropubic prostatectomy: impact on pathologic outcome, anastomotic strictures, and continence. *Urology* 1998; **51**: 73–8.
8 Surya BV, Provet J, Johanson K-E, Brown J. Anastomotic strictures following radical prostatectomy: risk factors and management. *J Urol* 1990; **143**: 755–80.
9 Iselin CE, Robertson JE, Paulson DF. Radical perineal prostatectomy: oncological outcome during 20-year period. *J Urol* 1999; **161**: 163–8.
10 Boccon-Gibod L, Ravery V, Vordos D, Toublanc M, Delmas V, Boccon-Gibod L. Radical prostatectomy for prostate cancer: the perineal approach increases the risk of surgically induced positive margins and capsular incisions. *J Urol* 1998; **160**: 1383–5.
11 Schaeff B, Paolucci V, Thomopoulos J. Port site recurrences after laparoscopic surgery: a review. *Dig Surg* 1998; **15**: 124–34.
12 Schuessler WW, Schulam PG, Clayman RV, Kavoussi LR. Laparoscopic radical prostatectomy: initial short-term experience. *Urology* 1997; **50**: 854–7.
13 Guillonneau B, Vallancien G. Laparoscopic radical prostatectomy: the Montsouris experience. *J Urol* 2000; **163**: 418–22.
14 Ohori M, Abbas F, Wheeler TM, Kattan MW, Scardino PT, Lerner SP. Pathological features and prognostic significance of prostate cancer in the apical section determined by whole mount histology. *J Urol* 1999; **161**: 500–4.
15 Haese A, Huland E, Graefen M, Huland H. Supersensitive PSA-analysis after radical prostatectomy: a powerful tool to reduce the time gap between surgery and evidence of biochemical failure. *Anticancer Res* 1999; **19**: 2641–4.
16 Partin AW, Pound CR, Clemens JQ, Epstein JI, Walsh PC. Serum PSA after anatomic radical prostatectomy. *Urol Clin North Am* 1993; **20**: 713–18.
17 Quinlan DM, Epstein JI, Carter BS, Walsh PC. Sexual function following radical prostatectomy: influence of preservation of neurovascular bundles. *J Urol* 1991; **145**: 998–1002.
18 Geary ES, Dendiger TE, Freiha FS, Stamey TA. Nerve sparing radical prostatectomy: a different view. *J Urol* 1995; **154**: 145–9.
19 Popken G, Sommerkamp H, Schultze-Seemann W, Wetterauer U, Katzenwadel A. Anastomotic stricture after radical prostatectomy: incidence, findings and treatment. *Eur Urol* 1998; **33**: 382–6.
20 Tomschi W, Suster G, Holtl W. Bladder neck strictures after radical retropubic prostatectomy: still an unsolved problem. *Br J Urol* 1998; **81**: 823–6.
21 Van Kampen M, De Weerdt W, Van Poppel H, Baert L. Urinary incontinence following transurethral, transvesical and radical prostatectomy: retrospective study of 489 patients. *Acta Urol Belg* 1997; **65**: 1–7.

22 Montorsi F, Guazzoni G, Barbieri L *et al.* Recovery of spontaneous erectile function after nerve sparing radical prostatectomy with and without early intracavernous injections of prostaglandin E1: results of a prospective randomized trial. *J Urol* 1996; **155** (Suppl.): 468a (Abstract 628).

23 Costabile RA, Spevak M, Fishman IJ *et al.* Efficacy and safety of transurethral alprostadil in patients with erectile dysfunction following radical prostatectomy. *J Urol* 1998; **160**: 1325–8.

24 Zippe CD, Kedia AW, Kedia K, Nelson DR, Agarwal A. Treatment of erectile dysfunction after radical prostatectomy with sildenafil citrate (Viagra). *Urology* 1998; **52**: 963–6.

25 Quinlan DM, Nelson RJ, Walsh PC. Cavernous nerve grafts restore erectile function in denervated rats. *J Urol* 1991; **145**: 380–3.

26 Kim ED, Scardino PT, Hampel O, Mills NL, Wheeler TM, Nath RK. Interposition of sural nerves restores function of cavernous nerves resected during radical prostatectomy. *J Urol* 1999; **161**: 188–92.

27 Karakiewicz PI, Bazinet M, Zvara P *et al.* Inhibitors of lipid peroxidation may successfully reduce impotence following radical prostatectomy: a rat model. *J Urol* 1996; **155** (Suppl.): 617a (Abstract 1226).

28 Bugel H, Pfister C, Sibert L, Cappele O, Khalaf A, Grise P. Intraurethral macroplastique injections in the treatment of urinary incontinence after prostatic surgery. *Prog Urol* 1999; **9**: 1068–76.

29 Smith DN, Appell RA, Rackley RR, Winters JC. Collagen injection therapy for post-prostatectomy incontinence. *J Urol* 1998; **160**: 364–7.

15: The Case against Radical Surgery for Early Prostate Cancer

Leslie E. F. Moffat

Introduction

> 'At first sight, it seems illogical to consider deferred treatment in any condition whether malignant or not. . . . Further thought suggests that particularly in the elderly, conditions may be monitored rather than treated if the risk of treatment is high, the toxicity considerable, or the likely benefit small.'

Thus wrote Philip Smith in 1990 [1] discussing the case for no initial treatment of localized prostate cancer. This was written in the UK against a background of a low number of urologists per head of population. Treatment for prostate cancer, where given, was by hormone treatment, either orchiectomy or oestrogens, although luteinizing hormone-releasing hormone (LHRH) analogues were being introduced and anti-androgens were available.

The pattern of treatment in the USA was different. Radical prostatectomy was much more popular and surgical treatment received a further boost with the description of nerve sparing radical prostatectomy by Schlegel & Walsh [2] in 1982. The presentation of prostate cancer about 10 years earlier in the North American black population added to the number of patients seen in the USA [3].

Acid phosphatase was a useful marker, but it was not until prostate specific antigen (PSA) became available that more patients with early disease were seen in the UK and, combined with the advent of transrectal ultrasound (TRUS) biopsy, urologists were forced to address the issue of treatment differences between the USA and the UK.

The prevailing climate of opinion reflected the views of Smith and it was probably the Medical Research Council study of immediate vs. deferred hormone treatment that made urologists in the UK fully aware of the true death rate from cancer of the prostate [4].

Conservative treatment is also referred to as 'expectant treatment' or 'watchful waiting' [5]. The second term is used to acknowledge that treatment will be given on an *ad hoc* basis when or if required. Walsh [6] takes a more robust view of these options, calling them 'treatment with no curative intent'.

Despite the wealth of literature on prostate cancer, with over 7000 publications between 1996 and 1999, there remains uncertainty about the

264

clinical course of prostate cancer in all patients. Patterns became more evident after McNeal *et al.* [7] examined patterns of spread. It is becoming easier to predict local invasion [8], but calculating probability of survival is still an inexact science.

In older men with a limited life expectancy, independent of their prostate cancer, conservative treatment is favoured. There would be little debate about conservative management of a 90-year-old man with a tiny focus of prostate cancer in one prostatic chip with a Gleason score of 2. But what about a man of 35?

The current debate focuses on the efficacy of treatment and the morbidity of any such treatment.

Natural history

About 16%, or 1 in 6, of all men will develop clinically evident prostate cancer [9]. Although the prevalence of undiagnosed prostate cancer is known to be high in the elderly, there is much less data about its prevalence in younger men. In order to assess the natural history of untreated disease we must rely on observational studies. One of the first was a study by Whitmore [10] in 1984. He found long survival times without progression in a selected group of patients with stage B (T1–2) prostate cancer.

George [11] in the UK reported a prospective study in 1988. He followed 120 patients with early localized cancer. They were elderly, with a mean age of 74.8 years. All had histologically confirmed disease and negative bone scans. Local tumour progressed in 100 patients but metastases developed in only 13. Actuarial prostate cancer specific survival was 80% at 5 years and 75% at 7 years. He makes the point that earlier investigators lacked bone scans and could not distinguish metastatic disease accurately. It was also pointed out that earlier studies included patients in the non-treatment arm if they were too old or too ill [12,13].

In 1989, Johansson *et al.* [14] reported a series of 229 patients with T0–2 tumours of all grades. They reported 37% deaths at follow-up with only 7% from prostate cancer.

In 1992, Adolfsson and his colleagues [15] reported 122 patients followed prospectively and given deferred treatment. Most patients had low-volume tumours but a number of patients with larger tumours who did not wish treatment were included. At 5 years, only two patients were dead from prostate cancer and 21 had died from other illnesses. Adolfsson *et al.* calculated that the risk of dying from prostate cancer was 1% at 5 years and 16% at 10 years.

Also in 1992, Johansson *et al.* [16] reported further on his series of patients with early-stage untreated prostate cancer. He reported that 8.5% died from prostate cancer at a mean follow-up of 123 months. Of the total of 124 deaths, 105 (85%) were reckoned to be from other causes. In a subgroup considered eligible for, but not given or wishing, radical surgery the progression free 10-year survival rate was 53.1% (95% confidence interval 44–62%).

Jones [17], also in 1992, reviewed 233 patients with stages A or B prostate cancer who had conservative management. He pointed out that the probability of survival of the total cohort was comparable with similarly aged US males. The author makes the point that surveillance requires patient compliance and attendance. Since the advent of PSA and TRUS, 'determination of progression and/or activity of the disease [occurs] significantly earlier than waiting for the patient to register pain, weight loss, or lethargy'.

Aus [18] reported in 1994 on a retrospective analysis of a series of 503 patients with prostate cancer. In patients with no metastases at diagnosis and who survived more than 10 years, 63% had died from prostate cancer. In men aged less than 65 years at diagnosis, 75% died from prostate cancer.

Results of studies with patients undergoing conservative management for localized disease are summarized in Tables 15.1 and 15.2.

Many of the reported series were published prior to the development of PSA. The patient groups are heterogeneous and the staging of disease may be inaccurate. In an attempt to address this, Carter and Walsh measured PSA in normal men and men with benign prostatic hyperplasia (BPH), localized or malignant prostates using sera stored for an average of 17 years prior to diagnosis [19]. Men with final metastatic disease had PSA levels significantly greater than controls, their yearly change in PSA was higher, and at an average of 9 years prior to diagnosis the PSA was increasing exponentially [20]. Walsh [6] concludes that men with eventual metastatic disease harboured unrecognized advanced disease at least 10 years prior to diagnosis. Using figures from Gann *et al.* [3], he concluded that the lead-time in diagnosis associated with PSA testing is 4–5 years [20].

Gleason scores and survival

Gleason devised a histological grading system summing the two most predominant areas of Gleason grades observed at low microscopic power [21]. Albertsen *et al.* [22], publishing in 1995, carried out a competing risk analysis of men aged 55–74 years at diagnosis in a total of 767 men. Of 451 patients with T1 or T2 tumours treated with non-curative intent (immediate or delayed hormonal therapy only), he found that death from prostate cancer increased with Gleason score. This was a retrospective cohort study and did not measure patients' PSA. He concluded that men with a Gleason score of 2–4 had a minimal risk of cancer specific death from their disease within 15 years from diagnosis. Men with Gleason scores of 5 or 6 had a modest risk of cancer

Table 15.1 Outcome of studies with patients undergoing conservative management for localized disease (after Selley *et al.* [5])

Reference	Year	No. of patients	Clinical stage	Mean age at diagnosis (years)*	Mean follow-up (years)*	Observed survival (%)			Progression free survival (%)			Disease specific survival (%)	
						5 years	10 years	15 years	5 years	10 years	15 years	5 years	10 years
15	1992	122	T1–2	68	7.5	80	50	–	–	–	–	–	–
16	1992	223	T0–2	72	12.5	67	42	–	67	56	–	–	–
47	1987	44	T1–2			61	34	–	–	–	–	–	–
43	1990	50	VACURG I–II			70	55	32	–	–	–	–	–
15	1992	122	T1–2			51	–	–	–	–	–	99	84
48	1993	52	A1–B			–	–	–	–	–	–	–	75
49	1993	34	T0–2			67	34	–	–	–	–	89	87
25	1972	28	T1–2			–	–	–	–	–	–	70	–

* Lack of entry indicates data not reported.

Table 15.2 Outcome of studies with patients undergoing conservative management for localized disease (after Selley *et al.* [5]) [Data for final three columns still to come from author]

Study, country, year	Study design*	No. of patients	Mean age at diagnosis	Length of follow-up (months)	Clinical stage	Disease progression (%)	Metastases (%)	Died of prostate cancer (%)	Died of other causes (%)
Whitmore, USA, 1994 [50]	R	75	B1 (T2a,b): 65 (54–77) B2 (T2c): 67 (58–82) B3: 69 (63–81)	B1: 133 (24–222) B2: 130 (36–298) B3: 108 (26–197)	B1: 29 B2: 37 B3†: 9	B1: 65.5 B2: 78 B3: 44	B1: 6 B2: 17 B3: 2	B1: 10 B2: 43 B3: 0	B1: 13 B2: 46 B3: 33
Jones, USA, 1992 [17]	R	233	Unspecified	264	A1–B2 (T1–2)	A1: 0.4 A2: 3	B1: 1 B2: 3	A1: 6 A2: 5	B1: 2 B2: 6
Johansson *et al.*, Sweden, 1992 [16]	P	223	Unspecified	120	T0–2	34	12	8.5	47
Adolfsson *et al.*, Sweden, 1992 [15]	P	122	Median: 86 (38–89)	Median: 91 (8–127)	T1–2	55	14	7	31
Waaler and Stenwig, Norway, 1972 [25]	R	94	73 (52–90)	108	T0–2	T0: 1 T0 (focal): 2 T0 (diffuse): 7	T0: 0 T0 (focal): 7 T0 (diffuse): 6	T0: 0 T0 (focal): 3 T0 (diffuse): 6	33
George, UK, 1988 [11]	P	120	74 (62–90)	84	Unspecified	84	11	4	3.6
Zhang *et al.*, USA, 1991 [51]	R	132	72	96	T1a	10			2.2
Epstein *et al.*, USA, 1986 [52]	R	94	Died <4 years (75 years) Survived 4 years (65 years)	120 (96–216)	A1 (T1–2)	8		6	

*R, retrospective; P, prospective.

†Four patients were lost to follow-up.

specific death but men with Gleason scores of 7–10 have a high risk of cancer specific death when treated conservatively.

In most men with localized prostate cancer who present with moderately differentiated tumours, half will die from prostate cancer if they live for 15 years [23].

The case for less aggressive treatment has also been made [24–26], most persuasively by Chodak *et al.* [27]. Chodak *et al.* performed a pooled analysis of six non-randomized studies published since 1985 of 828 case records of men treated conservatively for clinically localized prostate cancer. A Cox regression analysis [28] was performed to determine which factors influenced survival in patients who did not die of causes other than prostate cancer, i.e. disease specific survival. Their reason for using pooled analysis was that Stewart and Parmar [29] showed that meta-analysis is less biased if data from individual patients are combined and the analysis is not confined to published figures.

The expected life expectancy was determined from standard life tables from the USA and Sweden. Chodak *et al.* verified that the proportional hazards model was appropriate and they then compared observed survival with Sweden's published life tables for the age of 70 using Cox regression and by a similar method compared survival with US life tables. Disease specific survival was calculated. Mortality at 10 years among men with grades 1 or 2 disease was 13% as compared with 66% among men with grade 3 disease.

Chodak and colleagues concluded that watchful waiting was justified in men with grade 1 or 2 clinically localized disease, especially if their life expectancy was less than 10 years. They suggest that whether a higher rate of disease free survival and metastasis free survival is worth the risk of complications of aggressive therapy should be left to the patient to decide.

They also conclude that in grade 3 cancers, neither radical surgery nor radiotherapy lowers the high rates of metastases and mortality seen with conservative treatments.

Treatment options

There is a wide variation in the incidence of radical treatment, even within men of similar socio-economic groups and identical ethnicity. It has been observed that a Caucasian male in Seattle has a 6.4% chance of having had radical prostatectomy by the age of 75 against a 1.3% chance in Connecticut [30].

Radical prostatectomy

Radical prostatectomy would normally be carried out in patients who have at least a 10-year life expectancy. The operation is not without side-effects: up to 25% of patients have some degree of incontinence, and up to 50% become impotent, despite the use of nerve sparing prostatectomy [31]. Although these figures are bettered in certain centres, the overall complication rate is high. There is also a 0.9% chance of peri-operative death. Exposure to non-autologous blood may be detrimental to cancer survival [32].

In those patients who have organ confined prostate cancer, about 90% are free of PSA relapse at 5 years after radical prostatectomy, as are about 70% of men with only focal prostate cancersular penetration. Prior to PSA testing, many patients were found to have positive lymph nodes, but the trend is now to operate in patients with low PSA levels, and focus on those patients who can theoretically be cured. Zincke *et al.* [33] reports the largest series, of over 3000 patients, with 5% dying of their disease at 5 years but 8.8% dying from other causes. Partin [8] has developed predictive tables to combine PSA levels, Gleason score and clinical stage to predict pathological stage and these may assist in patient selection. In the USA, where radical treatment is more common than in the UK, the death rate from prostate cancer has gone down, despite an increasing incidence. Surgeons attribute this to early surgery but it may be due to lead-time bias. The side-effects of radical surgery are detailed in Middleton *et al.* [34] using complication rates from numerous centres [34]. There is a wide range in the incidence of complications.

Selection bias in surgical series

Randomized trials are the only reliable way of minimizing selection bias towards one treatment or another. Surgery may be biased towards patients with more favourable disease and possibly with lower volume disease. Larger tumours, which have surgery, are more liable to be upstaged to T3 [35].

The British Association of Urological Surgeons Working Party states that 'there is good reason to question the current results of radical prostatectomy' [36], and that 'even in the best departments, positive margin rates are obtained which would be unacceptable in other types of tumour' [37,38].

Radiotherapy, conformal radiotherapy and brachytherapy

Radiotherapy has been difficult to evaluate in the treatment of early CAP. Many series include advanced local disease (T3). It is known that biopsy post-radiation therapy yields between 21% and 65% positive biopsies, but the series quoted tend to have a higher proportion of T2 and T3 disease [37].

Long-term results of 1500 patients in the Radiation Oncology Group (RTOG) show patients with early disease, defined in their analysis Gleason

Scores 2–5 with any stage as having a 5, 10 and 15 year disease-specific survival of 97, 85 and 71 years respectively [38]. These data confirm the efficacy of radiotherapy in early disease treatment and show that local control, which is known to be effective, leads to improved survival.

Comparison with srugical series is difficult. PSA levels post radiotherapy can be used as a treatment end point but do not distinguish between local failure and distant metastases. PSA levels are not necessarily predictive of disease-specific survival [37]. It remains to be seen whether conformal radiotherapy which is under trial [39] will improve these results or indeed whether brachytherapy (implantation of radioactive seeds into the prostate under ultrasound control) will produce better results [41,42].

Comparison of treatments

In order to assess therapy, the natural history of the disease needs to be determined.

In an age of evidence-based medicine there is a hierarchy of evidence [42]. The best situation is a meta-analysis of various large trials.

The VACURG trial is the only randomized controlled trial of radical prostatectomy vs. conservative management. No survival difference was demonstrated, but the study was under-powered and could not have demonstrated any expected small variance [43]. If large trials are not available, we must examine the available data.

Lu-Yao and Greenberg [44] reviewed the SEER database of 60 000 patients and reported treatment outcomes. Radical treatments were associated with better relative survival than an age matched population, but disease specific survival was unaffected by management policy. The investigators were unable to control for co-morbidity and tumour related variables such as tumour size and presenting PSA [35]. Central pathology review allows more accurate and more homogeneous interpretation of histology [45].

There have been no completed randomized controlled trials with sufficient power to detect any improvement in mortality from intervention. There are two trials evaluating randomized treatment of prostate cancer after detection, namely the PIVOT study in the USA and a smaller Scandinavian study [23]. The MRC study PR06, which intended to address this problem, had to be closed because of insufficient recruitment [46]. The first two trials will mature in the earlier part of the new millennium, but until then we must use the information which is already to hand. Middleton and his colleagues [34] attempted to compare different treatments in published reports using a systematic review. They concluded that valid comparisons of treatment could not be performed and that meta-analysis was inappropriate. They had to resort to presenting treatment alternatives with a range of treatment options.

Conclusion

The absence of large prospective randomized trials of the management of early prostate cancer hampers the decision making process about the need for treatment, and the age and stage at which it should be selected. It would appear that early prostate cancer with Gleason scores of 2–4 have a low risk of progression, although the longer the life expectancy, the higher the risk of eventual progression [22]. The presence of co-morbid conditions makes any benefit of radical treatment in elderly patients much less likely to confer benefit. It is known that patients with high-grade tumours (Gleason scores 7–10) have a high risk of their disease progressing and this may be independent of treatment [22].

The precise benefit of radical surgery is being redefined, and patients must be given guidance to interpret the wealth of literature on this topic, preferably given by a neutral person. The case for radical surgery is therefore based on the need to do something, and surgeons will oblige an anxious patient. It is imperative that further studies are conducted to demonstrate whether radical surgery produces measurable benefit. At present the detractors have powerful evidence that radical surgery does not benefit populations, and refinement of surgical and non-surgical treatments will be required before the sceptics are satisfied.

References

1   Smith P. The case for no initial treatment of localized prostate cancer. *Urol Clin North Am* 1990; **17**: 827–34.
2   Schlegel PN, Walsh PC. Neuroanatomical approach to radical cystoprostatectomy with preservation of sexual function. *J Urol* 1987; **138**: 1402–6.
3   Gann PH, Hennekens CH, Stampfer MJ. A prospective evaluation of plasma prostate-specific antigen for detection of prostate cancer. *JAMA* 1995; **273**: 289–94.
4   Medical Research Council Prostate Cancer Working Party Investigators Group. Immediate versus deferred treatment for advanced prostatic cancer: initial results of the Medical Research Council Trial. *Br J Urol* 1997; **79**: 235–46.
5   Selley S, Donovan J, Faulkner A, Coast J, Gillatt D. Diagnosis, management and screening of early localised prostate cancer. *Health Technol Assess* 1997; **1**: 1–96.
6   Walsh PC. The natural history of localized prostate cancer: a guide to therapy. In: Walsh PC, Retik AB, Vaughan ED, Wein AJ, eds. *Campbell's Urology*, Vol. 3, 7th edn. Philadelphia: WB Saunders, 1997: 2539–46.
7   McNeal JE, Kindrachuk RA, Freiha FS, Bostwick DG, Redwine EA, Stamey TA. Patterns of progression in prostate cancer. *Lancet* 1986; **1**: 60–3.
8   Partin AW, Subong EN, Walsh P *et al*. Combination of prostate-specific antigen, clinical stage, and Gleason score to predict pathological stage of localized prostate cancer. *JAMA* 1997; **277**: 1445–51.
9   Bostwick DG. Staging prostate cancer: current methods and limitations. *Eur Urol* 1997; **32** (Suppl. 3): 2–14.
10 Whitmore WF. Natural history and staging of prostate cancer. *Urol Clin North Am* 1984; **11**: 205–20.

11 George NJR. Natural history of localised prostatic cancer managed by conservative therapy alone. *Lancet* 1988; **1**: 494–7.

12 Blackard CE, Mellinger GT, Gleason DF. Treatment of stage I carcinoma of the prostate: a preliminary report. *J Urol* 1971; **106**: 729–33.

13 Byar DP, the Veterans Administrative Cooperative Urological Research Group. Survival of patients with incidentally found microscopic cancer of the prostate: results of a clinical trial of conservative treatment. *J Urol* 1972; **108**: 908–13.

14 Johansson JE, Andersson SO, Krusemo UB. Natural history of localised prostatic cancer. *Lancet* 1989; **1**: 799–803.

15 Adolfsson A, Carstensen J, Lowhagen T. Deferred treatment in clinically localised prostatic carcinoma. *Br J Urol* 1992; **69**: 183–7.

16 Johansson JE, Adami HO, Andersson SO, Bergstrom R, Holmberg L, Krusemo UB. High 10-year survival rate in patients with early, untreated prostatic cancer. *JAMA* 1992; **267**: 2191–6.

17 Jones GW. Prospective, conservative management of localized prostate cancer. *Cancer* 1992; **70**: 307–10.

18 Aus G. Prostate cancer: mortality and morbidity after non-curative treatment with aspects on diagnosis and treatment. *Scand J Urol Nephrol* 1994; **167** (Suppl.): 1–41.

19 Carter HB, Morrell CH, Pearson JD *et al*. Estimation of prostatic growth using serial prostate-specific antigen measurements in men with and without prostate disease. *Cancer Res* 1992; **52**: 3323–8.

20 Carter HB, Pearson JD, Metter EJ *et al*. Longitudinal evaluation of prostate-specific antigen levels in men with and without prostate disease. *JAMA* 1992; **267**: 2215–20.

21 Gleason D, Mellinger G, the Veterans Administrative Cooperative Urological Research Group. Prediction of prognosis for prostatic adenocarcinoma by combined histological grading and clinical staging. *J Urol* 1974; **111**: 58–64.

22 Albertsen PC, Fryback DG, Storer BE, Kolon TF, Fine J. Long-term survival among men with conservatively treated localized prostate cancer. *JAMA* 1995; **274**: 626–31.

23 Wilt TJ. Can randomized treatment trials in early stage prostate cancer be completed? *Clin Oncol* 1998; **10**: 141–3.

24 Wasson J, Cushman C, Bruskewitz RC *et al*. A structured literature review of treatment for localized prostate cancer. *Arch Fam Med* 1993; **2**: 487–93.

25 Waaler G, Stenwig AE. Prognosis of localised prostatic cancer managed by 'watch and wait' policy. *Br J Urol* 1972; **72**: 214–19.

26 Whitmore WF Jr, Warner JA, Thompson IM Jr. Expectant management of localized prostatic cancer. *Cancer* 1991; **67**: 1091–6.

27 Chodak GW, Thirsted RA, Gerber GS *et al*. Results of conservative management of clinically localized prostate cancer. *New Engl J Med* 1994; **330**: 242–8.

28 Cox DR. Regression models and life tables. *J Stat Soc [B]* 1972; **34**: 187–220.

29 Stewart LA, Parmar MKB. Meta-analysis of the literature or of individual patient data: is there a difference? *Lancet* 1993; **341**: 418–22.

30 Lu-Yao GL, Yao S. Population based study of long-term survival in patients with clinically localised prostate cancer. *Lancet* 1997; **349**: 892–3.

31 Walsh PC. Anatomic radical prostatectomy: evolution of the surgical technique. *J Urol* 1998; **160**: 2418–24.

32 McClinton S, Moffat LEF, Scott S, Urbaniak S, Kerridge D. Blood transfusion and survival following surgery for prostatic carcinoma. *Br J Surg* 1990; **77**: 140–2.

33 Zincke H, Oesterling JE, Blute ML *et al*. Long-term (15 years) results after radical prostatectomy for clinically localized (stage T2c or lower) prostate cancer. *J Urol* 1994; **152**: 1850–7.

34 Middleton RG, Thompson IM, Austenfeld MS *et al*. Prostate cancer clinical guidelines

panel summary report on the management of clinically localized prostate cancer. *J Urol* 1995; **154**: 2144–8.

35 Gerberg GS, Thisted RA, Scardino PT *et al*. Results of radical prostatectomy in men with clinically localized prostate cancer: multi-institutional pooled analysis. *JAMA* 1996; **276**: 615–61.

36 Dearnaley DP, Kirby RS, Kirk D, Malone P, Simpson RJ, Williams G. Diagnosis and management of early prostate cancer. (Report of a British Association of Urological Surgeons Working Party.) *BJU Int* 1999; **83**: 18–33.

37 Speight JL, Roach M III, In: Tanagho EA, McAninch JW, eds, *Smith's General Urology*, 15th edn. New York: Lange Medical Books, 2000.

38 Roach M *et al*. Long term survival after radiotherapy alone. Radiation Therapy Oncology Group. *J Urol* 1999; **161**: 864.

39 Dearnaley DP, Khoo VS, Norman AR *et al*. Comparison of radiation side effects of conformal and conventional radiotherapy in prostate cancer: a randomised trial. *Lancet* 1999; **353**: 267–72.

40 Ragde H, Elgamal AA, Snow PB *et al*. Ten-year disease free survival after transperineal sonography-guided iodine-125 brachytherapy with or without 45-gray external beam irradiation in the treatment of patients with clinically localized, low to high Gleason grade prostate carcinoma. *Cancer* 1998; **83**: 989–1001.

41 Ragde H, Blasko JC, Grimm PD *et al*. Brachytherapy for clinically localized prostate cancer: results at 7- and 8-year follow-up. *Semin Surg Oncol* 1997; **13**: 438–43.

42 Evidence-based Medicine Working Group. Evidence-based medicine: a new approach to teaching the practice of medicine. *JAMA* 1992; **268**: 2420–5.

43 Graversen PH, Nielsen KT, Gasser TC *et al*. Radical prostatectomy versus expectant primary treatment in stages 1 and 2 prostatic cancer. *Urology* 1990; **36**: 493–8.

44 Lu-Yao GL, Greenberg ER. Changes in prostate cancer incidence and treatment in USA. *Lancet* 1994; **343**: 251–4.

45 Ohori M, Goad JR, Wheeler TM, Eastham JA, Thompson TC, Scardino PT. Can radical prostatectomy alter the progression of poorly differentiated prostate cancer? *J Urol* 1994; **152**: 1843–9.

46 Moffat LEF. Randomised controlled trials in early prostate cancer: requiem or renaissance? *Clin Oncol* 2000; **12**: 213–14.

47 Moskowitz B, Nitecki A, Richter Levin D. Cancer of the prostate: is there a need for aggressive treatment? *Urol Int* 1987; **42**: 49–52.

48 Egawa S, Go M, Kuwao S, Shoji K, Uchida T, Koshiba K. Longterm impact of conservative management of localized prostate cancer: a twenty-year experience in Japan. *Urology* 1993; **42**: 520–6.

49 Stenzl A, Studer U. Outcome of patients with untreated cancer of the prostate. *Eur Urol* 1993; **24**: 1–6.

50 Whitmore WF. Expectant management of clinically localized prostatic cancer. *Semin Oncol* 1994; **21**: 560–8.

51 Zhang G, Wasserman NF, Sidi AA, Reinberg Y, Reddy PK. Long-term follow up results after expectant management of stage A1 prostatic cancer. *J Urol* 1991; **146**: 99–103.

52 Epstein JI, Paull G, Eggleston JC, Walsh PC. Prognosis of untreated stage A1 prostatic carcinoma: a study of 94 cases with extended follow up. *J Urol* 1986; **136**: 837–9.

Prostate Cancer: Commentary

J. Waxman

There has been considerable interest generated in the last decade in prostate cancer biology. Ten years ago the number of research papers in this area was very small, but now a mass of literature abounds.

The major scientific problem in prostate cancer — the problem that attracts the most significant attention from the scientific community — is the development of hormonal independence. The focus has been on the molecular changes within the gene encoding the androgen receptor, but there has also been much attention paid to oncogenes and differentiation markers.

The management of localized small bulk prostate cancer remains controversial, because of the lack of a significant randomized trial comparing observation, radiotherapy and surgery. Although the consensus now appears to be that radical surgery offers the best prospect for the patient with a poorly differentiated tumour, there is no major evidence from randomized data supporting this view. The excellent chapters by Tim Christmas and Alan Doherty, Leslie Moffat, and Drs Lewanski and Stewart describe the issues that are of note in this area.

The treatment of advanced prostatic cancer has disadvantages resulting from androgen deficiency. David Kirk, in his excellent chapter, describes the pros and cons of deferring treatment and concludes that this is a feasible and safe possibility for those patients with localized disease who are carefully monitored.

Over the last 20 years there has been significant change in the treatment of advanced prostatic cancer. Treatments have become more humane and chemotherapy has been developed which palliates symptoms and causes no significant toxicity. Drs Knox and Moore describe the benefits of chemotherapy for patients with hormone refractory prostate cancer. It is hoped that over the next 20 years advances in the molecular biology and treatment of prostate cancer will be such that there will be significant improvements in outpatients' chances of survival.

Part 4
Testicular Cancer

16: Genetics of Adult Male Germ Cell Tumours

J. Houldsworth, G. J. Bosl & R. S. K. Chaganti

Introduction

Adult human male germ cell tumours (GCTs) offer a unique system in which to study the transformation of a germ cell (GC) that would otherwise be destined to undergo a differentiation program leading to gametogenesis and, upon fertilization, to embryogenesis. GCTs retain a variable capacity for differentiation as evidenced by the array of undifferentiated and differentiated cell types observed within the tumours that mimic normal human developmental differentiation patterns. Thus, transformed male GCs exhibit the potential to elicit molecular events that resemble in part those occurring in the developing human embryo, albeit in a spatially and temporally aberrant manner and without the contribution of a maternal complement. Uniquely then, GCTs and derived cell lines lend themselves for studies aimed at understanding the biological mechanisms of many facets of embryogenesis, such as loss of regulators of GC totipotentiality, proliferation vs. cell/fate lineage decisions, and genomic imprinting.

Genetic analyses of these tumours have yielded important information regarding the underlying genetic lesions of GC transformation, which can now be tested in murine models. Notably, genes which are mapped to chromosome 12p which are present in higher than normal copy number in all GCTs, and which are thought to function early in GC tumorigenesis are targeted for study. Such an oncogene under study is that encoding cyclin D2. Historically, GCTs have been suggested to arise by transformation of a genocyte, based upon common histological features, immunohistochemical markers, and epidemiological studies. However, another model that incorporates genetic data has been postulated whereby GCTs arise by rescue of GCs in which an aberrant recombinational event has occurred during pachytene phase of meiosis, normally leading to apoptotic cell death. The two proposed models will be discussed.

Overall, GCTs display a remarkable cure rate, in that over 90% of newly diagnosed patients are cured either by surgery alone or in combination with radiation/chemotherapy treatments. Thus, they provide an excellent system in which cellular factors portending sensitivity to chemotherapeutic agents can be studied. Various genetic lesions associated with resistance of GCTs to cisplatin-based chemotherapy have now been identified, and knowledge gained from such studies could aid in the understanding of acquired resistance to therapy in other tumour systems.

Recent studies have identified molecular lesions associated with GC transformation, differentiation, and resistance to treatment. These studies will be reviewed and discussed in the context of GC and tumour biology, and of their relevance to the treatment of cancer. Insights gained from these studies into the genetic events controlling GCT biology have prompted the development of models as will be discussed, which serve as starting points for experimental approaches aimed at unravelling the unique biology of these tumours.

Pathobiology

Adult male GCTs are broadly subdivided into two groups: seminomas and non-seminomas [1]. Seminomas exhibit a morphology resembling undifferentiated spermatogonial germ cells, and account for approximately 20–50% of adult GCTs [1]. They are usually cured by a combination of surgery and radiation therapy [2]. Non-seminomas, on the other hand, are sensitive to cisplatin-based chemotherapy, and are cured at a high rate by combination surgery and chemotherapy [2]. They can display a variety of histopathologies mimicking various extents of differentiation ranging from early postzygotic (embryonal carcinomas), to extra-embryonic (yolk sac tumours, choriocarcinomas), and to embryonic somatic differentiation patterns (teratomas). Non-seminomas displaying one pure histology are less common (10–20%) than mixed GCTs which exhibit more than one non-seminomatous histology, and account for about one-third of all GCTs [1]. Combined GCTs show both seminomatous and non-seminomatous histologies. Teratomatous lesions can occasionally undergo further malignant transformation exhibiting aggressive proliferation and histological differentiation into non-GC malignancies such as sarcoma, leukaemia, and carcinoma. In this case, tumours can respond to treatment appropriate for the transformed histology, rather than to cisplatin-based treatment [3].

Carcinoma *in situ* (CIS) or intratubular germ cell neoplasia (ITGCN) is the first lesion pathologically recognized in the testis, and is generally accepted as the common precursor for all invasive GCTs [1]. Malignant germ cells are contained within the seminiferous tubules. While 90% of GCTs present in this manner in the testis, a minority present at extragonadal sites such as the anterior mediastinum, retroperitoneum, and the pineal gland. Seminoma arising at these sites are highly curable, but those with a non-seminomatous histology exhibit a low likelihood of cure with cisplatin-based chemotherapy, the underlying genetic basis of which is unknown [2].

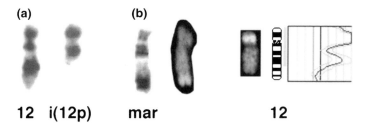

(a)   **(b)**

12   i(12p)   mar   12

Figure 16.1 Increased 12p copies are evident in all adult male GCTs. Extra copies of 12p are present as an i(12p) (a) or as tandem duplications embedded within marker chromosomes (b). In this case, tumour 287A, a marker chromosome (mar) contained 12p sequences as revealed by FISH with a chromosome 12p-specific painting probe (b). An additional subregional amplification of 12p11.2–p12 was also observed in this tumour by comparative genomic hybridization analysis (b). The dark line in the ratio profile represents the mean of 8–10 chromosomes, and the light lines represent standard deviations. The vertical bar on the right of the ideogram indicates the threshold value of 1.20 for gain.

Genetics of transformation

It is now over 15 years since the original identification of the characteristic cytogenetic marker of adult male GCTs, an isochromosome of the short arm of chromosome 12 [4]. This gain of extra copies of 12p is observed as such in 85% of tumours, and in the remaining as tandem duplications embedded within chromosomes [5] (Fig. 16.1). The presence of this abnormality, as assessed by fluorescence *in situ* hybridization (FISH) of interphase tumour cells using a 12p painting probe, is now used in a diagnostic setting to confirm GCT origin. In addition, extra copies of 12p are evident as early as CIS, and thus represent an early, if not the earliest, genetic lesion associated with GC transformation [6].

Recent studies have focused on identifying the oncogene on 12p that could play such a role. One study took a candidate gene approach, which indicated that the cyclin D2 gene (*CCND2*), mapped to 12p13 and present in higher than normal copy number in GCTs, is a good oncogenic candidate [7]. Aberrant expression of cyclin D2 was detected in the malignant cells of CIS, with little or no expression detected in normal GCs. In addition, biochemical studies on GCT-derived cell lines indicated that the expressed cyclin D2 was in an active complex with the cyclin-dependent kinases 4/6 [7]. The role of the D-type cyclins in both regulation and deregulation of the normal cell cycle has been well described [8]. In the latter case, amplification/overexpression of D-type cyclins has been observed in multiple tumour types and has been thought to represent an early genetic lesion that can deregulate normal cell cycling thus portending genomic instability [8]. In keeping with this model, aberrant cyclin D2 expression was detected in all 10 CIS specimens studied, in seminomas and non-seminomas with varying patterns, and was up/down-regulated in teratomas dependent on the histologies present [7].

Other studies aimed at identifying the driver gene on 12p have focused attention on genes mapped to 12p11.2–p12. Such studies have been prompted by the observation that a minority of GCTs display, in addition to extra copies of the whole 12p arm, a subregional amplification of genetic material derived from this region [9,10] (Fig. 16.1). The smallest region of overlap of amplification within such a group of GCTs was estimated to be between 1750 and 3000 kbp in length and contains three candidate genes (*KRAS2*, *SOX5*, and *JAW1*) [9]. The functional roles of these genes in GCT development remain to be determined. It is conceivable that other as yet unidentified genes mapped to this region may be involved.

Karyotypic analyses of these tumours also revealed that they are predominantly near-triploid, with various recurrent chromosomal abnormalities, some of which are associated with histological subtypes [11]. In particular, breakpoints involving 1p32–p36 and 7q11.2 were significantly associated with a teratomatous histology, and 1p22 with yolk sac tumours. Deletion/rearrangement at 12q, 1p32–p36, and 7q, and deletion at 6q13–q25 comprise the most frequently observed non-random chromosomal aberrations. Few GCTs have been reported to exhibit cytological evidence for gene amplification in the form of double minute chromosomes and/or homogeneously staining regions [12,13]. These studies also indicated that GCTs that underwent malignant transformation exhibited chromosomal changes previously reported to be non-randomly associated with *de novo* tumours with the same histological characteristics [11]. These include 2q37 rearrangements in rhabdomyosarcoma, +8 and del(5q) in myeloid leukaemia, and t(11;22)(q24;q12) in primitive neuroectodermal tumour [14].

It has been widely accepted that GCTs presenting at mediastinal and pineal sites arise by transformation of a GC misplaced during migration in the developing embryo. This view is held despite the failure of morphological studies to locate misplaced GCs in murine and human embryos [15,16], and more recent evidence that such GCs undergo apoptotic cell death [17]. In addition, comparison of the chromosomal abnormalities in extragonadal-presenting GCTs with those of gonadal-presenting GCTs reveals no difference in the presence of increased copies of 12p and incidence of recurring chromosomal breaks [18]. Thus, it is possible that these so-called extragonadal GCTs arise through reverse migration of occult CIS gonadal lesions [18].

Overall, these conventional cytogenetic analyses have guided subsequent molecular genetic studies. Of particular note is the further molecular examination of 12q aberrations. Restriction fragment length polymorphism analysis (RFLP) of GCTs identified two sites of loss of heterozygosity (LOH) along the long arm of chromosome 12 (12q13 and 12q22), indicative of two putative tumour suppressor gene (TSG) sites [19]. Further detailed genomic analysis of 12q22 has now determined a minimally deleted region in GCTs of 830 kbp that is covered by a high resolution BAC/PAC contig [20]. Expressed sequences within this region can now be tested as candidates for the putative TSG mapped to this locus. More traditional LOH studies of the whole chromosomal complement performed on these tumours revealed a number of sites with a high frequency of LOH. These included sites of known TSGs (*RB1*, *DCC*, and *NME*), of previously known chromosomal regions (1p, 3p, 5q, 9p, 10q, 11p, 11q, and 17p), and of several novel sites (1q, 2q, 3q, 5p, 9q, 12q, 18p, and 20p) [21]. Additional molecular genetic studies are required to not only identify the putative TSGs at these loci but also determine their functional roles in GCT biology.

While the cell of origin of these tumours is undoubtedly a GC, the stage in the life of a GC at which transformation occurs has been a subject for conjecture. Two models have been proposed (Fig. 16.2). The first, by Skakkebaek and colleagues [22], is based primarily on immunocytological marker expression, and endocrinological and epidemiological considerations. In this model, gonocytes within the developing male embryo that fail to undergo spermatogonial differentiation are considered the cells of origin (Fig. 16.2, Model A). At this early stage in normal GC biology, the gonocytes express kit receptor responsive to the growth factor SCF expressed by Sertoli cells [23]. During spermatogonial differentiation, kit receptor is normally down-regulated. Thus a gonocyte with continued expression of kit receptor is presumably at risk for continued growth stimulation and abnormal cell cycling, a prerequisite for transformation. Evidence for this model comes from kit receptor/SCF expression patterns in GCT lesions and in the testes of patients with syndromes that predispose to GC transformation [24,25]. Postnatal and pubertal endocrine activities have been implicated as mediators of invasion of malignant GCs [22] (Fig. 16.2). This model as yet remains to be experimentally tested.

The second model of GC transformation, proposed by us, takes into account cytogenetic, molecular genetic, and immunocytological properties of GCTs [26] (Fig. 16.2, Model B). These include triploid–tetraploid chromosome numbers, increased 12p copy number, cyclin D2 expression in CIS, and abundant expression of wild type (wt) p53 [4–7,11,27,28]. In this model, the target cell is a pachytene spermatocyte, which has replicated chromosomes, expresses wt p53, and has DNA breaks associated with normal stage-specific recombinational events [29] (Fig. 16.2). Such cells in which aberrant chromatid exchanges occur would normally be eliminated by apoptosis, except perhaps in the case of an event leading to increased 12p, where resulting expression of cyclin D2 leads to aberrant re-initiation of a mitotic cell cycle. Data supportive of such a model come from the studies of mice with a homozygously inactivated *Ccnd2* locus [30]. Null females were sterile, as a

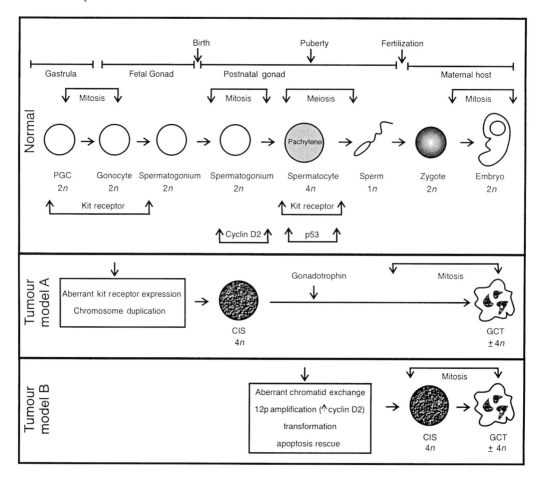

Figure 16.2 A diagrammatic representation of male GC development during a normal lifespan, and the proposed models of GC transformation. GCT development is depicted in the context of normal germ cell biology as discussed in the text. Model A is that proposed by Skakkebaek *et al.* [22] and Model B that proposed by Chaganti & Houldsworth [26].

result of a disrupted ovarian granulosa cell proliferative response to follicle-stimulating hormone (FSH), mediated by cyclin D2. Null males, however, while not sterile, did have testes of smaller weight and reduced sperm counts evident only after sexual maturation [30]. Other studies of normal mice have shown that cyclin D2 is specifically expressed in postnatal testes in GCs that are undergoing mitotic expansion [31, and unpublished observations]. Expression is down-regulated and rarely observed in the adult murine or human testis [7,31]. Thus, cyclin D2 does play an important role in normal GC development, and its subversion may well have oncogenic consequences as evidenced by abnormal expression in GCTs and ovarian granulosa cell tumours [7,30]. A GC with a 4*n* DNA content re-entering into a mitotic cell cycle has obvious potential to suffer further genetic insult such as loss of genetic material arising from genomic instability. Transgenic murine models are currently being utilized to test this model.

Genetics of differentiation

Unique to GCTs is the observed array of histopathological entities resembling different stages of normal human embryogenesis. By their very nature, GCs are totipotential cells that normally upon fertilization with a maternal complement initiate a series of spatially and temporally regulated cell divisions and fate/lineage decisions. Adult male transformed GCs also have this capacity, though in an aberrant form and without a maternal contribution. Seminomas can be viewed as mitotically dividing transformed GCs that, like normal GCs prior to fertilization, are under inhibitory control for zygotic-like differentiation. Non-seminomas, then, have been released from this control as for normal GCs after fertilization. The underlying genetic basis of these seminal events in mammalian development remains largely unknown, and studies of GCTs refractory to such embryological switches may aid in the elucidation of the genetic mechanisms involved.

An additional embryological switch that can be well studied in GCTs is that governing cell proliferation vs. cell differentiation. In this context, LOH studies have already indicated that a higher overall loss of genetic material is associated with highly differentiated teratomas compared with less differentiated embryonal carcinomas [21]. The genes at such chromosomal sites whose function is altered by loss/mutation may well act as effector genes in regulating these events. Notable among the genes deleted in teratomas were *NME1* and *NME2*, for which there is evidence of function as a transcription factor to negatively regulate differentiation [32]. Further studies determined that the levels of Nm23 proteins were 4- to 5-fold lower in teratomas than in embryonal carcinomas [33]. The functional consequence of this observation needs to be further investigated.

Derived human embryonal carcinoma cell lines provide a useful resource for identification of cellular effectors of cell fate/lineage decision events. Some embryonal carcinoma cell lines display the ability to differentiate along somatic lineages and extra-embryonic endodermal lineages, placing them as equivalents of cells derived from the inner cell mass in the developing embryo [34]. One such cell line, NT2/D1, which differentiates along a neuronal lineage in response to all-*trans*-retinoic acid, is being utilized for studies aimed at analysing the roles of different retinoid receptors in this differentiation programme [35]. Recently it has also been used as a source of differentiated neuronal cells that would otherwise be unavailable or difficult to obtain [36]. Other GCT-derived cell lines exhibit the additional ability to differentiate into trophoblastic cells, placing them at an earlier stage in embryogenesis to trophoectodermal fate decision [34]. Embryonal (teratoma) vs. extra-embryonal (yolk sac tumour, choriocarcinoma) commitment mechanisms can be identified in such cell lines. By contrast, other embryonal carcinoma cell lines lack the ability to undergo differentiation [34]. These cell lines provide an ideal system in which master regulators of differentiation induction and cell fate decision can be identified.

As already mentioned, GCTs can undergo an embryonal-like developmental programme without a maternal contribution. This has obvious implications to genomic imprinting wherein parental imprints are erased prior to meiosis, and new patterns laid down during gametogenesis and embryogenesis [37,38]. Recent studies have demonstrated biallelic expression in GCTs of *H19* and *IGF2* which normally exhibit monoallelic expression in post-fertilization somatic cells [39]. These results are consistent with our model, which suggests a pachytene spermatocyte (imprint-erased) as the cell of origin for these tumours.

Genetics of resistance

Since the curative potential of cisplatin-based chemotherapy of male GCTs has been recognized, many studies have been undertaken to distinguish between patients most likely to be rendered free of disease and cured (good-risk) and those least likely to be cured (poor-risk). Clinico-pathological features associated with a poor outcome include mediastinal non-seminomatous primary tumours, and those exhibiting hepatic, osseous, and/or brain metastases [2]. In addition, patients with high serum levels of lactate dehydrogenase (LDH), alpha fetoprotein (AFP), or chorionic gonadotrophin (HCG) are also considered to have a low likelihood of complete remission [2]. Surgical resection of residual masses after chemotherapy has often revealed the presence of teratoma in the specimens, reflective of the relative resistance of this tumour histology to cisplatin-based chemotherapy [2].

While over 90% of newly diagnosed patients and 70–80% of those who present with metastatic disease are cured, there remain 20–30% presenting with metastatic disease which exhibits clinical resistance to treatment. Recent studies have focused on identifying the causative genetic lesions. As previously noted, GCTs as a whole express high levels of wt p53 [27,28], a key regulator in the cellular response of a cell to agents such as those used in chemotherapy [40]. While mutations of p53 are common in 50% of other tumours, this genetic lesion has been detected in only a subset of GCT specimens that exhibited a clinical resistance to cisplatin-based chemotherapy [41–43]. Thus within this subset, the simplest explanation for the observed clinical resistance is the inability of the tumour cells to mount the appropriate

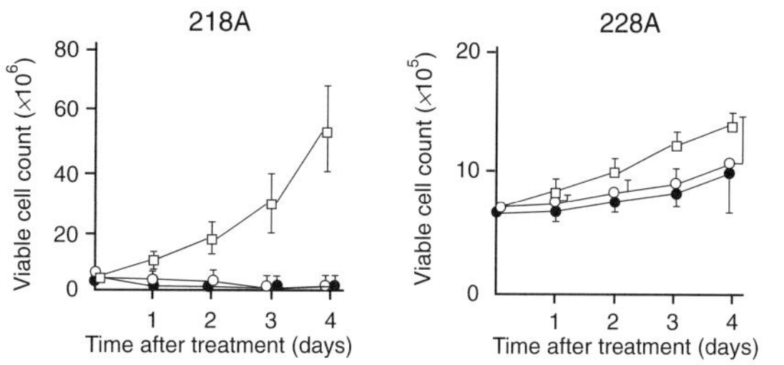

Apoptotic Cells

218A Cisplatin	218A 5 h	228A Cisplatin	228A 5 h	*P* value
0 μg/ml	3.2% ± 2.1%	0 μg/ml	1.8% ± 1.3%	0.4 > *P* > 0.3
4 μg/ml	7.7% ± 4.3%	4 μg/ml	2.4% ± 1.6%	0.2 > *P* > 0.1
8 μg/ml	9.6% ± 5.7%	8 μg/ml	2.8% ± 1.9%	0.2 > *P* > 0.1
	24 h		24 h	
0 μg/ml	3.8% ± 1.3%	0 μg/ml	2.5% ± 1.8%	0.4 > *P* > 0.3
4 μg/ml	16.8% ± 3.1%	4 μg/ml	3.1% ± 2.1%	0.1 > *P* > 0.05
8 μg/ml	16.9% ± 6.6%	8 μg/ml	3.1% ± 2.0%	0.01 > *P* > 0.005

(a)

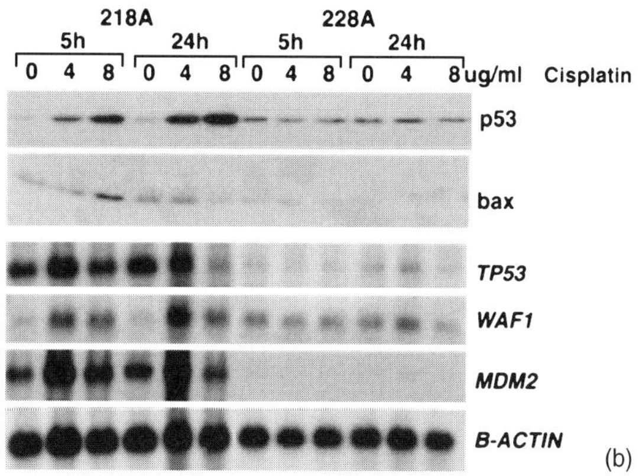

(b)

Figure 16.3 The relative resistance of a GCT cell line 228A (with a p53 mutation) after cisplatin exposure, compared with GCT cell line 218A (wt p53). After exposure to cisplatin (□, 0; ○, 4; ●, 8 μg/mL cisplatin), viable cell counts and cells undergoing apoptosis were determined by trypan blue and Hoescht 33528 staining, respectively (a) [43]. Standard deviations are shown. The steady state levels of the indicated mRNAs and proteins were assessed in the two cell lines following exposure to cisplatin (b). β-Actin was used to control for RNA loading. Reproduced with permission from *Oncogene* [43].

cellular response, namely apoptosis, after therapy because of inactivating p53 mutations.

In vitro studies have indeed confirmed this conclusion [43]. In this study, cell lines derived from a clinically resistant GCT with a p53 mutation, and from a sensitive GCT with wt p53, were treated with cisplatin and the cellular response evaluated (Fig. 16.3). The resistant cell line exhibited a much reduced number of cells undergoing cell death by apoptosis and little or no induction of the levels of p53 and p53-responsive genes compared with the sensitive cell line [43] (Fig. 16.3). Thus the extreme sensitivity of GCTs to cisplatin-based chemotherapy is rooted in a p53-dependent pathway mutation, which results in clinical resistance. Curiously, the GCT specimens that exhibited the p53 mutations were mainly teratomas. Immunohistochemical analysis of p53 expression in GCTs has indicated a lower level of expression in more differentiated teratomatous lesions, possibly predisposing a cellular setting for selective pressure for p53 mutation [44].

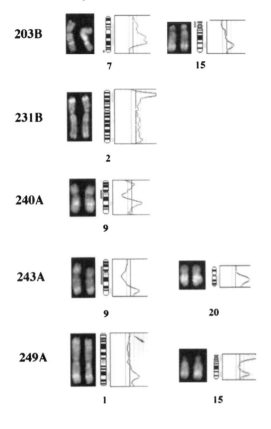

203B 7 15

231B 2

240A 9

Figure 16.4 Partial CGH karyotypes (left) and corresponding ratio profiles (right) illustrating high level amplification of chromosomal regions (other than 12p) in five resistant GCTs. The vertical bars on the left and right of the ideogram indicate threshold values of 0.80 and 1.20 for loss and gain, respectively. The ratio profiles are as described in Fig. 16.1. Reproduced with permission from *Cancer Research* [10].

243A 9 20

249A 1 15

Gene amplification is another genetic lesion often associated with tumour progression and resistance to treatment [45]. Traditional cytogenetic analyses have identified few GCT specimens with cytological evidence of gene amplification [12,13]. Recurring gains, losses, and high level amplification of genetic material in male GCTs have now been assessed by comparative genomic hybridization (CGH) [10,46,47]. As expected, 12p DNA sequences were over-represented in all cases, with subregional amplification of 12p11.2–p12 in a subset of both cured tumours and those with a resistant phenotype [10,46]. While one report suggested that loss of 6q15–q21 in two residual tumours may be associated with resistance to chemotherapy [46], another noted that gain of 6q21–q24 was more prevalent in resistant cases [47]. However, the most striking difference noted between sensitive and resistant GCTs was the exclusive presence of high level amplification of chromosomal sites other than 12p in a subset of cases within the resistant cohort [10]. Eight sites were amplified in 5 out of 17 resistant tumours, with one site (15q23–q24) being amplified in two tumours (Fig. 16.4). The identity of the amplified and presumably overexpressed genes at these loci remain unknown at present, but

(a)   (b)

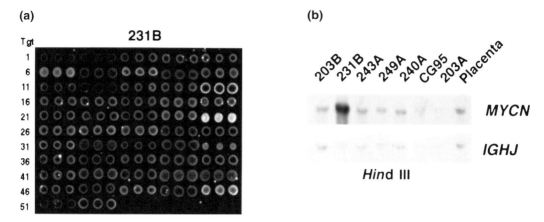

Figure 16.5 Microarray hybridization of 51 genes with GCT 231B DNA. The image obtained for the microarray hybridization with control placenta DNA (red) and GCT 231B DNA (green) is shown (a). Each gene is arrayed three times, and in this case the target gene showing excess green signal is *MYCN*. Amplification of *MYCN* in GCT 231B was confirmed by Southern hybridization (b). *IGHJ* was used to control for DNA loading. (Shown in colour, Plate 9, facing p. 178.)

application of microarray CGH and microarray expression technologies should markedly enhance this search (Fig. 16.5).

Several studies have clearly shown that the cellular response of GCT cell lines to DNA-damaging agents such as those used in chemotherapy is p53-mediated apoptosis [43,48], with few exceptions [49]. It has been suggested that the exquisite sensitivity of these tumours to such treatment could additionally arise because of a reduced ability of GCT-derived cell lines to repair DNA damage induced by chemotherapeutic agents [50]. Indeed, low levels of a protein involved in DNA damage recognition and facilitation of DNA repair complex assembly, XPA, have been reported in GCT-derived cell lines, and could account for these observations [51]. The precise biochemical link between the induction of physical damage in DNA, reduced repair, and the cellular apoptotic response to it is unclear at present. Further downstream in the cellular response, the apoptotic/survival decision could be switched to that of cell survival through alterations of the levels of the individual bcl-2 family of proteins. In GCTs, proapoptotic members such as bax have been noted to be at higher levels than the anti-apoptotic members such as bcl-2 [48], thus favouring an apoptotic response. Recent *in vitro* evidence indicates that bcl-X_L, another anti-apoptotic bcl-2 family member, may actually have a controlling role in maintaining the apoptotic response to DNA-damaging agents, rather than bcl-2 [52]. Thus, it is conceivable that resistance to chemotherapy in GCTs could also be acquired through imbalance in the levels of the bcl-2 family members, though this pathway of resistance has yet to be fully explored in GCTs.

Conclusion

Transformation of a cell within the germ line leads to the formation of a biologically fascinating tumour that can be utilized to study many facets of normal human embryological development. In this chapter we have discussed how studies performed within tumours could help identify master regulators of several aspects of human development. Murine modelling of human GC transformation itself is now within study, and will elucidate the precise stage in normal GC development and genetic lesions required for this event to occur. With the advent of cisplatin-based chemotherapy in the treatment of adult male GCTs, the scientific challenge becomes the identification of the underlying biochemical features of the extreme sensitivity of these tumours to such treatment and of the genetic lesions portending resistance. The knowledge gained from such studies may also be of significance to the understanding of therapy resistance in other tumour systems.

References

1   Ulbright TM. Germ cell neoplasms of the testis. *Am J Surg Pathol* 1993; **17**: 1075–91.
2   Bosl GJ, Motzer RJ. Testicular germ-cell cancer. *N Engl J Med* 1997; **337**: 242–53.
3   Motzer RJ, Amsterdam A, Prieto V *et al*. Teratoma with malignant transformation: diverse malignant histologies arising in men with germ cell tumors. *J Urol* 1998; **159**: 133–8.
4   Atken NB, Baker MC. i(12p): Specific chromosomal marker in seminoma and malignant teratoma of the testis? *Cancer Genet Cytogenet* 1983; **10**: 199–204.
5   Rodriguez E, Houldsworth J, Reuter VE *et al*. Molecular cytogenetic analysis of i(12p)-negative human male germ cell tumors. *Genes Chromo Cancer* 1993; **8**: 230–6.
6   Vos AM, Oosterhuis JW, de Jong B *et al*. Cytogenetics of carcinoma in situ of the testis. *Cancer Genet Cytogenet* 1990; **46**: 75–81.
7   Houldsworth J, Reuter V, Bosl GJ *et al*. Aberrant expression of cyclin D2 is an early event in human male germ cell tumorigenesis. *Cell Growth Differ* 1997; **8**: 293–9.
8   Weinberg RA. The retinoblastoma protein and cell cycle control. *Cell* 1995; **81**: 323–30.
9   Mostert MC, Verkerk AJ, van de Pol M *et al*. Identification of the critical region of 12p over-representation in testicular germ cell tumors of adolescents and adults. *Oncogene* 1998; **16**: 2617–27.
10 Rao PH, Houldsworth J, Palanisamy N *et al*. Chromosomal amplification is associated with cisplatin resistance of human male germ cell tumors. *Cancer Res* 1998; **58**: 4260–3.
11 Rodriguez E, Mathew S, Reuter V *et al*. Cytogenetic analysis of 124 prospectively ascertained male germ cell tumors. *Cancer Res* 1992; **52**: 2285–91.
12 Samaniego F, Rodriguez E, Houldsworth J *et al*. Cytogenetic and molecular analysis of human male germ cell tumors: chromosome 12 abnormalities and gene amplification. *Gene Chromo Cancer* 1990; **1**: 289–300.
13 Albrecht S, Armstrong DL, Mahoney DH *et al*. Cytogenetic demonstration of gene amplification in a primary intracranial germ cell tumor. *Gene Chromo Cancer* 1993; **6**: 61–3.
14 Chaganti RSK, Klein EA. Cytogenetic basis for molecular analysis of leukemia, lymphoma, and solid tumors. In: Cosman J, ed. *Molecular Genetics in Clinical Diagnosis*. New York: Elsevier Publishing, 1991: 73–104.

15 Chiquoine AD. The identification, origin, and migration of the primordial germ cells in the mouse embryo. *Anat Rec* 1954; **118**: 135–46.

16 Witschi E. Migration of the germ cells of human embryos from the yolk sac to the primitive gonadal folds. *Contr Embryol Carnegie Inst* 1948; **32**: 67–80.

17 Pesce M, Farrace MG, Piacentini M *et al.* Stem cell factor and leukemia inhibitory factor promote primordial germ cell survival by suppressing programmed cell death (apoptosis). *Develop* 1993; **118**: 1089–94.

18 Chaganti RSK, Rodriguez E, Mathew S. Origin of adult male mediastinal germ-cell tumours. *Lancet* 1994; **343**: 1130–2.

19 Murty VVVS, Houldsworth J, Baldwin S *et al.* Allelic deletions in the long arm of chromosome 12 identify sites of candidate tumor suppressor genes in male germ cell tumors. *Proc Natl Acad Sci USA* 1992; **89**: 11006–10.

20 Murty VVVS, Montgomery K, Dutta S *et al.* A 3-Mb high-resolution BAC/PAC contig of 12q22 encompassing the 830-kb consensus minimal deletion in male germ cell tumors. *Genome Res* 1999; **9**: 662–71.

21 Murty VVVS, Bosl G, Houldsworth J *et al.* Allelic loss and somatic differentiation in human male germ cell tumors. *Oncogene* 1994; **9**: 2245–51.

22 Skakkebaek NE, Rajpert-de Meyts E, Jorgensen N *et al.* Germ cell cancer and disorders of spermatogenesis: an environmental connection? *APMIS* 1998; **106**: 3–12.

23 Loveland KL, Schlatt S. Stem cell factor and c-kit in the mammalian testis: lessons originating from Mother Nature's gene knockouts. *J Endocrinol* 1997; **153**: 337–44.

24 Rajpert-de Meyts E, Skakkebaek NE. Expression of the *c-kit* protein product in carcinoma-in-situ and invasive testicular germ cell tumours. *Int J Androl* 1994; **17**: 85–92.

25 Rajpert-de Meyts E, Jorgensen N, Brondum-Nielsen K *et al.* Developmental arrest of germ cells in the pathogenesis of germ cell neoplasia. *APMIS* 1998; **106**: 198–206.

26 Chaganti RSK, Houldsworth J. The cytogenetic theory of the pathogenesis of human adult male germ cell tumors. *APMIS* 1998; **106**: 80–4.

27 Bartkova J, Bartek J, Lukas J *et al.* P53 protein alterations in human testicular cancer including pre-invasive intratubular germ-cell neoplasia. *Int J Cancer* 1991; **49**: 196–202.

28 Schenkman NS, Sesterhenn IA, Washington L *et al.* Increased p53 protein does not correlate to p53 gene mutations in microdissected testicular germ cell tumors. *J Urol* 1995; **154**: 617–21.

29 Schwartz D, Goldfinger N, Rotter V. Expression of p53 protein in spermatogenesis is confined to the tetraploid pachytene primary spermatocytes. *Oncogene* 1993; **8**: 1487–94.

30 Sicinski P, Donaher JL, Geneg Y *et al.* Cyclin D2 is an FSH-responsive gene involved in gonadal cell proliferation and oncogenesis. *Nature* 1996; **384**: 470–4.

31 Nakayama H, Nishiyama H, Higuchi T *et al.* Change in cyclin D2 mRNA expression during murine testis development detected by fragmented cDNA subtraction method. *Dev Growth Differ* 1996; **38**: 141–51.

32 Postel EH, Berberich SJ, Flint SJ *et al.* Human *c-myc* transcription factor PuF identified as nm23 H2 nucleoside diphosphate kinase, a candidate suppressor of tumor metastasis. *Science* 1993; **261**: 478–80.

33 Backer JM, Murty VVVS, Potla L *et al.* Loss of heterozygosity and decreased expression of NME genes correlate with teratomatous differentiation in human male germ cell tumors. *Biochem Biophys Res Commun* 1994; **202**: 1096–103.

34 Andrews PW. Teratocarcinomas and human embryology: pluripotent human EC cell lines. A review. *APMIS* 1998; **106**: 158–68.

35 Moasser MM, Reuter VE, Dmitrovsky E. Overexpression of the retinoic acid receptor γ directly induces terminal differentiation of human embryonal carcinoma cells. *Oncogene* 1995; **10**: 1537–43.

36   Hong CS, Caromile L, Nomata Y *et al.* Contrasting role of presenilin-1 and presenilin-2 in neuronal differentiation in vitro. *J Neurosci* 1999; **19**: 637–43.

37   Barlow D. Imprinting: a gamete's point of view. *Trends Genet* 1994; **10**: 194–9.

38   Lyon MF. Epigenetic inheritance in mammals. *Trends Genet* 1993; **9**: 123–8.

39   Looijenga LHJ, Verkerk AJMH, Dekker MC *et al.* Genomic imprinting in testicular germ cell tumors. *APMIS* 1998; **106**: 187–97.

40   Levine AJ. p53, the cellular gatekeeper for growth and division. *Cell* 1997; **88**: 323–31.

41   Heimdal K, Lothe LA, Lystad S *et al.* No germline *P53* mutations detected in familial and bilateral testicular cancer. *Genes Chromo Cancer* 1993; **6**: 92–7.

42   Peng H-Q, Hogg D, Malkin D *et al.* Mutations of the *p53* gene do not occur in testis cancer. *Cancer Res* 1993; **53**: 3574–8.

43   Houldsworth J, Xiao H, Murty VVVS *et al.* Human male germ cell tumor resistance to cisplatin is linked to TP53 gene mutation. *Oncogene* 1998; **16**: 2345–9.

44   Heidenreich A, Schenkman NS, Sesterhenn IA *et al.* Immunohistochemical and mutational analysis of the p53 tumor suppressor gene and the bcl-2 oncogene in primary testicular germ cell tumors. *APMIS* 1998; **106**: 90–100.

45   Schwab M, Amler LC. Amplification of cellular oncogenes: a predictor of clinical outcome in human cancer. *Genes Chromo Cancer* 1990; **1**: 181–93.

46   Mostert MM, van de Pol M, Olde Welghuis D *et al.* Comparative genomic hybridization of germ cell tumors of the adult testis: confirmation of karyotypic findings and identification of 12p-amplicon. *Cancer Genet Cytogenet* 1996; **89**: 146–52.

47   Summersgill B, Goker H, Weber-Hall S *et al.* Molecular cytogenetic analysis of adult testicular germ cell tumors and identification of regions of consensus copy number change. *Br J Cancer* 1998; **77**: 305–13.

48   Chresta CM, Masters JRW, Hickman JA. Hypersensitivity of human testicular tumors to etoposide-induced apoptosis is associated with functional p53 and a high bax:bcl-2 ratio. *Cancer Res* 1996; **56**: 1834–41.

49   Burger H, Nooter K, Boersma AW *et al.* Distinct p53-independent apoptotic cell death signalling pathways in testicular germ cell tumor cell lines. *Int J Cancer* 1999; **81**: 620–8.

50   Koberle B, Grimaldi KA, Sunters A *et al.* DNA repair capacity and cisplatin sensitivity of human testis tumor cells. *Int J Cancer* 1997; **70**: 551–5.

51   Koberle B, Masters JRW, Hartley JA *et al.* Defective repair of cisplatin-induced DNA damage caused by reduced XPA protein in testicular germ cell tumors. *Current Biol* 1999; **9**: 273–6.

52   Arriola EL, Rodriguez-Lopez AM, Hickman JA *et al.* Bcl-2 overexpression results in reciprocal downregulation of Bcl-X(L) and sensitizes human testicular germ cell tumors to chemotherapy-induced apoptosis. *Oncogene* 1999; **18**: 1457–64.

17: Surveillance, Chemotherapy, and Radiotherapy for Stage 1 Testicular Germ Cell Tumours

D. H. Palmer & M. H. Cullen

Introduction

At the beginning of the twentieth century, cure rates for early stage non-seminomatous germ cell tumours of the testis were approximately 10% [1]. Now, most patients are cured. Treatment has improved dramatically, but so has the detection of metastases through staging investigations. The introduction of routine chest radiographs, CT scanning and tumour marker (AFP, HCG) analysis brought progressively narrower definitions of stage 1 disease and hence better outcomes for cases labelled as such.

The first elective treatment to positively affect outcome was the routine prophylactic treatment of para-aortic lymph nodes. Traditionally, in the US and most of Europe this comprised retroperitoneal lymph node dissection (RPLND), whereas in the UK radiotherapy was used. Neither method is without long-term side-effects. RPLND frequently resulted in loss of seminal emission, whereas radiotherapy can cause radiation enteritis and stricture in up to 10% of cases [2]. Radiotherapy may also reduce bone marrow tolerance to subsequent chemotherapy and may be associated with the development of second malignancies within the radiation field [3].

In the late 1970s the introduction of cisplatin-based combination chemotherapy revolutionized the treatment of testicular tumours, resulting in cure of most patients even with advanced disease [4]. This allowed the consideration of no prophylactic treatment for carefully investigated and monitored patients with stage 1 disease since those who relapsed could be salvaged using chemotherapy.

Surveillance for stage 1 non-seminomatous germ cell tumours

At the end of the 1970s several groups began to employ a policy of no prophylactic treatment for patients with stage 1 non-seminomatous germ cell tumours, reserving chemotherapy for those patients who subsequently recurred. From 1982, several studies of patients managed in this manner reported recurrence rates of between 17% and 24% [5,6]. Recurrence usually occurred within 12 months of orchidectomy and patients were successfully salvaged using chemotherapy. This led to Medical Research Council (MRC) studies of a policy of surveillance in the management of stage 1 non-seminomatous germ cell tumours.

In 1984, a retrospective analysis of patients managed in a surveillance programme was undertaken [7]. Two hundred and fifty-nine patients treated by orchidectomy alone and followed for a median of 30 months were identified. There were 70 (27%) recurrences, 53 occurring within the first year. As well as examining recurrence rates, a detailed histological review of all tumours was undertaken. Each tumour was assessed, without knowledge of outcome, and scored with respect to histological stage and tumour classification. The relationship between these variables and recurrence was then investigated using univariate and multivariate analyses. The most important independent predictor of recurrence was invasion of testicular veins. Other independent predictors were invasion of lymphatics, absence of yolk sac elements, and presence of undifferentiated tumour. A simple index based on the number of these features present enabled identification of patients at higher risk of recurrence. This is summarized in Fig. 17.1. Fifty-five patients had three or four of these risk factors, and 58% of these relapsed within 2 years of orchidectomy. The addition of further variables did not enhance the predictive model.

Following on from the retrospective analysis, a prospective study of surveillance was undertaken [8]. The aims of this study were to determine recurrence rate and to verify the validity of the histological index as a tool to predict risk of recurrence. Surveillance involved follow-up attendance at monthly intervals for the first year, every 2 months for the second, every 3 months for the third, and so on, often up to 10 years or more. At each visit clinical examination, chest radiograph, and tumour marker assays were

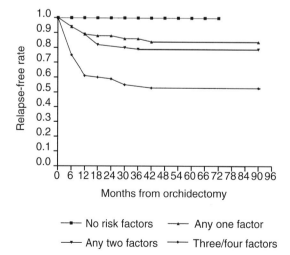

Figure 17.1 Number of prognostic factors and risk of relapse following orchidectomy.

undertaken. CT scanning of the thorax and abdomen was performed 4–6 times in the first year, 0–2 times in the second, and according to clinical indication thereafter. Data from 373 patients with a median follow-up of 5 years were analysed. The recurrence rate was 27%. Of these, 80% recurred within the first year. Following treatment for recurrence with combination cisplatin-containing chemotherapy, 5-year survival exceeded 98%. The prognostic index defined in the retrospective study was applied to this patient population. The ability to define groups at varying risks of recurrence was confirmed. Again a group of patients with any three or all four of the factors listed above were shown to be at a significantly higher risk of recurrence (46% after 2 years).

Similar results have been reported in a recent retrospective analysis of patients with clinical stage 1 non-seminomatous germ cell tumours managed with orchidectomy and RPLND. Two hundred and ninety-two patients were followed for a minimum of 2 years. Risk of metastases was defined as those patients with pathological stage 1 disease who subsequently developed recurrence or those patients with pathological stage 2 disease following RPLND. Embryonal carcinoma predominance (defined as the presence of embryonal carcinoma at a level greater than any other histological type) and vascular invasion (venous and/or lymphatic) were identified as independent risk factors for risk of metastases. Patients without these factors had a metastasis rate of 16%, those with either one had a metastasis rate of 30%, and those with both had a metastasis rate of 62% [9].

Both the retrospective and the prospective MRC surveillance studies demonstrated an overall recurrence rate of 25–30%, with most occurring during the first year after orchidectomy. Nearly all patients with recurrence were salvaged with chemotherapy, resulting in a 5-year survival rate of 98%. These data are consistent with other surveillance studies, and the survival figures compare favourably with the best series for RPLND [10–12]. Thus careful surveillance plus chemotherapy at the earliest sign of recurrence is an effective management approach to patients with stage 1 non-seminomatous germ cell tumours.

Such a policy might appear to offer the perfect management strategy since the majority of patients avoid any further treatment, and those who develop recurrence are detected at an early stage and cured with chemotherapy. However, there are drawbacks. For some patients, frequent hospital attendance, physical examination, blood tests, and CT scans can be stressful and serve as a constant reminder of their cancer history and ongoing risk of recurrence. This has been referred to as the Damocles syndrome. Surveillance also depends critically on excellent patient compliance. This can be a problem for young patients who may have a less well-developed sense of responsibility for their own health. They are more inclined to move to different localities and can experience difficulties with employment, mortgages, life insurance, or adoption while undergoing surveillance.

Adjuvant chemotherapy for stage 1 non-seminomatous germ cell tumours

The MRC studies of surveillance for stage 1 non-seminomatous germ cell tumours reported a histological prognostic index capable of identifying a group of patients with a higher risk of recurrence, approaching 50% after 2 years. This group accounted for 23% of all patients with stage 1 disease [8]. With the success of chemotherapy in the management of advanced non-seminomatous germ cell tumours it was proposed that such high-risk patients may be suitable candidates to receive adjuvant chemotherapy.

Analysis of prognostic factors in disseminated non-seminomatous germ cell tumours has shown that chemotherapy is most effective with minimal tumour burden. This should be relevant to the treatment of subclinical microscopic disease in the adjuvant context.

When using cisplatin-based chemotherapy short-term tolerance decreases with an increasing number of courses. Similarly, long-term toxicity increases with increasing total dose. Using chemotherapy in the adjuvant setting would mean that, even in a high-risk group, about half the patients would be receiving unnecessary treatment. It is therefore vital that the minimum treatment required to eradicate the small tumour burden should be given.

In a trial of adjuvant chemotherapy following RPLND for stage 2 non-seminomatous germ cell tumours, 195 patients were randomized between surveillance or two courses of cisplatin-based chemotherapy [13]. The recurrence rates were 49% and 6% in the respective arms. Five of the six patients who recurred in the chemotherapy arm did so prior to receiving the treatment. A further trial randomized 191 patients with stage 2b non-seminomatous germ cell tumours at RPLND to receive either two or four courses of cisplatin, vincristine, and bleomycin (PVB) chemotherapy [14]. Recurrence rates were equivalent in the two arms. Furthermore, toxicity was reported as 'tolerable' in 84% of patients receiving two courses compared with 53% of patients receiving four courses.

In summary, two courses of adjuvant chemotherapy appear to be sufficient to eradicate residual disease in nearly all cases of stage 2 non-seminomatous germ cell tumours following RPLND, and such treatment is generally well tolerated.

Extrapolating from these data, the MRC designed a prospective study offering two courses of bleomycin, etoposide, and cisplatin (BEP) chemotherapy to patients with high-risk stage 1 non-seminomatous germ cell tumours [15]. The aim of the study was to evaluate the efficacy and long-term toxicity of adjuvant chemotherapy. Since survival was expected to approach 100% the study was non-randomized, but was monitored closely with strict stopping rules should the recurrence rate exceed 5%.

One hundred and fourteen patients were treated and followed up for a median of 4 years. The 2-year recurrence-free survival was 98%. The 95% confidence interval excluded a true recurrence rate of more than 5%. Two patients developed recurrence, one of whom, following histological review, was found to have adenocarcinoma of the rete testis rather than a germ cell tumour. Long-term toxicity was assessed by pre- and post-treatment analysis of renal function, lung function, semen analysis, and audiometry. No major, clinically significant changes were observed. This demonstrates that the major toxicities associated with BEP chemotherapy were mild or absent following just two courses of treatment.

In order to refine and reduce further the toxicity of adjuvant chemotherapy, the MRC set up a pilot study substituting BOP for BEP chemotherapy, in which etoposide is replaced by vincristine [16]. For this study the definition of 'high risk' was broadened to include all patients with 'vascular' (i.e. lymphatic and/or venous) invasion. This was prompted by the difficulties in clearly distinguishing veins and lymphatics histologically, and in assessing the significance of yolk sac elements. Furthermore, there is now more universal acceptance of vascular invasion as the key prognostic factor [17]. This change increases somewhat the 2-year recurrence-free survival of the high-risk group (from 53% to 60%), but also substantially increases the overall proportion of high-risk patients from less than 25% to just over 50%. One hundred and fifteen patients were treated and have been followed for a median of 14 months so far. The 12-month recurrence-free survival was 98.3%. There was less complete alopecia but it was still a significant problem, affecting 20% of cases despite the use of vincristine in place of etoposide.

These studies demonstrated the use of adjuvant chemotherapy to be a safe and effective approach to the management of high-risk stage 1 non-seminomatous germ cell tumours. Since cure is not guaranteed patients cannot be discharged immediately from follow-up. However, a much less intensive surveillance programme can be adopted for patients with recurrence-free survival of 98% at 2 years.

A prospective randomized trial of chemotherapy in good prognosis metastatic non-seminomatous germ cell tumours has compared BEP with BEC in which cisplatin was replaced by the less toxic analogue carboplatin [18]. This study demonstrated cisplatin-based chemotherapy to be superior to the carboplatin-based regime. This suggests that the toxicity of adjuvant chemotherapy could not be further reduced by using carboplatin in place of cisplatin without potentially compromising efficacy.

The MRC currently recommends two courses of BEP for adjuvant chemotherapy for stage 1 patients with vascular invasion.

Management preferences in stage 1 non-seminomatous germ cell tumours

With the advent of safe and effective adjuvant chemotherapy, patients with stage 1 non-seminomatous germ cell tumours, especially those at high risk of recurrence, now have a choice of management options. They may select two courses of adjuvant chemotherapy immediately following orchidectomy, or they may enter an intensive surveillance programme, with three or four courses of chemotherapy only in the event of recurrence. These options achieve the same outcome, with cure rates approaching 100%.

To investigate which approach patients may prefer, a questionnaire survey was undertaken [19]. Questionnaires were sent to patients with newly diagnosed non-seminomatous germ cell tumours, to patients with previous experience of surveillance and/or chemotherapy, and to three groups of healthy controls including oncologists with an interest in testicular tumours. The choice of immediate adjuvant chemotherapy, or surveillance, or for the physician to decide on management was offered for different risks of relapse ranging from 10% to 90%. Two hundred and seven completed questionnaires were analysed. As might be expected, more respondents opted for adjuvant chemotherapy as risk of recurrence increased. This trend was observed in all groups, although there was wide variability in thresholds at which chemotherapy was chosen. In each group, some patients chose adjuvant chemotherapy even at the lowest (10%) level of risk. Patients previously treated with adjuvant chemotherapy were more likely to choose chemotherapy at a lower risk. Patients who had previously undergone surveillance required a higher risk before choosing chemotherapy. Newly diagnosed patients for whom this was a real-life scenario were more likely to defer the decision to their physician than those for whom the question was hypothetical.

This study provided insight into the degree of patient understanding of statistical information and of patient involvement in decision-making. It highlighted that factors such as differences in personality as well as knowledge and experience influence decision-making.

In summary, patients with stage 1 non-seminomatous germ cell tumours can be successfully managed either by a policy of surveillance with chemotherapy only in the event of recurrence, or by treatment with two courses of adjuvant chemotherapy. Both options result in the same excellent survival prospects but with different shortcomings. It may be the case therefore that there is no one single best treatment approach, rather an optimum plan for each individual. This emphasizes the importance of offering clear information about different treatment options to patients, accepting that some will wish their physician to decide.

Management of stage 1 seminoma

Surveillance for stage 1 seminoma

Non-seminomatous germ cell tumour provides an ideal model for surveillance. Early detection of recurrence is facilitated by the use of reliable tumour markers and the vast majority of patients recur within 12 months of orchidectomy, thus allowing a relatively limited period of intense surveillance. The same is not true for seminoma. Studies of patients with stage 1 seminoma managed by orchidectomy alone report a recurrence rate of approximately 20% at 2 years [20]. However, recurrences are occasionally reported more than 8 years after orchidectomy. Furthermore, tumour markers are only rarely a reliable means of detecting recurrence, leading to an increased reliance on the use of clinical and radiological examination. These factors make surveillance a less attractive option for the management of stage 1 seminoma.

Radiotherapy for stage 1 seminoma

Surveillance studies of patients with stage 1 seminoma report a recurrence rate of approximately 20%. Because of the practical and psychological difficulties associated with surveillance, adjuvant treatment following orchidectomy is desirable. Since those patients who do have recurrence are nearly always cured by salvage treatment, it is vital that any adjuvant treatment has acceptable short- and long-term toxicities.

   Traditionally, adjuvant treatment has comprised radiotherapy to the para-aortic and ipsilateral iliac lymph nodes ('dog-leg' field). This approach reduces the recurrence rate from 20% to 3%. Although long-term toxicity is low, clinically significant acute gastrointestinal toxicity is reported in up to 60% of patients, and moderately severe chronic gastrointestinal toxicity in up to 5% [21]. Further, there may be a risk of developing a second malignancy, especially of the upper gastrointestinal tract or bladder [22], or leukaemia due to irradiation of pelvic bone marrow [23]. Analysis of patterns of recurrence has shown that the vast majority occur in the para-aortic lymph nodes, with iliac node recurrence being very rare, as might be predicted given the propensity for lymphatic spread and the anatomy of testicular lymphatic drainage [20]. This suggests a role for reduction in target volume to the para-aortic region, omitting pelvic irradiation, with the aim of reducing toxicity whilst maintaining efficacy.

The MRC therefore undertook a randomized trial comparing 'dog-leg' with para-aortic node radiotherapy. A dose of 30 Gy in 15 fractions was used. Data regarding survival, recurrence pattern and toxicity were analysed. Four hundred and seventy-eight patients were randomized and followed for a median of 4.5 years. During this time there were 18 recurrences, nine in each group. The 3-year recurrence-free survival was 96% in both arms. There were four pelvic recurrences, all in the group receiving para-aortic radiotherapy. Although this difference was statistically significant, the 95% confidence interval for differences in pelvic recurrence rate excluded a true increase in pelvic recurrence of more than 4%.

Acute gastrointestinal toxicity and acute myelotoxicity were seen less often and were less pronounced in the group receiving para-aortic treatment. Chronic gastrointestinal toxicity, specifically peptic ulcer disease, had an equal incidence in both groups. Sperm counts were higher in the para-aortic group, particularly in the first 2 years after treatment. Although the difference narrowed after 2 years owing to recovery of spermatogenesis in the 'dog-leg' group, this may still be clinically relevant in that patients, whose median age was 38 years, may not wish to delay plans for fathering children for several years. Three second malignancies were reported, but the follow-up period is so far too short to assess any difference between the two groups.

In conclusion, this study showed that para-aortic radiotherapy can be safely adopted as routine treatment for patients with stage 1 seminoma (except in cases of prior pelvic, scrotal, or inguinal surgery which may have disrupted normal lymphatic drainage) [24].

A further MRC randomized trial of adjuvant radiotherapy is ongoing in which patients are allocated to receive either 30 Gy in 15 fractions or 20 Gy in 10 fractions in an effort to further reduce toxicity without compromising efficacy. The results of this trial are awaited.

Adjuvant chemotherapy for stage 1 seminoma

By the early 1980s there were reports of increasingly good results with the use of single agent cisplatin chemotherapy for patients with metastatic seminoma. In fact, when matched stage for stage, chemotherapy resulted in longer disease-free survival than radiotherapy [25]. Use of the less toxic platinum analogue carboplatin in patients with metastatic seminoma has also produced successful results [26]. However, the majority of patients who were not cured by carboplatin could be rescued using cisplatin-based chemotherapy, suggesting that carboplatin may be less effective as first line therapy.

The success of chemotherapy in the management of metastatic seminoma prompted the investigation of its use in the adjuvant setting. Chemotherapy has several potential advantages over radiotherapy in this context. In particular, it can be administered more conveniently as a single outpatient treatment compared to the more intensive 10–15 sessions of radiotherapy. Further, the early toxicity of carboplatin chemotherapy is well recognized and easily managed. No significant long-term toxicity has been seen following the use of carboplatin in patients with metastatic disease, even up to 10 years after treatment. Several pilot studies using one or two courses of carboplatin as adjuvant treatment for stage 1 seminoma have been performed. Of around 250 patients who have been studied there have been only three recurrences reported so far, although given the natural history of seminoma further late recurrences are possible [27]. These initial data also suggest that chemotherapy is well tolerated.

Following on from this, the MRC has launched a large, randomized trial comparing a single course of carboplatin with standard radiotherapy for patients with stage 1 seminoma. This trial aims to compare recurrence rates between the two treatment modalities. It also aims to compare quality of life, immediate and delayed toxicity and the relative cost of each treatment. It will also be important to demonstrate that the use of adjuvant chemotherapy does not compromise salvage chemotherapy in the event of recurrence. The trial opened in June 1996 and with current accrual rates will achieve its target of 1200 patients during 2000. This number will allow the exclusion of a difference in survival of 3% or more, with 90% power.

Since this trial aims to substitute one form of adjuvant treatment for another it has not been necessary to identify those patients at a higher risk of recurrence as has been done in patients with non-seminomatous germ cell tumours receiving adjuvant chemotherapy. However, a recent analysis of three large seminoma surveillance studies looked at 549 patients followed for a median of 7 years, during which time 101 patients developed recurrences [28]. Tumour size and rete testis invasion were identified as prognostic factors for recurrence. This suggests that it may be possible to make rational decisions on the management of stage 1 seminoma based on the risk of recurrence, although such prognostic factors must first be validated prospectively.

Conclusion

When studying the use of adjuvant chemotherapy for patients with a curable malignancy the primary endpoint is recurrence rate. However, several other factors must also be considered. It is important to know how many patients are being treated unnecessarily. Such information can come only from analysis of prognostic factors in large numbers of patients. It is also important to recognize the possibility of late toxicity of chemotherapy since this is the potential price to be paid in order to avoid intensive surveillance.

The ultimate aim of managing early stage testicular tumours is to achieve cure with minimal side-effects of treatment and minimal follow-up.

In the case of stage 1 non-seminomatous germ cell tumours adjuvant chemotherapy does not achieve a 100% cure rate, although recurrence-free survival after 2 years is 98%. Further recurrences after this time are unlikely. Chemotherapy therefore offers a realistic alternative to surveillance and may be the preferred treatment for some patients.

For patients with stage 1 seminoma, surveillance is not a satisfactory option since there is no reliable tumour marker to aid early detection of recurrence, and there is an increased incidence of late recurrences compared with non-seminomatous germ cell tumours. The use of adjuvant radiotherapy reduces the recurrence rate from about 20% to 3% with few long-term toxicities. The introduction of carboplatin offers safe treatment that can be given on an outpatient basis with mild, easily controlled acute toxicity. If the current MRC trial comparing a single course of carboplatin with radiotherapy shows an equivalence of disease control then chemotherapy is likely to replace radiotherapy and become standard treatment because of the advantages offered in terms of economy, convenience and lesser toxicity.

References

1   Oliver RTD, Read G, Jones WG. Justification for a policy of surveillance in the management of stage 1 testicular teratoma. In: Denis L, Murphy GP, Prout GR, Shroder F, eds. *Controlled Clinical Trials in Urological Oncology.* New York: Raven Press, 1984: 73–8.

2   Whitmore WF. Surgical treatment of clinical stage 1 non-seminomatous germ cell tumours of the testis. *Cancer Treat Report* 1982; **66**: 5–10.

3   Glatstein E. Optimal management of clinical stage 1 nonseminomatous testicular carcinoma: one oncologist's view. *Cancer Treat Report* 1982; **66**: 11–18.

4   Einhorn LH, Donohue JP. Cis-diaminedichloroplatinum, vinblastine and bleomycin combination chemotherapy in disseminated testicular cancer. *Ann Intern Med* 1977; **87**: 293–8.

5   Peckham MJ, Barrett A, Husband JE, Hendry WF. Orchidectomy alone in testicular stage 1 non-seminomatous germ-cell tumours. *Lancet* 1982; **2**: 678–80.

6   Read G, Johnson RJ, Wilkinson PM, Eddleston B. Prospective study of follow-up alone in stage 1 teratoma of the testis. *Br Med J* 1983; **287**: 1503–5.

7   Freedman LS, Parkinson MC, Jones W *et al.* Histopathology in the prediction of relapse of patients with stage 1 testicular teratoma treated by orchidectomy alone: a Medical Research Council collaborative study. *Lancet* 1987; **2**: 294–8.

8   Read G, Stenning SP, Cullen MH *et al.* Medical Research Council prospective study of surveillance for stage 1 testicular teratoma. *J Clin Oncol* 1992; **10**: 1762–8.

9   Sweeney CJ, Hermans BP, Heilman DK, Foster RS, Donohue JP, Einhorn LH. Results and outcome of retroperitoneal lymph node dissection for clinical stage 1 embryonal carcinoma-predominant testis cancer. *J Clin Oncol* 2000; **18**: 358–62.

10 Donohue JP. Retroperitoneal lymphadenopathy: the anterior approach including bilateral supra-renal hilar dissection. *Urol Clin North Am* 1977; **44**: 509–23.

11 Staubitz WJ, Early KS, Magoss IV *et al*. The surgical treatment of non-seminomatous germinal testis tumours. *Cancer* 1973; **32**: 1206–11.

12 Richie JP. Modified retroperitoneal lymphadenectomy for patients with clinical stage 1 testicular cancer. *Semin Urol* 1988; **6**: 216–22.

13 Williams SD, Stablein DM, Einhorn LH *et al*. Immediate adjuvant chemotherapy versus observation with treatment at relapse in pathological stage 2 testicular cancer. *N Engl J Med* 1987; **317**: 1433–8.

14 Hartlapp JH, Weissbach L, Horstman-Dubral B. Stage 2 non-seminomatous testicular tumours: necessity and extent of adjuvant chemotherapy. *Proc Eur Conf Clin Oncol* 1987; **4**: 183.

15 Cullen MH, Stenning SP, Parkinson MC *et al*. Short course adjuvant chemotherapy in high-risk stage 1 non-seminomatous germ cell tumours of the testis: a Medical Research Council report. *J Clin Oncol* 1996; **14**: 1106–13.

16 Dearnaley SD, Fossa SD, Kaye SB *et al*. Adjuvant bleomycin, vincristine, and cisplatin (BOP) for high risk clinical stage 1 (HRCS1) non-seminomatous germ cell tumours (NSGCT) – a Medical Research Council (MRC) pilot study. *Proc ASCO* 1998; **17**: 1189 (309a).

17 Pont J, Albrecht W, Postner G, Sellner F, Angel K, Holtl W. Adjuvant chemotherapy for high-risk clinical stage 1 nonseminomatous testicular germ cell cancer: long-term results of a prospective trial. *J Clin Oncol* 1996; **14**: 441–8.

18 Horwich A, Sleijfer DT, Fossa SD *et al*. Randomised trial of bleomycin, etoposide, and cisplatin compared with bleomycin, etoposide, and carboplatin in good-prognosis metastatic non-seminomatous germ cell cancer: a multi-institutional Medical Research Council/European Organisation for Research and Treatment of Cancer trial. *J Clin Oncol* 1997; **15**: 1844–52.

19 Cullen MH, Billingham LJ, Cook J, Woodroffe CM. Management preferences in stage 1 non-seminomatous germ cell tumours of the testis: an investigation among patients, controls, and oncologists. *Br J Cancer* 1996; **74**: 1487–91.

20 Horwich A, Alsanjary NA, Hern R, Nicholls J. Surveillance following orchidectomy for stage 1 testicular seminoma. *Br J Cancer* 1992; **65**: 775–8.

21 Fossa SD, Aass N, Kaalhus O. Radiotherapy for testicular seminoma stage 1: treatment results and long-term post-irradiation morbidity in 365 patients. *Int J Radiat Oncol Biol Phys* 1989; **16**: 383–8.

22 Hoff Wanderas E, Fossa SD, Tretli S. Risk of subsequent non-germ cell cancer after treatment of germ cell cancer in 2006 Norwegian male patients. *Eur J Cancer* 1997; **33**: 253–62.

23 Horwich A, Bell J. Mortality and cancer incidence following treatment for seminoma of the testis. *Radiother Oncol* 1994; **30**: 193–8.

24 Fossa SD, Horwich A, Russell JT *et al*. Optimal planning target volume for stage 1 testicular seminoma: a Medical Research Council randomised trial. *J Clin Oncol* 1999; **17**: 1146–54.

25 Oliver RTD. Limitations to the use of surveillance as an option in the management of stage 1 seminoma. *Int J Androl* 1987; **19**: 263–8.

26 Peckham MJ, Hendry WF. Advanced seminoma: treatment with cisplatinum-based combination chemotherapy or carboplatin (JM8). *Br J Cancer* 1985; **1**: 7–13.

27   Oliver RTD, Edmonds PM, Ong JYH *et al*. Pilot study of 1 and 2 course carboplatin as adjuvant for stage 1 seminoma: Should it be tested in a randomised trial against radiotherapy? *Int J Radiat Oncol Biol Phys* 1994; **29**: 2–8.
28   Wade P, von der Maase H, Horwich A *et al*. Prognostic factors for relapse in stage 1 seminoma managed by surveillance. *Proc ASCO* 1998; **17**: 1188 (309a).

18: Chemotherapy of Testicular Cancer

I. A. Burney & G. M. Mead

Introduction

One of the major advances in oncology during the last 25 years has been the achievement of cure for over 80% of patients with metastatic testicular germ cell tumours (GCTs) [1]. This chapter will review the initial management with chemotherapy of patients with metastatic disease. The emphasis throughout will be on treatment results in randomized trials, either completed or currently in progress, and an attempt will be made to define current best standard practice.

Over the past few years, attempts have been made to refine chemotherapy with the aim of reducing treatment toxicity in those patients anticipated to have a good prognosis, and increasing cure rates in patients with adverse presenting features. An important recent advance has been the definition of various prognostic groups in patients with metastatic disease. Over the last 15 years, multiple prognostic factor based classifications have been developed [2–8]. Although these were based on similar prognostic variables, such as tumour bulk and tumour markers, the classifications varied in the patient details within the different prognostic groups. This controversy was resolved with the development of the International Germ Cell Consensus Classification (IGCCC) [9]. This validated prognostic factor-based classification, shown in Table 18.1, has been widely adopted. However, it should be noted that any description of the effects of chemotherapy is muddied by the fact that this classification is not always applied to every chemotherapy study completed before the IGCCC was agreed.

Management of metastatic non-seminomatous GCT

Good prognosis disease

In the IGCCC study, 56% of patients with non-seminoma fell into a good prognosis group; they were found to have a 5-year progression-free survival rate of 89% and an overall survival rate of 92%. The combination of bleomycin, etoposide and cisplatin (BEP) is the standard treatment for these patients, against which new treatments should be compared [10]. BEP

Table 18.1 International Germ Cell Consensus Classification (IGCCC) (International Germ Cell Consensus Group [9])

Risk category	Seminoma	Non-seminomatous germ cell tumour
Good	Any LDH Any HCG Any primary site Non-pulmonary visceral metastases absent	LDH < 1.5 × ULN HCG < 5000 mIU/mL AFP < 1000 ng/mL Gonadal or retroperitoneal primary Non-pulmonary visceral metastases absent
Intermediate	Any LDH Any HCG Any primary site Non-pulmonary visceral metastases present	LDH 1.5–10.0 × ULN HCG 5000–50 000 mIU/mL AFP 1000–10 000 ng/mL Gonadal or retroperitoneal primary Non-pulmonary visceral metastases absent
Poor	—	LDH > 10 × ULN HCG > 50 000 mIU/mL AFP > 10 000 ng/mL Mediastinal primary site Non-pulmonary visceral metastases present

AFP, alpha-fetoprotein; HCG, human chorionic gonadotrophin; LDH, lactate dehydrogenase; ULN, upper limit of normal.

became the standard of care following the Southeastern Cancer Study Group (SECSG) trial in which BEP was compared with the then standard chemotherapy regimen, PVB (cisplatin, vinblastine and bleomycin), and was found to have equivalent response and survival rates with significantly less toxicity [10]. Over the past few years, attempts have been made to minimize the toxicity of BEP, in particular the pulmonary toxicity related to bleomycin exposure, and the neurotoxicity and nephrotoxicity caused by cisplatin.

ELIMINATION OF BLEOMYCIN

Four randomized trials have addressed the value of bleomycin in chemotherapy programmes [11–14]. Bosl and colleagues [11] randomized patients to four cycles of etoposide and cisplatin (EP) vs. three cycles of vinblastine, bleomycin, cisplatin, cyclophosphamide and dactinomycin (VAB-6). VAB-6 and EP provided equivalent long-term disease-free survival; however, EP proved the less toxic regimen. The Australasian Germ Cell Trial Group randomized patients to receive cisplatin and vinblastine with or without bleomycin (PV vs. PVB) [12]. Despite a higher rate of toxic death in the three-drug arm, more patients died of progressive disease in the two-drug arm.

Table 18.2 Randomized trials: omission of bleomycin

Reference	Regimen	Cycles	Complete remission (%)	Comments
11	VAB-6	3	85	Equivalent in efficacy
	EP	4	82	Two-drug regimen less nephrotoxic and myelosuppressive
12	PVB	4	94	Two drugs inferior
	PV	4	89	More relapses (15% vs. 5%) in PV arm
				More toxic deaths with PVB
13	BEP	4	94	Two drugs inferior
	EP	4	88	More treatment failures in BEP arm
				Toxicities comparable
14	BEP	4	95	Two drugs inferior
	EP	4	87	Long-term survival equal
				More toxicity in BEP arm

BEP, bleomycin, etoposide, cisplatin; EP, etoposide, cisplatin; PV, cisplatin, vinblastine; PVB, cisplatin, vinblastine, bleomycin; VAB-6, vinblastine, bleomycin, cisplatin, cyclophosphamide, dactinomycin.

The Eastern Cooperative Oncology Group, following a study showing equivalence of three vs. four cycles of BEP (etoposide dose $500 \, mg/m^2$ per course), randomized patients to receive three courses of cisplatin and etoposide with or without bleomycin (EP vs. BEP) [13]. This study was discontinued when inferior complete remission (CR), failure-free survival (FFS) and overall survival (OS) rates were found in the group treated without bleomycin. More recently, the European Organization for Research and Treatment of Cancer (EORTC) reported the results of a large randomized trial which compared cisplatin and etoposide dose ($360 \, mg/m^2$ per course) with or without bleomycin (EP vs. BEP) in 419 patients [14]. Although the incidence of pulmonary and neurotoxicity and Raynaud's phenomenon was increased in the three-drug arm, failure-free survival was reduced, and it was concluded that bleomycin could not be deleted without compromising treatment efficacy. The results of these trials are summarized in Table 18.2.

Although the four trials differ in the use of vinblastine or etoposide, and the dose of etoposide used, they did demonstrate that the elimination of bleomycin resulted in inferior CR rates and in many cases compromised the FFS and OS. Hence, at the moment, the recommendation is to use bleomycin at a dose of 30 000 units weekly. More recent studies in good prognosis disease have used bleomycin to a total dose of 270 000 units—a level that has rarely been associated with bleomycin lung in younger patients. Concerns remain, however, about older patients (>40 years) [15], in whom four cycles of BEP with a reduced dose of bleomycin (see below) may be preferable.

REDUCING THE DURATION OF CHEMOTHERAPY

In an attempt to reduce toxicity without compromising efficacy, the SECSG conducted a randomized prospective trial comparing BEP (etoposide dose 500 mg/m^2 per course) given for four cycles over 12 weeks with three cycles over 9 weeks [16]. After a median follow-up of 10.1 years there was no significant difference in survival between the two treatment groups [17]. The statistical validity of this study of 184 patients has been criticized because of the relatively wide confidence intervals. The EORTC and the Medical Research Council (MRC) recently completed a large phase III trial including 812 patients in which this question was re-examined [18]. This study was designed to rule out a 5% reduction in 2-year FFS; preliminary results suggest this aim has been achieved, but the final analysis is awaited.

Taken together these two trials suggest that three cycles of BEP (etoposide 500 mg/m^2 per course) are as effective as four cycles in terms of achieving CR and long-term FFS in the good prognosis group. The omission of bleomycin appears to compromise the short- and long-term CR rates in good prognosis GCT either when three courses of treatment are used or when etoposide is used at reduced dose for four courses. It is suggested, however, that three cycles of BEP and four cycles of EP (etoposide dose 500 mg/m^2 per course in both regimes) may be equally effective—certainly patients treated by the Memorial Group have achieved a durable CR rate of 88% following four cycles of EP [19]. Recently, the French Federation of Cancer Centres reported the results of the first randomized trial addressing this issue in abstract form. They compared three cycles of BEP with four cycles of EP in good prognosis patients. The preliminary results confirmed equivalent efficacy and toxicity for both treatment regimens [20].

SUBSTITUTION OF CARBOPLATIN FOR CISPLATIN

Another important issue that has been addressed in the past few years has been the possibility of the substitution of carboplatin for cisplatin, thereby reducing the nephrotoxicity and neurotoxicity of treatment. These efforts are summarized in Table 18.3. Carboplatin is an analogue of cisplatin which has a substantially lower gastrointestinal, renal and neurological toxicity profile and may be given in an outpatient setting.

A multi-institutional trial in the USA randomized patients prospectively to either etoposide and cisplatin (EP) cycled every 21 days or etoposide and carboplatin (EC) cycled every 28 days [21]. Carboplatin was administered at a dose of 500 mg/m^2. Although the CR rates were comparable in the two groups, the relapse-free survival was inferior for the patients treated with EC. Mature survival data have not been reported. Subsequently the German

Table 18.3 Randomized trials: substitution of carboplatin for cisplatin

Reference	Regimen	Cycles	Complete remission (%)	Comments
21	EP	4	90	More relapses (12% vs. 3%) in EC arm
	EC	4	88	Relapse-free survival inferior for EC; overall survival similar
22	BEP	4	81	More relapses (32% vs. 13%) in CEB arm
	CEB	4	76	More adverse events in CEB arm
23	BEP	4	94	More treatment failures in CEB arm
	CEB	4	87	More deaths in CEB arm

BEP, bleomycin, etoposide, cisplatin; CEB, bleomycin, etoposide, carboplatin; EC, etoposide, carboplatin, cycled every 4 weeks; EP, etoposide, cisplatin, cycled every 3 weeks.

Testicular Cancer Study Group compared a combination of carboplatin, etoposide and bleomycin (CEB) with BEP [22]. Both combinations were repeated every 21 days and the carboplatin dose was calculated to an area under the curve (AUC) of 5. The CR rates in the two groups were comparable; however, more patients relapsed in the CEB arm (32% vs. 13%).

More recently, the MRC/EORTC groups have reported a large randomized multicentred trial comparing four cycles of BEP with four cycles of CEB [23]. Carboplatin was given at a dose of AUC 5 and was escalated subject to the depth of nadir blood counts; the treatment was repeated at 21-day intervals. Etoposide was given at a dose of 360 mg/m^2 per course in both arms of the study and, unusually, bleomycin was given at a dose of 30 000 units every 3 weeks for four courses. A significantly larger number of patients who were allocated to receive BEP achieved CR. The FFS at 1 year was also significantly superior for the BEP group (91% vs. 77%). Indeed this result was comparable to those achieved with either BEP × 3 or EP × 4. Currently in the UK the standard regimen is BEP × 3 (etoposide 500 mg/m^2), but the consensus view is that EP given for four courses [19,20] or BEP given for four courses (etoposide 360 mg/m^2 per course, with bleomycin 30 000 units per course) [23] will produce similar results.

Treatment of intermediate and poor risk GCT

About 40–45% of patients fall into the intermediate/poor risk groups. According to the IGCCC database the 5-year survival rates for the intermediate and poor risk groups are 79% and 48%, respectively [9]. Although the IGCCC stratifies patients in three risk groups, the management of intermediate and poor risk groups is usually considered together. Patients in these groups often present with clinically threatening disease which requires urgent treatment. A number of trials have addressed the issue of improving the outcome for these patients. These trials have investigated escalation of the cisplatin dose, dose intensity increase, dose intensity maintenance by colony stimulating factors, the substitution of bleomycin with more active agents such as ifosfamide, and also the use of first line high dose chemotherapy (HDCT). These studies will now be described.

DOSE ESCALATION OF CISPLATIN

Cisplatin is probably the most important drug in the management of advanced germ cell malignancy. In an attempt to see whether dose escalation of this drug would improve outcome, the SECSG and Southwest Oncology Group (SWOG) conducted a randomized trial comparing a cisplatin dose of either 20 mg/m^2 i.v. for 5 days, or 40 mg/m^2 i.v. for 5 days given as part of the BEP treatment programme [24]. Sixty-eight per cent of the patients in the high dose arm and 73% of patients in the standard dose arm achieved CR. The OS at the median follow-up of 24 months was 74% in each arm. The high dose cisplatin arm was far more toxic and the study group felt this could not be recommended.

IFOSFAMIDE BASED REGIMENS

Ifosfamide is clearly an active drug in advanced germ cell cancer and has been used to achieve durable remissions in 25–30% of patients with recurrent GCT [25]. In a prospective randomized trial, patients were allocated to receive either four cycles of conventional BEP or four cycles of etoposide, ifosfamide and cisplatin (VIP) [26]. The remission rate was 37% for VIP and 31% for BEP. FFS and OS for the two groups were 64% and 60% and 74% and 71%, respectively. The treatments were considered equivalent; however, VIP was far more toxic and BEP was therefore recommended as standard therapy for these patients.

The MRC/EORTC developed a similar phase III trial comparing an intensive sequential chemotherapy schedule (BOP/VIP-B) consisting of bleomycin, vincristine, cisplatin/etoposide, ifosfamide, cisplatin and bleomycin with four cycles of BEP followed by two cycles of EP [27]. Both groups received a total dose of cisplatin of 600 mg/m^2 and bleomycin 360 000 units. With a median follow-up of 3.1 years there was no significant difference in the FFS or OS between the two arms. Once again, however, myelosuppression, febrile neutropenia and weight loss were far more common in the BOP/VIP-B arm of the trial, and it was concluded that BEP/EP should remain the standard treatment.

In conclusion, neither ifosfamide nor cisplatin dose intensification have resulted in a survival advantage for patients with intermediate/poor prognosis disease but do cause increased toxicity. BEP remains the standard therapy.

USE OF COLONY STIMULATING FACTORS TO MAINTAIN
THE DOSE INTENSITY

A subset of patients in the MRC/EORTC study were further randomized to receive or not to receive granulocyte colony stimulating factor (G-CSF) (filgrastim) to try and maintain the dose intensity of the two chemotherapy arms and to determine whether this strategy would have a favourable impact on survival [28]. Filgrastim was administered at a dose of 5 µg/kg/day from days 3 to 9 after each cycle of BOP and from days 6 to 19 after each cycle of VIP, BEP or EP. Patients in the filgrastim arm achieved significantly higher dose intensities despite which the toxic death rate was reduced in patients receiving BOP/VIP-B (although not in the BEP arm). However, there was no overall beneficial effect on FFS or survival and it was concluded that there was no role for the routine use of filgrastim in these patients.

In a further study, Bajorin and colleagues randomized 104 patients being treated with ifosfamide based combinations to receive or not to receive granulocyte-macrophage colony stimulating factor (GM-CSF) [29]. Although they observed fewer clinically significant infections with the GM-CSF-treated arm during the first cycle of chemotherapy, a similar effect was not observed during the subsequent cycles.

The results of these two studies suggest that the routine use of colony stimulating factors cannot be justified outside clinical trials.

ROLE OF HIGH DOSE CHEMOTHERAPY

High dose chemotherapy in the modern era has focused on the drug combination carboplatin and etoposide (± cyclophosphamide or ifosfamide). The use of high dose therapy following initial standard treatment has been evaluated in two initial phase II trials from the Memorial Hospital.

In a preliminary study, patients with poor risk features who were found to have slow decline of alpha-fetoprotein (AFP) or beta-human chorionic gonadotrophin (BHCG) during standard therapy with VAB-6 were switched to treatment with high dose carboplatin and etoposide [30]. Comparison of the results of this study with historical controls suggested an increase in event-free and overall survival in favour of the high dose chemotherapy arm.

In a subsequent study [31], Motzer and colleagues similarly treated patients with poor prognosis disease with slow marker decline during VIP chemotherapy with high dose therapy — on this occasion using a combination of high dose carboplatin, etoposide and cyclophosphamide supplemented by stem cell and growth factor support. Again the authors concluded that this treatment approach may well have salvaged patients otherwise destined to develop progressive disease.

As a result of these studies a multi-institutional randomized phase III study is currently under way in the USA comparing four cycles of BEP with two cycles of BEP followed by two cycles of high dose cyclophosphamide, carboplatin and etoposide with stem cell support. Results are awaited with interest.

Bokemeyer and colleagues have taken a different approach to poor prognosis GCT. In an initial phase I/II dose finding study, they treated patients with escalating doses of VIP supported initially by growth factors, then by growth factors given together with previously harvested peripheral stem cells [32]. This approach proved feasible, and in a matched pair analysis [33] appeared more successful than standard chemotherapy with BEP or VIP. This treatment is currently being compared with standard BEP in a randomized EORTC trial in poor prognosis patients.

Following a successful phase II evaluation of paclitaxel [34] the EORTC has recently initiated a new trial in patients with intermediate prognosis disease comparing BEP with T-BEP (paclitaxel added to standard doses of BEP). The results of this study are awaited with interest.

In summary, for intermediate and poor prognosis patients BEP remains the 'best' current therapy.

Treatment of seminoma

The IGCCC classifies seminoma into either good (90% of cases) or intermediate (10% of cases) risk on the basis of the absence/presence of non-pulmonary visceral disease [9].

Currently chemotherapy is recommended for patients with stage IIC, III and IV disease or for patients who relapse following radiotherapy [35–37].

An important difference between patients with seminoma and non-seminoma is the age profile of the patient population. Patients with seminoma are older by a median of 10 years and therefore are more prone to chemotherapy toxicity, particularly with regard to bleomycin [15]. For this reason, and because of the great chemosensitivity of seminoma, a number of studies have examined the potential role of single agent chemotherapy, particularly with carboplatin [38,39]. These studies were considered sufficiently encouraging to proceed to a randomized trial, conducted by the MRC, in which 120 patients were randomized to receive either carboplatin (400 mg/m^2 every 21 days) or cisplatin and etoposide [40]. This study was prematurely terminated when it became apparent that carboplatin was inferior to cisplatin when used in a sister study in non-seminoma, as described previously [23]. In this study carboplatin proved to have an inferior FFS (76% vs. 82%) and survival (89% vs. 91%), although the differences were not statistically significant because of wide confidence intervals.

A similar comparative trial (carboplatin vs. cisplatin, etoposide and ifosfamide) has been completed in Germany but is as yet unpublished. Further data on seminoma are available from the EP vs. EC multi-institutional study previously described [21]. In this study 26% of randomized patients had pure seminoma and those that received EC (etoposide and carboplatin) had a significantly poorer failure-free survival than comparable patients receiving EP. Detailed results from the MRC/EORTC study comparing three BEP vs. four BEP [18] are awaited with interest. Twenty-five per cent of these patients had pure seminoma.

On the basis of the limited data available, the known chemosensitivity of disease and concern about the toxicity of bleomycin, four cycles of EP would seem a reasonable standard chemotherapy for advanced seminoma, although three cycles of BEP should produce equivalent results in younger patients.

Who should treat GCT

In the past few years there has been some debate regarding the optimal site of treatment for patients with GCT [41]. Given the exceptional chemosensitivity and high rates of cure which should be achievable in this condition, the Calman-Hine group has advised that these patients should be managed in Cancer Centres. Recent guidelines from the Scottish International Guidelines Network also recommended that such patients be referred to specialist centres. Additional support for this approach is provided by retrospective analysis of the previously described BEP vs. BOP/VIP-B study [42]. This showed that those treatment institutions entering smaller numbers of patients (<5 vs. >5 randomized) achieved inferior results, with lower CR rates, lower rates of surgery, higher rates of toxic death and lower survival. The treating institution appeared to be a prognostic factor of the same magnitude as the established pretreatment characteristics. Such data with regard to survival and treatment complications confirm the views of most oncologists in clinical practice, who argue strongly for centralization and specialization.

Conclusion

Remarkable improvements in survival have occurred in patients with metastatic GCT. Using the IGCCC criteria, patients with good prognosis disease can expect FFS rates of at least 90%, with cure rates in excess of 95%, if treated with BEP × 3 [18], EP × 4 [19,20] or BEP (low dose etoposide and bleomycin) × 4 [23]. Standard therapy for intermediate/poor prognosis disease remains four cycles of BEP, with bleomycin given to a dose of 360 000 units. These patients should achieve overall FFS rates of 60–65%, with cure rates of 70–75%.

References

1   Bosl G, Sheinfield J, Bajorin D *et al*. Cancer of the testis. In: Devita VT, Hellman S, Rosenberg SA, eds. *Cancer: Principles and Practice of Oncology*, 5th edn. New York: Lippincott-Raven, 1997: 1397–425.

2   Bajorin D, Katz A, Chan E *et al*. Comparison of criteria for assigning germ cell tumour patients to 'good risk' and 'poor risk' studies. *J Clin Oncol* 1988; **6**: 786–92.

3   Birch R, Williams S, Cone A *et al*. Prognostic factors for favourable outcome in disseminated germ cell tumours. *J Clin Oncol* 1986; **4**: 400–7.

4   Bosl GJ. Prognostic factors for metastatic testicular germ cell tumours: the Memorial Sloan-Kettering cancer model. *Eur Urol* 1993; **23**: 182–7.

5   Droz JP, Kramar A, Ghosn M *et al*. Prognostic factors in advanced non-seminomatous testicular cancer: a multivariate logistic regression analysis. *Cancer* 1988; **62**: 564–8.

6   Mead GM, Stenning SP, Parkinson MC *et al*. The second Medical Research Council study of prognostic factors in non-seminomatous germ cell tumours. (Medical Research Council Testicular Working Party.) *J Clin Oncol* 1992; **10**: 85–94.

7   Stoter G, Sleifer D, Kaye SB *et al*. Prognostic factors in metastatic non-seminomatous germ cell tumours: an interim analysis of the EORTC GU-Group experience. *Eur Urol* 1993; **23**: 202–6.

8   Gerl A, Clemm C, Lamerz R *et al*. Prognostic implications of tumour marker analysis in non-seminomatous germ cell tumours with poor prognosis metastatic disease. *Eur J Cancer* 1993; **7**: 961–5.

9   International Germ Cell Consensus Group. International Germ Cell Consensus Classification: A prognostic factor based staging system for metastatic germ cell cancers. *J Clin Oncol* 1997; **15**: 594–603.

10 Williams SD, Birch R, Einhorn LD *et al*. Treatment of disseminated germ cell tumours with cisplatin, bleomycin and either vinblastine or etoposide. *N Engl J Med* 1987; **316**: 1435–40.

11 Bosl GJ, Geller NL, Bajorin D *et al*. A randomised trial of etoposide + cisplatin vs vinblastine + bleomycin + cisplatin + cyclophosphamide + dactinomycin in patients with good prognosis germ cell tumours. *J Clin Oncol* 1988; **6**: 1231–8.

12 Levi JA, Raghavan D, Harvey V *et al*. The importance of bleomycin in combination chemotherapy for good prognosis germ cell carcinoma. *J Clin Oncol* 1993; **11**: 1300–5.

13 Loehrer PJ, Johnson DH, Elson P *et al*. Importance of bleomycin in favourable-prognosis disseminated germ cell tumours: an Eastern Co-operative Oncology Group trial. *J Clin Oncol* 1995; **13**: 470–6.

14 deWit R, Stoter G, Kaye SB *et al*. Importance of bleomycin in combination chemotherapy for good prognosis testicular nonseminoma: a randomised study of the European Organisation for Research and Treatment of Cancer genitourinary tract cooperative group. *J Clin Oncol* 1997; **15**: 1837–43.

15 Simpson AB, Paul J, Graham J, Kaye SB. Fatal bleomycin pulmonary toxicity in the west of Scotland 1991–5: a review of patients with germ cell tumours. *Br J Cancer* 1998; **78**: 1061–6.

16 Einhorn LH, Williams SD, Loehrer PH *et al*. Evaluation of optimal duration of chemotherapy in favourable prognosis disseminated germ cell tumours: a Southeastern Cancer Study Group protocol. *J Clin Oncol* 1989; **7**: 387–91.

17 Saxman SB, Finch D, Gonin R, Einhorn LH. Long term follow up of a phase III study of three versus four cycles of bleomycin, etoposide and cisplatin in favourable prognosis germ cell tumours: the Indiana University experience. *J Clin Oncol* 1998; **16**: 702–6.

18 deWit R, Roberts JT, Wilkinson P *et al*. Is 3BEP equivalent to 3BEP-1EP in good prognosis germ cell cancer? An EORTC/MRC phase III study. *Proc Am Soc Clin Oncol* 1999; **18**: 309a.

19 Xiao H, Maxumdar M, Bajorin D *et al*. Long term follow up of patients with good risk germ cell tumours treated with etoposide and cisplatin. *J Clin Oncol* 1997; **15**: 2553–8.

20 Culine S, Kerbrat P, Bouzy J *et al*. Are 3 cycles of bleomycin, etoposide and cisplatin (3BEP) or 4 cycles of etoposide and cisplatin (4EP) equivalent regimens for patients with good risk metastatic seminomatous germ cell tumours (NSGCT)? Preliminary results of a randomised trial. *Proc Am Soc Clin Oncol* 1999; **18**: 309a.

21 Bajorin DF, Sarosdy MF, Pfister DG *et al*. Randomised trial of etoposide and cisplatin versus etoposide and carboplatin in patients with good risk germ cell tumours: a multi-institutional study. *J Clin Oncol* 1993; **11**: 598–606.

22 Bokemeyer C, Kohrmann O, Tischler J *et al*. A randomised trial of cisplatin, etoposide and bleomycin (PEB) versus carboplatin, etoposide and bleomycin (CEB) for patients with good risk metastatic nonseminomatous germ cell tumours. *Ann Oncol* 1996; **7**: 1015–21.

23 Horwich A, Sleifer D, Fossa S *et al*. Randomised trial of bleomycin, etoposide and cisplatin compared with bleomycin, etoposide, and carboplatin in good prognosis metastatic non-seminomatous germ cell cancer: a multiinstitutional Medical Research Council/European Organisation for Research and Treatment of Cancer trial. *J Clin Oncol* 1997; **15**: 1844–52.

24 Nichols CR, Williams SD, Loehrer PJ *et al*. Randomised study of cisplatin dose intensity in poor risk germ cell tumours: a Southeastern Cancer Study Group and Southwest Oncology Group protocol. *J Clin Oncol* 1991; **9**: 1163–72.

25 Motzer RJ, Cooper K, Geller NL *et al*. The role of ifosfamide plus cisplatin based chemotherapy as salvage therapy for patients with refractory germ cell tumours. *Cancer* 1990; **66**: 2476–81.

26 Nichols CR, Catalano PJ, Crawford ED *et al*. Randomised comparison of cisplatin and etoposide and either bleomycin or ifosfamide in treatment of advanced disseminated germ cell tumours: an Eastern Cooperative Oncology Group, Southwest Oncology Group, and Cancer and Leukaemia Group B study. *J Clin Oncol* 1998; **16**: 1287–93.

27 Kaye SB, Fossa S, Mead GM *et al*. Intensive induction-sequential chemotherapy with BOP/VIP-B compared with treatment with BEP/EP for poor prognostic metastatic nonseminomatous germ cell tumour: a randomised Medical Research Council/European Organisation for Research and Treatment of Cancer study. *J Clin Oncol* 1998; **16**: 692–701.

28 Fossa SD, Kaye SB, Mead GM *et al*. Filgrastim during combination chemotherapy of patients with poor prognosis metastatic germ cell malignancy. *J Clin Oncol* 1998; **16**: 716–24.

29 Bajorin DF, Nichols CR, Schmoll HJ *et al*. Recombinant human granulocyte-macrophage colony stimulating factor as an adjunct to conventional dose ifosfamide based chemotherapy for patients with advanced or relapsed germ cell tumours: a randomised trial. *J Clin Oncol* 1995; **12**: 79–86.

30 Motzer RJ, Maxumdar M, Gulati SC *et al*. Phase II trial of high dose carboplatin and etoposide with autologous bone marrow transplantation in first line therapy for patients with poor risk germ cell tumours. *J Natl Cancer Inst* 1993; **85**: 1828–35.

31   Motzer RJ, Mazumdar M, Bajorin DF *et al*. High dose carboplatin, etoposide and cyclophosphamide with autologous bone marrow transplantation in first line therapy for patients with poor risk germ cell tumours. *J Clin Oncol* 1997; **15**: 2546–52.

32   Bokemeyer C, Horstrick A, Beyer J *et al*. The use of dose intensified chemotherapy in the treatment of metastatic nonseminomatous testicular germ cell tumours: German Testicular Cancer Study Group. *Semin Oncol* 1990; **25**: 24–32.

33   Bokemeyer C, Kollmannsberger C, Meisner C *et al*. First line high dose chemotherapy compared with standard dose PEB/VIP chemotherapy in patients with advanced germ cell tumours: a multivariate and matched-pair analysis. *J Clin Oncol* 1999; **17**: 340–56.

34   Bokemeyer C, Beyer J, Metzner B *et al*. Phase II study of paclitaxel in patients with relapsed or cisplatin-refractory testicular cancer. *Ann Oncol* 1996; **7**: 31–4.

35   Einhorn LH, Williams SD. Chemotherapy of disseminated seminoma. *Cancer Clin Trials* 1980; **3**: 307–13.

36   Horwich A, Dearnaley DP. Treatment of seminoma. *Semin Oncol* 1992; **19**: 171–80.

37   Mencel PJ, Motzer RJ, Mazumdar M *et al*. Advanced seminoma: results, survival and prognostic factors in 142 patients. *J Clin Oncol* 1994; **12**: 120–6.

38   Horwich A, Dearnaley DP, Duchesne G *et al*. Simple nontoxic treatment of advanced metastatic seminoma with carboplatin. *J Clin Oncol* 1989; **7**: 1150–6.

39   Schmoll HJ, Harstrick A, Bokemeyer C *et al*. Single agent carboplatinum for advanced seminoma. *Cancer* 1993; **72**: 237–47.

40   Horwich A, Oliver TD, Fossa SD *et al*. A randomised MRC trial comparing single agent carboplatin with etoposide and cisplatin in patients with advanced metastatic seminoma. *Proc ASCO* 1996: Abstract 668.

41   Mead GM. Who should manage germ cell tumours of the testis. *Br J Urol* 1999; **84**: 61–7.

42   Collette L, Sylvester RJ, Stenning SP *et al*. Impact of treating institution on survival of patients with poor prognosis metastatic nonseminoma. *J Natl Cancer Inst* 1999; **91**: 839–46.

19: Salvage Chemotherapy Regimens for Relapsing Germ Cell Cancer

M. L. Harvey & G. M. Mead

Introduction

Although the majority of patients with metastatic germ cell cancer are cured, for the small group of patients requiring salvage chemotherapy the overall chance of survival is relatively poor, ranging between 25% and 30% [1–4]. Yet for these patients, survival is a significant prospect. In this chapter we define this group and describe their prospects.

Definitions

Patients with primary chemorefractory or relapsing germ cell cancer are a heterogeneous group requiring careful definition. Confirmation of relapse is required, and is diagnosed on the basis of rising tumour markers or biopsy proof of residual unresectable viable germ cell cancer. This group should be distinguished from patients with stable markers at the end of chemotherapy, who generally present initially with very high human chorionic gonadotrophin (HCG) levels. This is because 45% of these patients will have HCG levels which will gradually return to normal without further therapy [5]. Patients with rising markers need also to be classified separately from those patients with growing tumour masses and normal serum markers who usually have differentiated teratoma or occasionally a second non-germ cell malignancy and whose treatment of choice will usually be surgery rather than chemotherapy [6,7]. Finally within this heterogeneous group are those patients with brain metastases at relapse who present with one of two different clinical pictures with differing prognoses. Isolated relapse in the brain may occur as a sanctuary site phenomenon following the completion of chemotherapy. Cure is possible in as many as 39% of these cases with surgery and/or irradiation [8]. By contrast, patients with intra-cerebral and systemic relapse usually have an appalling prognosis and are often better managed palliatively.

Prognostic variables

The majority of relapses occur early after the completion of chemotherapy.

In a recent Medical Research Council study, 57% of relapses occurred in <1 year, 20% in 1–2 years and only 23% in >2 years [4]. However, late relapse at over 2 years occurred in 2.9% of the total cases originally commencing chemotherapy, a figure identical to that found by the Indiana group [9]. The prognostic variables defined by the majority of studies include the type of initial chemotherapy and the primary site of the original cancer.

It is widely accepted that cisplatin remains the key drug in both the initial and salvage management of germ cell cancers. The failure of a tumour to respond to cisplatin is in itself a major prognostic variable. This failure is defined as evidence of relapse of cancer within 4 weeks of the last cisplatin dose and is associated with a very adverse outcome [10].

Potentially curative treatments in the setting of recurrent disease include conventional dose salvage therapy, high-dose chemotherapy with autologous stem cell transplantation (ASCT), surgery or any combination of these treatments. Although surgery is ordinarily avoided in patients with rising tumour markers at the time of first relapse, there is no doubt that this treatment can be curative in selected patients failing second or third line chemotherapy ('desperation surgery') and should be considered in all cases with resectable lesions [11].

The literature describing salvage chemotherapy for germ cell cancers is extremely heterogeneous, largely comprising the referral treatment experience of larger Cancer Centres and thereby affected by selection bias. No randomized trials have yet been reported. The great majority of patients will require salvage treatment with either conventional dose or high-dose chemotherapy. These treatments are associated with significant toxicity and, in this context, the identification of the prognostic factors which determine outlook is extremely significant for individual patients.

For patients receiving their first tranche of salvage chemotherapy, adverse prognostic factors include primary refractory disease, duration of interval between complete response and relapse, and the level of serum markers at relapse (variably HCG, alpha-fetoprotein (AFP) and lactate dehydrogenase (LDH)) [1–4].

In two recent series good and poor prognostic groups were identified (Table 19.1). Gerl *et al.* [3] were able to identify 42% of patients in relapse who had a 5-year survival of 72% compared with 11% 5-year survival in the remaining patients. Similarly, Fossa *et al.* [4], in the largest series published to date, identified a good prognosis group constituting 76% of cases with a 5-year survival of 47% and a poor prognosis group with a 3-year survival of 0%. Fossa *et al.* concluded that the good prognosis patients could reasonably be treated with conventional dose salvage therapy but suggested that high-dose therapy would be considered for remaining patients.

Table 19.1 Prognostic factors at first relapse of germ cell cancer treated with conventional dose salvage chemotherapy

Gerl *et al.* [3]
Adverse factors:
  Age ≤ 35 years
  Complete response to initial treatment
  Relapse-free interval > 3 months
67 patients
No risk factors ($n = 28, 42\%$) 5-year survival 72%
  (54–90%)
Any risk factors ($n = 39, 58\%$) 5-year survival 11% (0–22%)

Fossa *et al.* [4]
Adverse factors:
  Progression-free survival < 2 years
  < Complete response to induction chemotherapy
  High markers (AFP > 100 kU/L or HCG > 100 IU/L)
124 patients
One or two factors ($n = 94, 76\%$) 5-year survival 47%
Three factors ($n = 30, 24\%$) 3-year survival 0%

Beyer *et al.* [10] assessed prognostic factors in 310 patients undergoing high-dose chemotherapy at four Centres. Wide variations between Centres were found in the treatment given prior to high-dose therapy and in the drug combinations, dosages and schedules used for this treatment. After multivariate analysis, the factors found to be associated with a poor prognosis were scored and three prognostic groups identified (Table 19.2).

Conventional salvage therapies

Single agents

In the early 1980s, etoposide was shown to be highly active in patients who failed the then standard chemotherapy regimens [12]. This agent was then incorporated into first line therapy and shown to be a highly effective substitute for vinblastine in the bleomycin, etoposide, cisplatin (BEP) regimen [13]. Etoposide is now less frequently used in conventional dose at the time of first relapse, but certainly has a role as a component of high-dose therapy (see below) [14,15]. Etoposide has also been evaluated as an oral agent, either as a maintenance therapy following salvage high-dose chemotherapy or as palliative therapy in patients deemed incurable with chemotherapy or surgery [16,17].

The next agent to be systematically evaluated after etoposide was ifosfamide. This was first used as a single agent in heavily pretreated patients with an overall response rate of 23% in patients with cisplatin refractory disease

Table 19.2 Prognostic variables at the time of salvage high-dose chemotherapy
(Beyer *et al.* [10])

Factor	Score
1 Progressive disease before high-dose chemotherapy	1
2 Mediastinal primary non-seminoma	1
3 Cisplatin refractory disease (stable or responding disease on cisplatin with failure < 4 weeks)	1
4 Absolute cisplatin refractory disease (progression within 4 weeks of cisplatin, no stable disease or response)	2
5 HCG before high-dose chemotherapy > 1000 IU/L	2

	No.	Two-year failure-free survival (%)	Two-year overall survival (%)
Good (score 0)	118	51	61
Intermediate (score 1 or 2)	92	27	34
Poor (score > 2)	19	5	8

[18]. It has not been confirmed that there is a role for ifosfamide in initial therapy but this agent remains a frequently used component of standard second line chemotherapy [19].

Methotrexate has also been evaluated. This is a highly active drug in gestation trophoblastic disease and probably has some activity in male germ cell cancers [20]. However, a conflicting report found little activity for methotrexate used at moderately high dose ($1 \, g/m^2$) [21]. No responses were seen in 12 heavily pretreated patients. The anthracyclines appear to have little activity as second line therapy. Both doxorubicin and epirubicin have been evaluated and found to be inactive [22,23].

New drugs

The testing of new chemotherapy agents in patients with refractory germ cell cancer has become increasingly difficult as the overall prognosis has improved. New agents do, however, continue to be identified and are currently undergoing evaluation.

Encouragingly, both gemcitabine, a deoxycytidine analogue, and paclitaxel, a taxane, have recently shown activity as single agents in salvage therapy.

Paclitaxel has been evaluated in two phase II studies. Motzer *et al.* [24] gave single agent paclitaxel $250 \, mg/m^2$ by 24 h infusion to 31 patients who had received either one cisplatin based regimen or ≤6 cycles of cisplatin based therapy. Remarkably, eight patients (26%) achieved partial or complete remission. This group included patients with primary refractory disease and mediastinal primary cancer. In a second report, 18 patients were treated with paclitaxel at a dose of 170 mg/m^2 by 24 h infusion. Two patients (11%) responded. This patient group was more heavily pretreated [25].

Gemcitabine has also been recently evaluated, again with encouraging results. Bokemeyer *et al.* [26] treated 35 heavily pretreated patients with gemcitabine at a dose of 1 g/m^2 i.v. weekly for 3 out of each 4 weeks, and 6 of 31 evaluable patients (19%) responded. Einhorn *et al.* [27] treated 21 patients at slightly higher dose (1.2 g/m^2) using the same schedule. This was a very heavily treated group of patients, in spite of which 3 (15%) responded.

As a result of these observations, paclitaxel is currently being tested as a component of initial chemotherapy in combination with BEP (T-BEP) by the European Organization for Research and Treatment of Cancer. A combination of paclitaxel and gemcitabine is currently being tested by the Eastern Co-operative Oncology Group in patients with refractory germ cell cancers.

Drug combinations—standard-dose therapy

It is widely accepted that VeIP (vinblastine, ifosfamide and cisplatin) is the standard conventional dose combination chemotherapy regimen for patients failing BEP. VeIP has been widely evaluated. The most comprehensive experience to date is that of the Indiana group [28]. They treated 135 patients with VeIP, all of whom developed progressive disease after initial chemotherapy with cisplatin/etoposide based combinations. Patients progressing within 3 weeks of previous cisplatin therapy were excluded from the study. Fifty per cent of patients in this study achieved complete remission with chemotherapy plus, in some, surgery. Twenty-four per cent of patients were continuously free of disease and a further 8% alive following this treatment. Strikingly, no patient with extragonadal non-seminomatous tumour was rendered permanently disease free—compared with 30% of patients with gonadal primaries. This regimen was, however, reported as being substantially toxic. Seventy-one per cent of patients were hospitalized for neutropenic fever and 27% required platelet transfusions. However, no growth factors were used during the period of this study.

A number of other authors have reported experience with VeIP and achieved results comparable with the Indiana experience [15,29].

Four cycles of VeIP currently forms one arm of an ongoing randomized French trial of first salvage chemotherapy for germ cell cancer. The other arm comprises 3 cycles of VeIP followed by a single cycle of high-dose chemotherapy. This study is not as yet complete, and the results are awaited with interest.

A number of other regimens have been used as first line salvage. Levi *et al.* [30] reported on the use of etoposide, dactinomycin and methotrexate given intravenously at 21 day intervals. Twenty-nine per cent of patients remained failure free following this treatment with or without surgery. Surprisingly, no relapses were reported. One confounding feature of this study is the inclusion of patients with residual masses with neither biopsy proof of cancer nor raised serum markers. Ledermann *et al.* [31] also reported on the use of POMB-ACE (cisplatin, vincristine, methotrexate, bleomycin/dactinomycin, cyclophosphamide and etoposide) or EP-OMB (etoposide and cisplatin/vincristine methotrexate and bleomycin) chemotherapy, achieving overall survival of 46% with a median follow-up of 4 years. More recently, Shamash *et al.* [32] reported use of m-BOP (methotrexate, bleomycin, vincristine and cisplatin), which when used together with surgery achieved a failure-free survival of 45%. The results from these small series have not been confirmed by other groups.

The newer investigational agents introduced into practice in the 1990s have been incorporated into standard-dose second line regimens—usually with growth factor support. Motzer *et al.* [7], in a preliminary report, described the treatment of 24 patients with good prognostic features (testicular primary site, complete response with prior chemotherapy regimen) with paclitaxel (escalating dose to $250 \, \text{mg/m}^2$ by 24 h infusion), ifosfamide ($1.2 \, \text{g/m}^2$ days 2–6 with mesna) and cisplatin ($20 \, \text{mg/m}^2$ days 2–6). At the time of the report 21 patients were evaluable, with 15 (57%) achieving a favourable response which was complete in 14. Twelve of these patients remained progression free at a median follow-up time of 15 months.

High-dose chemotherapy of metastatic germ cell cancer

Germ cell cancers are highly chemosensitive and rarely involve the bone marrow. They are therefore ideal candidates for high-dose chemotherapy. Whilst cisplatin is the most effective chemotherapy agent in initial chemotherapy, it is not possible to dose escalate this drug because of renal and neurological toxicity. All modern studies of high-dose salvage chemotherapy have substituted carboplatin for cisplatin because it is well tolerated at high dose. Fortunately etoposide can easily be escalated with tolerable toxicity. In the majority of studies, cyclophosphamide has been most commonly used as the third agent, although occasionally ifosfamide, which is less well tolerated, has been administered.

The first reports of high-dose therapy used autologous bone marrow transplantation (ABMT) and single agent chemotherapy with cyclophosphamide or etoposide [33,34]. However, high-dose therapy became a widely used treatment modality only when the combination of high-dose carboplatin and etoposide with autologous marrow support was established and cure became a possibility. The initial experience with this regimen was sobering. Only 6 of 40 patients treated consecutively with one or two cycles of this treatment at Indiana University between 1986 and 1989 achieved prolonged remission. There was a treatment associated mortality of 10%. No patient with relapse of mediastinal germ cell cancer achieved long-term remission [35].

These results were confirmed in an Eastern Co-operative Oncology Group study in which a further 40 patients received high-dose chemotherapy with carboplatin and etoposide. Five patients achieved a sustained remission and a further 5 patients died of treatment related toxicity [36]. Simultaneously with these studies, Siegert *et al.* developed a high-dose carboplatin, etoposide and ifosfamide regimen given for one cycle with either autologous marrow or peripheral blood progenitor cell support. Event-free survival was achieved in 35% of patients, with two (3%) toxic deaths. Only 1 of 23 patients with cisplatin refractory disease survived compared with 24 of 45 (53%) of patients with sensitive disease [37]. Comparable results to these were achieved by Lotz *et al.* [38] from France using two cycles of high-dose carboplatin, etoposide and ifosfamide and Motzer *et al.* [39] using two cycles of high-dose carboplatin, etoposide and cyclophosphamide. In the majority of these trials, patients received ABMT with or without haematopoietic growth factor support. A second cycle of high-dose chemotherapy was administered only to responding patients who recovered satisfactorily from their first high-dose treatment.

More recently, peripheral blood stem cells (PBSCs) have replaced autologous marrow rescue because of their convenience compared with standard ABMT [40]. This, and the appreciation that early intervention with high-dose chemotherapy was very much better tolerated, has led to the early incorporation of high-dose chemotherapy into treatment regimens [41].

Broun *et al.* [42] treated 25 patients relapsing after only one platinum based regimen with one or two cycles of high-dose carboplatin and etoposide using either ABMT or PBSC ('tandem' therapy). The majority of these patients had received conventional dose salvage chemotherapy with VeIP or other regimens, although four patients received no salvage chemotherapy prior to high-dose chemotherapy. At the time of reporting, 13 of 25 patients (52%) were continuously progression free. The authors concluded that this treatment approach was promising and well tolerated.

Whilst many studies used one or two cycles of high-dose chemotherapy, the advantage of more cycles of treatment has been evaluated, although not in a salvage setting. Rodenhuis *et al.* [43] administered up to three cycles of high-dose chemotherapy with a combination of cyclophosphamide, thiotepa and carboplatin to patients with germ cell cancer. This group clearly demonstrated that they were able to harvest sufficient stem cells to support this approach. However, toxicity increased markedly as each cycle was delivered [43]. Rodenhuis *et al.* [44] described 35 patients with relapsing germ cell cancer who initially underwent stem cell harvesting, then received an initial cycle of high-dose carboplatin and etoposide without stem cell support. Treatment was followed by two courses of high-dose carboplatin, thiotepa and cyclophosphamide, and 26 patients managed to receive this entire treatment course. The second high-dose course was complicated by veno-occlusive disease in 4 patients. The 2-year event-free survival was 51%.

Long-term follow-up following high-dose therapy has been reported by many groups, and that of Beyer *et al.* [40] is representative of the collective experience. Not unexpectedly, late toxicities were common and included evidence of symptomatic peripheral neuropathy, renal damage and ototoxicity.

The management of patients relapsing after high-dose therapy is difficult and prognosis poor. A median survival of 6 months was reported recently; a third of the patients relapsing received further chemotherapy with occasional worthwhile responses to paclitaxel and ifosfamide containing combinations [45].

Late relapse of germ cell cancer

A small proportion (3%) of patients with germ cell malignancy will develop late relapse of their disease over 2 years after completing combination chemotherapy. Relapse can be due either to growth of differentiated teratoma, which should be treated surgically, or to undifferentiated cancer, and is characteristically manifest by an elevated AFP level. These relapses have been described as occurring over 20 years following initial combination chemotherapy.

Two large series have described late relapse and its management. Baniel *et al.* [9] described 47 patients relapsing over 5 years after their initial treatment. Sixty-nine per cent of these patients had been treated at first presentation with combination chemotherapy. Twenty-one patients (25.9%) achieved long-term remission. Sixty-five patients were treated for late relapse by chemotherapy. Strikingly, only two of these were rendered permanently disease free by this treatment alone, and 19 of 21 patients achieving long-term remission required surgery in addition.

In a comparable German study, Gerl *et al.* [46] succeeded in obtaining a substantial remission in 9 of 25 patients (36%). Six of these patients required surgical treatment in addition to chemotherap.

There is no reported experience of the use of high-dose chemotherapy in patients with late relapse, who have a very poor prognosis if found to have inoperable tumours before or after salvage chemotherapy.

Conclusion

Relapsing germ cell cancer is a heterogeneous disease and it is likely that published literature suffers from a referral and selection bias. It is absolutely mandatory to confirm that patients do indeed have progressive cancer. Overall, older series have consistently shown that 25–30% patients can expect to be rendered disease free by re-treatment. It is at present unclear whether patients should be treated at the time of first relapse with conventional dose chemotherapy or should receive tandem chemotherapy amalgamating both conventional and high-dose chemotherapy. In addition there is no clear evidence from clinical studies as to which high-dose chemotherapy regimen should be given and for how many cycles. Prognostic factors at relapse have been identified which can help select patients for these different treatment approaches.

A number of new chemotherapy drugs are under evaluation at present, and it is hoped that these will be successfully incorporated in salvage protocols and lead to an improvement in the current results of salvage therapy.

The numbers of patients requiring salvage chemotherapy are small and diminishing. It is essential that these patients are treated in large Centres and incorporated into trials in order that maximum information can be obtained for our future patient population.

References

1 Motzer RJ, Geller NL, Tan CCY *et al*. Salvage chemotherapy for patients with germ cell tumors. *Cancer* 1991; **67**: 1305–10.

2 Josefsen D, Ous S, Joie J *et al*. Salvage treatment in male patients with germ cell tumours. *Br J Cancer* 1993; **67**: 568–72.

3 Gerl A, Clemm C, Schmeller N *et al*. Prognosis after salvage treatment for unselected male patients with germ cell tumours. *Br J Cancer* 1995; **72**: 1026–32.

4 Fossa SD, Bokemeyer C, Gerl A *et al*. Treatment outcome of patients with brain metastases from malignant germ cell tumors. *Cancer* 1999; **85**: 988–97.

5 Zon R, Nichols C, Einhorn L. Management strategies and outcomes of germ cell tumor patients with very high human chorionic gonadotropin levels. *J Clin Oncol* 1998; **16**: 1294.

6 Jeffery GM, Theaker JM, Lee AHS *et al*. The growing teratoma syndrome. *Br J Urol* 1991; **67**: 195–202.

7 Motzer RJ, Amsterdam A, Prieto V *et al*. Teratoma with malignant transformation: diverse malignant histologies arising in men with germ cell tumors. *J Urol* 1998; **159**: 133–8.

8 Fossa SD, Stenning SP, Gerl A *et al*. Prognostic factors in patients progressing after cisplatin based chemotherapy for malignant non-seminomatous germ cell tumours. *Br J Cancer* 1999; **80**: 1392–9.

9 Baniel J, Foster RS, Gonin R *et al*. Late relapse of testicular cancer. *J Clin Oncol* 1995; **13**: 1170–6.

10 Beyer J, Kramar A, Mandanas R *et al*. High-dose chemotherapy as salvage treatment in germ cell tumours: a multivariate analysis of prognostic variables. *J Clin Oncol* 1996; **14**: 2638–45.

11   Murphy BR, Breeden ES, Donohoue JP *et al.* Surgical salvage of chemorefractory germ cell tumors. *J Clin Oncol* 1993; **11**: 324–9.

12   Fitzharris BM, Kaye SB, Saverymuttu S *et al.* VP16-213 as a single agent in advanced testicular tumors. *Eur J Cancer* 1980; **16**: 1193–7.

13   Williams SD, Birch R, Einhorn LH *et al.* Treatment of disseminated germ cell tumors with cisplatin, bleomycin, and either vinblastine or etoposide. *N Engl J Med* 1987; **316**: 1435–40.

14   Motzer RJ, Cooper K, Geller NL *et al.* The role of ifosfamide plus cisplatin based chemotherapy as salvage therapy for patients with refractory germ cell tumors. *Cancer* 1990; **66**: 2476–81.

15   Farhat F, Culine S, Theodore C *et al.* Cisplatin and ifosfamide with either vinblastine or etoposide as salvage therapy for refractory or relapsing germ cell tumor patients. *Cancer* 1996; **77**: 1193–7.

16   Greco FA, Johnson DH, Hainsworth JD. Chronic oral etoposide. *Cancer* 1991; **67**: 303–9.

17   Cooper MA, Einhorn LH. Maintenance chemotherapy with daily oral etoposide following salvage therapy in patients with germ cell tumors. *J Clin Oncol* 1995; **13**: 1167–9.

18   Wheeler BM, Loehrer PJ, Williams SD *et al.* Ifosfamide in refractory male germ cell tumors. *J Clin Oncol* 1986; **4**: 28–34.

19   Nichols CR, Catalano PJ, Crawford ED *et al.* Randomized comparison of cisplatin and etoposide and either bleomycin or ifosfamide in treatment of advanced disseminated germ cell tumors: an Eastern Cooperative Oncology Group, Southwest Oncology Group and Cancer and Leukemia Group study. *J Clin Oncol* 1998; **16**: 1287–93.

20   Smith D, Rustin G, Hitchins R *et al.* Single agent activity of methotrexate in advanced non-seminomatous testicular germ cell tumours. *Eur J Cancer* 1988; **24**: 1779–81.

21   Atkinson CH, Horwich A, Peckham MJ. Methotrexate for relapse of metastatic non-seminomatous germ cell tumour. *Med Oncol Tumour Pharmacother* 1987; **8**: 33–7.

22   O'Bryan RM, Luce JK, Talley RW *et al.* Phase II evaluation of adriamycin in human neoplasia. *Cancer* 1973; **32**: 1–8.

23   Stoter G, Akdas A, Fossa SD *et al.* High dose epirubicin in chemotherapy refractory non-seminomatous germ cell cancer: a phase II study. *Ann Oncol* 1992; **3**: 577–8.

24   Motzer RJ, Bajorin DF, Schwartz LH *et al.* Phase II trial of paclitaxel shows antitumour activity in patients with previously treated germ cell tumors. *J Clin Oncol* 1994; **12**: 2277–83.

25   Sandler AB, Cristou A, Fox S *et al.* A phase II trial of paclitaxel in refractory germ cell tumors. *Cancer* 1998; **82**: 1381–6.

26   Bokemeyer C, Gerl A, Schoffski P *et al.* Gemcitabine in patients with relapsed or cisplatin refractory testicular cancer. *J Clin Oncol* 1999; **17**: 2512–16.

27   Einhorn LH, Stender MJ, Williams SD. Phase II trial of gemcitabine in refractory germ cell tumors. *J Clin Oncol* 1999; **17**: 509–11.

28   Loehrer PJ, Gonin R, Nichols CR *et al.* Vinblastine plus ifosfamide plus cisplatin as initial salvage therapy in recurrent germ cell tumor. *J Clin Oncol* 1998; **16**: 2500–4.

29   Pizzocaro G, Salvioni R, Piva L *et al.* Modified cisplatin, etoposide (or vinblastine) and ifosfamide salvage therapy for male germ-cell tumors: long term results. *Ann Oncol* 1992; **3**: 211–16.

30   Levi JA, Thomson D, Harvey V *et al.* Effective salvage chemotherapy with etoposide, dactinomycin and methotrexate in refractory germ cell cancer. *J Clin Oncol* 1990; **8**: 27–32.

31   Ledermann JA, Holden L, Newlands ES *et al.* The longterm outcome of patients who relapse after chemotherapy for non-seminomatous germ cell tumours. *Br J Urol* 1994; **74**: 225–30.

32 Shamash J, Oliver RD, Ong J *et al.* Sixty percent salvage rate of germ cell tumours using sequential m-BOP, surgery and ifosfamide based chemotherapy. *Ann Oncol* 1999; **10**: 685–92.

33 Buckner CD, Clift RA, Fefer A *et al.* High dose cyclophosphamide (NSC-26271) for the treatment of metastatic testicular neoplasm. *Cancer Chemother Rep* 1974; **58**: 709–14.

34 Postmus PE, Mulder MH, Sleijfer DT *et al.* High dose etoposide for refractory malignancies: a phase I study. *Cancer Treat Rep* 1984; **68**: 1471–4.

35 Broun ER, Nichols CR, Kneebone P *et al.* Longterm outcome of patients with relapsed and refractory germ cell tumors treated with high dose chemotherapy and autologous bone marrow rescue. *Ann Int Med* 1992; **117**: 124–8.

36 Nichols CR, Anderson J, Lazarus HM *et al.* High dose carboplatin and etoposide with autologous bone marrow transplantation in refractory germ cell cancer: an Eastern Cooperative Oncology Group protocol. *J Clin Oncol* 1992; **10**: 558–63.

37 Siegert W, Beyer J, Strohscheer I *et al.* High dose treatment with carboplatin, etoposide and ifosfamide followed by autologous stem cell transplantation in relapsed or refractory germ cell cancer: a phase I/II study. *J Clin Oncol* 1994; **12**: 1223–31.

38 Lotz JP, Andre T, Donsimoni R *et al.* High dose chemotherapy with ifosfamide, carboplatin, and etoposide combined with autologous bone marrow transplantation for the treatment of poor prognosis germ cell tumors and metastatic trophoblastic disease in adults. *Cancer* 1995; **75**: 3.

39 Motzer RJ, Mazumdar M, Bosl GJ *et al.* High dose carboplatin, etoposide and cyclophosphamide for patients with refractory germ cell tumors: treatment results and prognostic factors for survival and toxicity. *J Clin Oncol* 1996; **14**: 1098–105.

40 Beyer J, Kingreen D, Krause M *et al.* Long term survival of patients with recurrent or refractory germ cell tumors after high dose chemotherapy. *Cancer* 1997; **79**: 161–8.

41 Motzer RJ, Gulati SC, Crown JP *et al.* High dose chemotherapy and autologous bone marrow rescue for patients with refractory germ cell tumors. *Cancer* 1992; **69**: 550–6.

42 Broun ER, Nichols CR, Cornetta K *et al.* Tandem high dose chemotherapy with autologous bone marrow transplantation for initial relapse of testicular germ cell cancer. *Cancer* 1997; **79**: 1605–10.

43 Rodenhuis S, Westermann A, Holtkamp MJ *et al.* Feasibility of multiple courses of high dose cyclophosphamide, thiotepa, and carboplatin for breast cancer or germ cell cancer. *J Clin Oncol* 1996; **14**: 1473–83.

44 Rodenhuis S, De Wit R, De Mulder PHM *et al.* A prospective multicentre trial of repeated high dose chemotherapy in relapsing germ cell cancer. *Proc ASCO* 1999: 1190.

45 Pont J, Bokemeyer C, Harstrick A *et al.* Chemotherapy for germ cell tumors relapsing after high dose chemotherapy and stem cell support: a retrospective multicenter study of the Austrian study group on urologic oncology. *Ann Oncol* 1997; **8**: 1229–34.

46 Gerl A, Clemm C, Schmeller N *et al.* Late relapse of germ cell tumors after cisplatin based chemotherapy. *Ann Oncol* 1997; **8**: 41–7.

20: Surgery for Testicular Cancer

W. F. Hendry

Introduction

Testicular tumours, silent, solid and sinister, typically afflict young men. They also weigh heavily upon the surgeon and oncologist who must look after them. First, the correct diagnosis must be made, as early in the course of the disease as possible, since the cure rate is dependent upon the extent of malignancy at presentation. Next, the primary tumour must be removed. Fastidious care is required if the patient is to avoid the nuisance of a haematoma or painful scar. After careful pathological examination of the excised testicle and serial measurement of markers, precise non-invasive imaging permits accurate staging.

The initial choice of treatment regimen must be correct for the stage of the disease: once a mistake in management has occurred which allows metastases to become bulky, the chance of cure is reduced [1]. After chemotherapy, surgical extirpation of residual masses may present a formidable challenge. Thereafter, cure is dependent upon vigilant follow-up, so that relapse can be detected early and treated promptly. The excellent results now being reported from specialist Cancer Centres depend upon effective collaboration between oncologist and urologist. The risk of dying is more than doubled if the patient is not managed in a specialist unit [2], and is especially high if they fall into a poor prognosis group [3]. Finally, it must never be forgotten that these young men and their partners are likely to have expectations of raising a family; any possible impact of therapy on reproductive function should be minimized, and any such risk must be fully understood.

The urologist should not tolerate delay in initial treatment. The most important variables affecting the outcome are tumour volume and serum marker levels at presentation, which correlate directly with delay from first symptom to start of treatment [4]. Sadly, many patients wait a long time before seeking medical advice [5]. Often, the delay does not stop there. The correct diagnosis may be established at the first consultation in as few as 43% of men [6]. With a history of less than 6 months, most patients with metastases have small volume disease and low serum marker levels, in contrast to those with a history of more than 6 months. Over 90% of patients with small volume metastases and low serum marker levels are alive at 3 years compared with only half of those with very bulky disease and high marker levels. Fortunately the latter group accounts for only 16% of patients with metastases [7].

Clinical diagnosis

The diagnosis of testicular tumours may be difficult. Although patients usually present with painless testicular enlargement, the commonest error is to mistake a tumour for epididymitis because the swollen testis is tender. In fact, a substantial number of patients with a testicular tumour complain of pain from the outset [8]. Many of these testes are found on pathological examination to show evidence of haemorrhage. A small bleed into or adjacent to the tumour not only causes pain and sudden swelling, but subsequent re-absorption. This re-absorption may account for later subsidence of the swelling, which may coincide with antibiotic therapy, thus reinforcing the wrong diagnosis of infection. Others have noted that pain was commonly a presenting feature, which led to the condition being treated as inflammatory for too long [9]. Again, delay was associated with higher stage disease and poorer results.

A history of trauma, recent or remote, is reported in some 20% of cases. This 'red-herring' should not be allowed to distract attention from the true underlying condition. Previous surgery to the testis or inguinal canal may make the findings more difficult to interpret, and may alter the pattern of lymphatic spread. Orchidopexy, for example, may deflect metastases to the inguinal or iliac lymph nodes; sometimes the resulting lymphoedema may lead to a swollen leg as the presenting feature.

Men with a history of cryptorchidism have a markedly increased chance of developing testicular malignancy. Indeed, approximately 10% of tumours occur in testes that are or have been maldescended. The risk is six times greater for abdominal testes than for lower-lying testes. One-quarter of patients with a history of bilateral maldescent who develop a tumour in one testis will go on to develop a contralateral tumour. When only one testis is maldescended, one in five of the tumours that develop occur in the contralateral, normally situated testicle [10]. It is not known for certain whether the age at treatment has an effect on the risk of cancer [11], although some authors found no tumours occurring in boys who had undergone orchidopexy before the age of 6 [12].

Tumours are more likely to occur in testes that are atrophic, whether following orchidopexy [13], torsion [14] or trauma [15]. The incidence of these abnormalities, and hence perhaps the risk of testicular tumours, is higher in males exposed prenatally to exogenous hormones (such as diethylstilboestrol) [16,17] or radiation [18].

Carcinoma *in situ* can be found in testicular biopsies from 2–3% of men treated for undescended testes [19,20], and in 5% of biopsy specimens taken from the contralateral testes of men with previous testicular tumours [21]. Positive findings are most common when the testis is atrophic or following maldescent [22]. Over 50% of men believed to have extragonadal germ cell tumours show carcinoma *in situ* on testicular biopsy [18]. At least half of the men with carcinoma *in situ* eventually develop testicular tumours [23]. A negative biopsy makes subsequent tumour development highly unlikely but not impossible [24]. Testicular biopsy is therefore offered to men who are known to be at high risk [25], since the carcinoma *in situ*, and the risk of development of malignancy, can be eliminated by a brief course of radiotherapy [26]. This inevitably induces sterility, and so sperm cryopreservation should be arranged prior to commencing such treatment [27,28].

The patient who has had a testicular tumour before represents a particular problem: it is his only testicle and he is usually acutely aware of any changes that may occur in it. Almost 3% of men attending the Testicular Tumour Clinic at the Royal Marsden Hospital (hereafter referred to simply as the Royal Marsden Hospital) developed tumour in the contralateral testis, in two instances synchronously and in the remainder at intervals from 4 months to 15 years [29]. All patients are therefore instructed to examine the remaining testicle at regular intervals, and tumours as small as 0.5 cm diameter have been self-diagnosed. In addition, biopsy is offered to all patients with infertility, a history of maldescent or an atrophic testis [25].

Careful clinical examination of the testis is the best method of detecting a tumour. Physical examination of the testes starts with the patient standing: a testis with a tumour usually lies lower than normal, whereas inflammatory lesions or torsion tend to raise the testis. Once the patient is lying down, the entire outline of the body of the testis can be defined between the thumb, index and middle fingers, gently sliding the organ from one examining hand to the other to assess its consistency and localize any induration. A tumour is identifiable first because it is a firm or hard swelling in the body of the testis, secondly because it enlarges the testicle, which may feel relatively heavy, and thirdly because it causes the testicle to lose its normal sensation on gently squeezing it. Abnormal firmness in the body of the testis is the most reliable finding; however, difficulty may arise when the tumour lies in the groove between the testis and epididymis.

Scrotal ultrasound [30,31] clearly elucidates the anatomy (Fig. 20.1), and differentiates cystic from solid lesions. Ultrasound, which is almost 100% sensitive in detecting tumours, can also pick up lesions that are too small to palpate [32]. Epidermoid cysts can sometimes be recognized and may be suitable for local excision. Microlithiasis may be demonstrated, which is associated with tumour in up to one-third of cases [33]. This condition is also commonly found with cryptorchidism, but its aetiology remains obscure [34].

If doubt persists, the best course of action is to explore the testicle. The

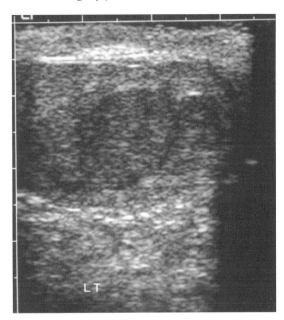

Figure 20.1 Ultrasound scan
showing small testicular
tumour.

differential diagnosis includes epididymitis, torsion, tuberculosis, gumma and granulomatous orchitis. No harm will come from exploring these conditions, and there is much to support the view that all non-transilluminable testicular swellings should be explored unless the swelling is strictly confined to the epididymis or there are pus cells in the urine to confirm the diagnosis of epididymitis. The technique of exploration is described in detail below.

Patients sometimes present with metastatic germ cell malignancy when no primary tumour can be palpated in either testis. Such patients often have advanced disease, presenting with abdominal pain and systemic symptoms [35]. The diagnosis may be established by the finding of high serum marker levels, or by biopsy of enlarged abdominal or cervical lymph nodes, or lung biopsy. Some have a history of testicular atrophy, and when the testicle is examined histologically there may be evidence of a microscopic primary tumour. In other cases, the primary tumour can disappear, leaving only a scar [36]; however, biopsy is likely to show the presence of carcinoma *in situ* [37].

Treatment of the primary tumour

Investigations which should precede orchidectomy

Either alpha-fetoprotein (AFP), beta-human chorionic gonadotrophin (BHCG) or both are elevated in half of patients with non-seminomatous germ cell tumours on presentation and in three-quarters of patients on relapse [38].

This information is invaluable for follow-up purposes, since these markers may rise, indicating recurrence, long before metastases are visible on X-ray or scanning; of course, this is the time that chemotherapy is most effective. It follows that blood should be taken for estimation of AFP and BHCG before the testicle is explored. There is really no need to delay for other investigations apart from a chest X-ray.

The technique of orchidectomy

The surgical approach should be through a standard or skin crease inguinal incision. If inspection and palpation confirm the presence of a firm area in the body of the testis, often associated with dilated overlying veins, the cord is divided between clamps and the testis is removed. Biopsy is necessary only with a solitary testicle. Under these circumstances, the testicle should be mobilized through an inguinal incision after applying a soft clamp to the cord. The testicle is then bisected and a frozen section biopsy taken from a firm area to obtain histological confirmation of the diagnosis before removing the testis.

If there is a hydrocele it should not be tapped: it should be explored with a view to examining the testis, especially if it occurs for no apparent reason in a young man; an operation for cure of the hydrocele can be done if the testis is normal. The temptation to needle the scrotum or to do trans-scrotal biopsy should be resisted, since the tunica albuginea will contain the primary tumour provided it is not surgically breached. It is perfectly reasonable to explore the testes through a scrotal incision in the first instance, to inspect them and establish the diagnosis; if a tumour is present, a second incision can easily be made in the groin to remove the testis and cord. Provided that the tunica albuginea has not been opened there is no increased risk of scrotal dissemination.

Once the testicle has been removed the patient can be referred for further treatment as soon as the pathology report is available. Further local surgery is not necessary after inguinal orchidectomy, but difficulties may arise if a scrotal orchidectomy has been done. Not uncommonly a firm nodule is left in the scrotum adjacent to the cut end of the cord, and there may be considerable concern as to whether this is due to ligature, haematoma or residual tumour. Residual tumour may be present after primary scrotal biopsy or orchidectomy [39], in which case it is best to excise the stump of the cord through an inguinal incision, extended as a 'tennis-racket' incision around the scrotum as a partial or hemiscrotectomy. There appears to be no adverse effect on prognosis after prompt and adequate local management in such cases [40]. Amongst a group of stage I patients at the Royal Marsden Hospital who had scrotal interference at or prior to removal of the primary tumour, none developed scrotal recurrence during surveillance, and the overall relapse rate was comparable to that observed in this group as a whole [41]. Thus, a slightly more liberal approach to scrotal orchidectomy may be acceptable in this era of effective chemotherapy, but electively a groin approach is preferable [42–44].

Staging after orchidectomy

Staging investigations include CT scan of chest, abdomen and pelvis. Blood tests include full blood count, liver function tests, serum calcium, urea and electrolytes, measurement of serum AFP, lactate dehydrogenase (LDH) and BHCG levels, and renal function tests (EDTA or creatinine clearance). Pulmonary function tests are done for patients receiving bleomycin. Semen analysis and sperm banking is requested if the sperm count is adequate and treatment is likely to compromise fertility. Positron emission tomography (PET) has the potential to improve clinical staging, but has limited sensitivity for small retroperitoneal lymph node metastases [45].

The staging classification, which is based on the results of these investigations, includes subgroups, since it has been recognized that the distribution and volume of metastases is of critical importance in planning the treatment strategy [46] (Table 20.1). In a minority of patients, widespread tumour dissemination makes intensive staging unnecessary, and pretreatment investigation is limited to serum marker assay, assessment of renal and hepatic function, chest X-ray and full blood count.

Early prospective studies of patients on surveillance indicated that careful examination of the orchidectomy specimen allowed recognition of certain histological features that were predictive of relapse. Lymphatic and/or vascular

Table 20.1 The Royal Marsden Hospital staging classification (Peckham [46])

	Stage:
I	No evidence of metastases
IM	Rising serum marker levels with no other evidence of metastases
II	Abdominal node metastases:
	A: < 2 cm in diameter
	B: 2–5 cm diameter
	C: > 5 cm diameter
III	Supradiaphragmatic node metastases:
	0: no abdominal node metastases
	A,B,C: abdominal node sizes as in stage II
IV	Extralymphatic metastases:
	Lung
	L1: ≤ 3 metastases
	L2: > 3 metastases all < 2 cm in diameter
	L3: > 3 metastases, 1 or more > 2 cm in diameter
H+	Liver metastases

invasion and histology (presence of malignant teratoma undifferentiated (MTU)) were factors that were independently significant [47]. Absence of these factors has been confirmed to give a correct prediction of low risk of relapse at the 90% level [48]. In patients with clinical stage I non-seminomatous germ cell tumours who underwent retroperitoneal lymph node dissection, multivariate analysis confirmed that vascular invasion and percentage of embryonal carcinoma were significant prognostic indicators, and by combining these two variables the presence of lymph node metastases could be correctly predicted in 86% of patients [49]. However, it should be noted that there is some variation in pathological interpretation of the nature of the tumour and the presence or absence of vascular invasion between pathologists, and careful review may be advisable before final therapeutic decisions are made [50].

Surveillance vs. retroperitoneal lymph node dissection after orchidectomy for clinical stage I non-seminomatous testicular tumours

After orchidectomy, there is a choice of management for stage I non-seminomatous germ cell tumours [51]. While some centres have recommended primary retroperitoneal lymph node dissection, surveillance has been preferred for the past 20 years at the Royal Marsden Hospital. The surveillance protocol consists of monthly visits for the first year, 3-monthly for the second year, 4-monthly for the third year, 6-monthly for the fourth year and annually thereafter. CT scans are performed 3-monthly in the first year, with a final scan at the end of the second year. Chest radiographs are done, and serum AFP and HCG levels are measured at each visit.

Collected results of recent published series of stage I non-seminomatous germ cell tumours treated by surveillance are shown in Table 20.2 [52–56]. Survival is almost, but not quite, 100%. The disease can be expected to recur in patients on surveillance, most often within 12 months of presentation. Although relapse is often first detected by elevation of tumour markers alone, the commonest sites have been defined in a large collaborative Medical Research Council study. The para-aortic nodes were the most common site of relapse (about 60% of cases), but one-quarter recurred in the lungs, while relapse in the mediastinal (7%) or supraclavicular (3%) nodes was much less common [57]. Operative removal of the para-aortic lymph nodes does not therefore prevent recurrence of this disease and does not lessen the need for careful follow-up. Indeed, there is such a high likelihood of relapse after retroperitoneal lymph node dissection with pathologic stage I disease when embryonal carcinoma predominates in the orchidectomy specimen that adjuvant chemotherapy is now recommended [58].

Table 20.2 Results of surveillance for stage I non-seminomatous germ cell tumours

Reference	Year	No.	% relapse	% died
52	1995	154	27.3	1.3
53	1998	105	25.7	2.8
54	1999	170	28.2	0.6
55	1999	248	28.0	2.0
56	2000	357*	25.0	1.4

*Excluding 61 high-risk patients who received adjuvant chemotherapy.

In our experience of over 400 men at the Royal Marsden Hospital with stage I non-seminomatous germ cell tumours on surveillance, abdominal relapse was reduced from 16% to 8% by adopting a selective approach of adjuvant chemotherapy for patients at high risk of relapse. When abdominal relapse did occur, it generally responded to chemotherapy. Para-aortic lymphadenectomy was required in less than 5% of the overall patient population, and pathological examination showed that the residual mass usually contained teratoma differentiated [56].

The need for retroperitoneal lymph node dissection in early stage testicular non-seminomatous germ cell tumours is clearly much less than previously thought. We believe that this operation should be used highly selectively after chemotherapy, and not before it. The latter approach has little to commend it, particularly since it does not prevent relapse in the retroperitoneum that may be difficult to cure [59,60].

Stage IIA and IIB non-seminomatous germ cell tumours

Chemotherapy is the treatment of choice for patients with bulky stage II (IIC) presentations and those with stage III and IV disease. There remains some controversy regarding the management of patients with stage IIA and IIB disease. In the United States radical lymph node dissection is the preferred initial treatment. Approximately 50% of patients managed by initial surgery eventually required chemotherapy. The overall survival rate was 98% [61]. A policy employing initial chemotherapy is equally effective. Amongst 118 patients treated at the Royal Marsden Hospital, 97% were disease free [62]. Para-aortic lymphadenectomy for post-chemotherapy residual masses was required for 17% of stage IIA and 39% of stage IIB patients. Clearly, equivalent results can be obtained in stage IIA and IIB patients employing either treatment method. The choice between them depends upon the relative toxicity of the two approaches and to some extent upon patterns of established practice.

Surgical excision of residual masses

Three-quarters of patients who complete chemotherapy for advanced disease can be expected to have residual masses in the para-aortic region or in the chest, or in both sites: when resected, this tissue may contain residual undifferentiated malignancy [63]. It has been our policy at the Royal Marsden Hospital for over 20 years to remove all substantial residual masses after chemotherapy. However, this has raised a number of questions over the years:

1   How much chemotherapy should be given prior to surgery?
2   Is there a place for preoperative radiotherapy?
3   When should the surgery be done in relation to completion of chemotherapy?
4   How should sequential serum marker studies affect the timing of surgery?
5   How large a mass should be considered significant?
6   How complete must the surgery be?
7   What complications may arise?

Analysis of 231 patients treated at the Royal Marsden Hospital provided some answers to these questions [64]. Four cycles of chemotherapy produced complete remission in 70–75% of patients with advanced stage disease [63,65]. To operate before completion of 4 cycles would require a considerable number of unnecessary operations on lumps that might ultimately have resolved spontaneously. It would appear that there was no gain in administering more than 4 cycles of chemotherapy if the serum markers had returned to normal. The addition of radiotherapy in a small, uncontrolled series of observations did not produce any reduction in the proportion of cases with residual active malignancy [66]. Our practice therefore has been to remove residual masses 4–6 weeks after completion of 4 cycles of chemotherapy provided that the serum marker levels have returned to normal. If the surgery is done while the serum markers are still elevated there was a very high likelihood that the excised mass would contain active tumour; however, even with normal marker levels, 14% of our cases had residual malignancy. Thus, normalization of serum markers was no guarantee that a residual mass was tumour free. Overall, 85% of patients whose marker levels were normal at surgery are alive and well, compared with only 55% whose serum markers were elevated [64].

There is no general agreement on the minimum size of post-chemotherapy mass that merits excision. Our practice has been to recommend excision of all masses greater than 1 cm in diameter. Recent predictive models based on international data sets of more than 700 patients indicate that masses less than 1 cm diameter have a 25% chance of containing mature teratoma, and a 5% chance of harbouring cancer [67]. Using a decision analysis model, the estimated gains in 5-year survival are 4.3% and 2.7% following excision of

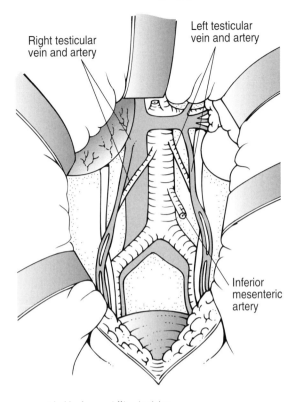

Right testicular
vein and artery

Left testicular
vein and artery

Inferior
mesenteric
artery

Figure 20.2 Access provided by long midline incision.

masses 1–2 cm and less than 1 cm diameter, respectively [68]. Our practice has been to excise thoroughly the residual mass itself, but not extend the dissection to the surrounding macroscopically normal nodes. This approach has gained general acceptance [69], although some surgeons prefer to use a modified template [70].

Excision of post-chemotherapy residual masses requires careful preoperative localization by CT scanning, so that the optimum surgical approach can be planned. This information is most conveniently presented in the form of a 'scanogram', relating the site of the residual mass to the surrounding vital structures. The relation of the mass to the renal vessels is of paramount importance: irrespective of the size of the mass, a long midline incision provides excellent access (Fig. 20.2) to tumours situated below this level (Fig. 20.3). However, if the mass extends above the renal vessels (Fig. 20.4), or if retrocrural or supradiaphragmatic structures are involved (Fig. 20.5), a thoracoabdominal incision provides much better access [71]. Metastases in the liver [72], neck [73] or lungs [74] may require synchronous or staged removal.

Metastases in the chest can be excised at the same time as abdominal nodes

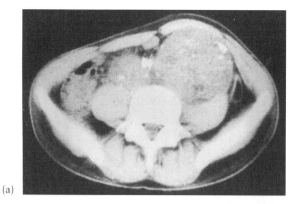

(a)

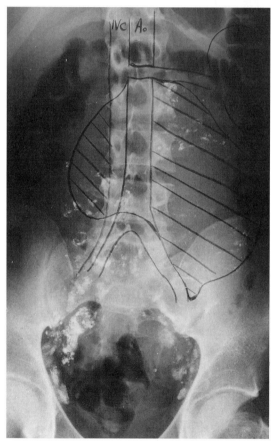

(b)

Figure 20.3 Large para-aortic lymph node mass lying below the renal vessels: (a) CT scan; (b) scanogram.

[75]. However, in some cases it may be wiser to plan a separate staged approach to widespread disease rather than trying to do too much through one incision, which may provide suboptimal access to difficult areas of tumour. Indeed, two recent patients have undergone no fewer than four separate procedures before achieving near-complete tumour clearance. The significance of

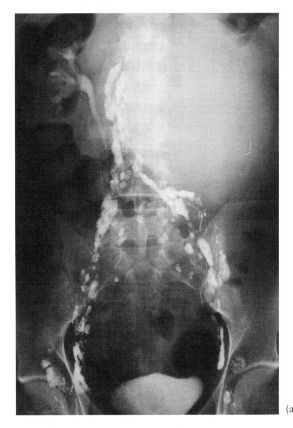

(a)

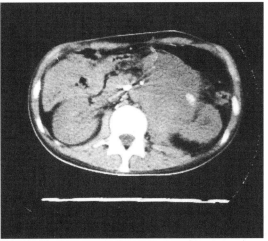

(b)

Figure 20.4 Left para-aortic mass extending above the renal vessels: (a) intravenous urogram; (b) CT scan.

leaving a small amount of differentiated teratoma behind is not clear, although there is evidence that this tissue is probably unstable [76,77]. Our present belief is that every effort should be made to remove it, a view shared by others [78].

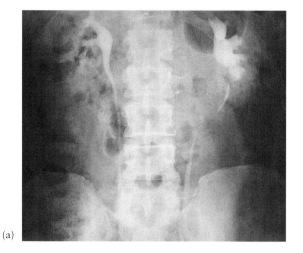

(a)

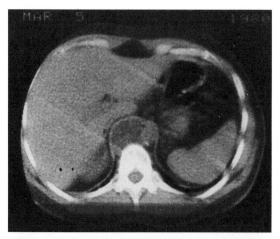

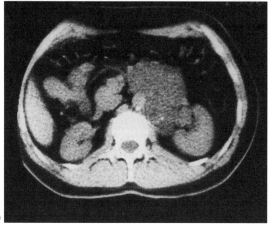

(b)

Figure 20.5 Left para-aortic mass with right retro-crural mass: (a) intravenous urogram; (b) CT scans; (c) scanogram.

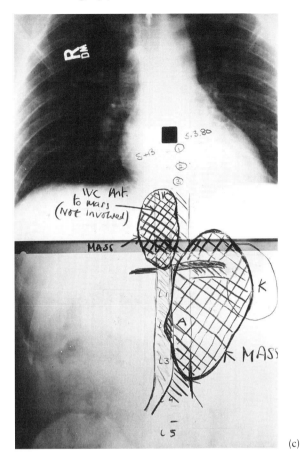

Figure 20.5 *Continued.*   (c)

Amongst 231 consecutive patients undergoing para-aortic lymphadenectomy after chemotherapy at the Royal Marsden Hospital, there was residual
undifferentiated teratoma (MTU) in 48 (21%), differentiated teratoma (TD)
in 131 (57%) and only fibrosis/necrosis in 52 (22%) [64] (Fig. 20.6). The incidence of residual MTU in this series is similar to that reported from other
centres [79]. The histological findings had a profound effect on prognosis,
as did completeness of surgical excision (Fig. 20.7). Multivariate analysis was
performed, and completeness of excision, pathology of the excised mass, elective vs. salvage surgery and year of treatment (before or after 1984) were
found to be independent prognostic variables. On the other hand, serum
markers at the time of surgery, and size of the mass did not provide any additional prognostic value once pathology and completeness of excision were
taken into account. Over 80% of these patients are long-term survivors.
Similar experience in over 800 patients reported from elsewhere indicates
that excellent long-term survival can be expected, although the presence of

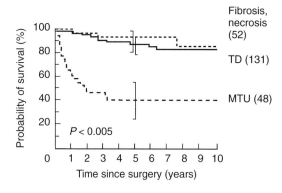

Figure 20.6 Survival after para-aortic lymphadenectomy related to histology of excised mass (Hendry *et al.* [64]).

undifferentiated tumour in the excised specimen and salvage surgery were recognized as adverse prognostic indicators [79].

The technical aspects of removal of these masses have been described elsewhere, and the potential hazards are well documented [80,81]. The problems encountered relate first to the sheer size of the mass, and secondly to involvement of adjacent structures. Ipsilateral kidneys may have to be removed (12.5% in our series), most of which are poorly functioning. The situation of the lymph node masses immediately adjacent to the great vessels means that care must be taken during dissection to avoid injury as far as possible. Pre-operative nuclear magnetic angiography is very helpful in distinguishing distortion of the great vessels from invasion [82]. In 7 cases the vena cava was invaded – no complications followed sleeve resection, an experience also reported by others [83–85]. The aorta or common iliac artery was resected and grafted in 10 cases, indicating that vascular experience and expertise should be immediately available [86]. Two patients died, one of respiratory failure after thoraco-abdominal surgery, and one of secondary haemorrhage 10 days after operation: our operative mortality of 0.9% may be compared with 0.8% recorded by Donohue [79,80]. Great care is required in the postoperative period in these patients who have received previous chemotherapy [45].

Impact of the disease and treatment on reproductive function

Sexual function is, in general, well preserved after treatment of testicular tumours [87,88]. However, many patients with testicular tumours have impaired fertility [27]. It is not clear whether this is due to inherent abnormality in the testicle, the effects of the tumour or a consequence of treatment [89]. Certainly there is often oligozoospermia at presentation before the orchidectomy, significantly different from the normal population, and from men presenting with other malignancy such as lymphoma [90]. After orchidectomy

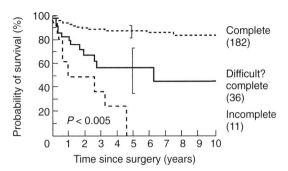

Figure 20.7 Survival after para-aortic lymphadenectomy related to completeness of surgical excision (Hendry *et al.* [64]).

and treatment, recovery of spermatogenesis does occur in some instances, even in patients who have received chemotherapy after an interval of 2 or more years [27]. It is therefore essential that reproductive function should be preserved as carefully as possible in these young men.

Loss of ejaculation may follow para-aortic lymph node dissection [91]. These patients may not only lose ejaculation but a minority may also suffer diminished libido, difficulty with orgasm and, in some cases, erectile dysfunction [87]. As a result of careful anatomical studies, the technique of primary retroperitoneal lymph node dissection was modified so that antegrade ejaculation is maintained in 70–90% of patients [92,93]. The technique is, however, painstaking and prolonged and may take anything up to 4 or 5h to complete. Some temporary loss of ejaculation is not uncommon but generally recovers over the months following the procedure. After para-aortic lymphadenectomy for post-chemotherapy residual nodal masses, loss of ejaculation occurred in 22% of the 186 Royal Marsden Hospital patients who were available for study [94]. Loss of ejaculation occurred significantly more often after bilateral (46%) than after unilateral (14%) lymphadenectomy, and it was related to the size of the excised mass (<4cm, 4%; 4–8cm, 19%; >8cm, 60%).

A nerve sparing operative technique led to a significant reduction in ejaculatory dysfunction, from 37% to 19% [94]. In an analysis of 192 patients undergoing post-chemotherapy retroperitoneal lymph node dissection elsewhere, antegrade ejaculation was preserved in 89% of patients following introduction of a nerve sparing technique, compared with only 11% previously observed with a modified bilateral template technique. There was no difference in survival rates and many of the men subsequently fathered children [95].

Loss of ejaculation is caused by division of the sympathetic nerves on both sides of the great vessels, or removal of the hypogastric plexus, which lies just below the bifurcation of the aorta [91]. Despite optimistic reports of return of ejaculation after the use of drugs such as ephedrine [96] or imipramine

[97,98], we have had little success in treating this complication, which probably should be regarded as permanent. However, success has been reported in these cases with electroejaculation [99]. It is most important to recognize patients at high risk of loss of ejaculation early in the course of their treatment so that seminal analysis and cryopreservation of semen can be arranged in suitable cases [100].

Surveillance with or without adjuvant chemotherapy does not impair fertility, a fact that has led to the birth of over 100 babies fathered by men with testicular tumours treated at our institution [56]. Similarly, 65% of 63 men trying to produce pregnancy after treatment of stage I tumours by surveillance were successful in a series reported from elsewhere [101]. Modern techniques of assisted reproduction such as *in vitro* fertilization and intra-cytoplasmic sperm injection allow production of pregnancy using only a few spermatozoa retrieved by electroejaculation or testicular sperm extraction [102]. It is therefore essential that spermatogenesis should be carefully safeguarded, and cryopreservation arranged prior to possibly toxic chemotherapy [103]. Increasingly successful therapy, a more open society and legal precedent all now demand that reproductive function and future fertility are kept in mind, and fully discussed with both patient and partner before, during and after treatment [104].

Conclusion

The management of testicular tumours requires close collaboration between surgeons and oncologists. The care of these patients requires specialist overview in Cancer Centres. Coordinated and collaborative care leads to improved results in terms of response rates and also in terms of minimizing treatment-related morbidity.

References

1   Mead GM, Stennings SP, Parkinson MC. The second Medical Research Council Study of prognostic factors in nonseminomatous germ cell tumors. *J Clin Oncol* 1992; **10**: 85–94.
2   Harding MJ, Paul J, Gillis CR, Kaye SB. Management of malignant teratoma: does referral to a specialist unit matter? *Lancet* 1993; **341**: 999–1002.
3   Collette L, Sylvester RJ, Stenning SP *et al.* Impact of the treating institution on survival of patients with "poor-prognosis" metastatic nonseminoma. (European Organization for Research and Treatment of Cancer Genito-Urinary Tract Cancer Collaborative Group and the Medical Research Council Testicular Cancer Working Party.) *J Natl Cancer Inst* 1999; **91**: 839–46.
4   Bosl GJ, Vogelzang NJ, Goldman A, Fraley EE, Lange PH, Levitt SH, Kennedy BJ. Impact of delay in diagnosis on clinical stage of testicular cancer. *Lancet* 1981; **2**: 970–3.
5   Thompson IM, Wear J, Almond C, Schewe EJ, Sala J. An analytical survey of one hundred and seventy-eight testicular tumours. *J Urol* 1961; **85**: 173–9.

6   Ekman P. Delay in the diagnosis of testicular cancer. *Lakartidningen* 1980; **77**: 4275–7.

7   Medical Research Council Working Party on Testicular Tumours. Prognostic factors in advanced nonseminomatous germ cell testicular tumours: results of a multicentre study. *Lancet* 1985; **1**: 8–11.

8   Stephen RA. The clinical presentation of testicular tumours. *Br J Urol* 1962; **34**: 448–50.

9   Sandeman JF. Symptoms and early management of germinal tumours of the testis. *Med J Aust* 1979; **2**: 281–4.

10 Martin DC. Malignancy and the undescended testis. In: Fonkalsrud EW, Mengel W, eds. *The Undescended Testis*. Chicago: Year Book Medical Publications, 1981: 144–56.

11 Pike MC, Chilvers C, Peckham MJ. Effect of age at orchidopexy on risk of testicular cancer. *Lancet* 1986; **1**: 1246–8.

12 Gehring GG, Rodriguez FR, Woodhead DM. Malignant degeneration of cryptorchid testes following orchidopexy. *J Urol* 1974; **112**: 354–6.

13 Giwercman A, Grindsted J, Hansen B, Jensen OM, Skakkebaek NE. Testicular cancer risk in boys with maldescended testis: a cohort study. *J Urol* 1987; **138**: 1214–16.

14 Chilvers CED, Pike MC, Peckham MJ. Torsion of the testis: a new risk factor for testicular cancer. *Br J Cancer* 1987; **55**: 105–6.

15 Hausfeld KF, Schrandt D. Malignancy of testis following atrophy: report of three cases. *J Urol* 1965; **94**: 69–72.

16 Gill WB, Schumacher GFB, Bibbo M. Pathological semen and anatomical abnormalities of the genital tract in human male subjects exposed to diethylstilboestrol in utero. *J Urol* 1977; **117**: 477–80.

17 Skakkebaek NE, Keiding N. Changes in semen and the testis. *Br Med J* 1994; **309**: 1316–19.

18 Loughlin JE, Robboy SJ, Morrison AS. Risk factors for cancer of the testis. *N Engl J Med* 1980; **303**: 112–13.

19 Krabbe S, Skakkebaek NE, Berthelsen JG *et al*. High incidence of undetected neoplasia in maldescended testes. *Lancet* 1979; **1**: 999.

20 Giwercman A, Bruun E, Frimodt-Moller C, Skakkebaek NE. Prevalence of carcinoma in situ and other histopathological abnormalities in testes of men with a history of cryptorchidism. *J Urol* 1989; **142**: 998–1002.

21 Berthelsen JG, Skakkebaek NE, von der Maase H, Sorensen BL, Mogensen P. Screening for carcinoma in situ of the contralateral testis in patients with germinal testicular cancer. *Br Med J* 1982; **285**: 1683–6.

22 Dieckmann KP, Loy V. Prevalence of contralateral testicular intraepithelial neoplasia in patients with testicular germ cell neoplasia. *J Clin Oncol* 1996; **14**: 3126–31.

23 Giwercman A, von der Maase H, Skakkebaek NE. Epidemiological and clinical aspects of carcinoma in situ of the testis. *Eur Urol* 1993; **23**: 104–14.

24 Dieckmann KP, Souchon R, Hahn E, Loy V. False negative biopsies for testicular intraepithelial neoplasia. *J Urol* 1999; **162**: 364–8.

25 Fordham MVP, Mason MD, Blackmore C, Hendry WF, Horwich A. Management of the contralateral testis in patients with testicular germ cell cancer. *Br J Urol* 1990; **65**: 290–3.

26 von der Maase H, Giwercman A, Skakkebaek NE. Radiation treatment of carcinoma in situ of the testis. *Lancet* 1986; **1**: 624–5.

27 Hendry WF, Stedronska J, Jones CR, Blackmore CA, Barrett A, Peckham MJ. Semen analysis in testicular cancer and Hodgkin's disease: pre- and post-treatment findings and implications for cryopreservation. *Br J Urol* 1983; **55**: 769–73.

28 Sibert L, Rives N, Rey D, Mace B, Grise P. Semen cryopreservation after orchidectomy in men with testicular cancer. *Br J Urol* 1999; **84**: 1038–42.

29 Sokal M, Peckham MJ, Hendry WF. Bilateral germ cell tumours of the testis. *Br J Urol* 1980; **52**: 158–62.

30 Vick CW, Brid KI, Rosenfield AT, Richter J, Taylor KJ. Ultrasound of the scrotal contents. *Urol Radiol* 1982; **4**: 147–53.

31 Tiptaft PC, Nicholls BM, Hately W, Blandy JP. The diagnosis of testicular swellings using water-path ultrasound. *Br J Urol* 1982; **54**: 759–64.

32 Horstman WG. Scrotal imaging. *Urol Clin North Am* 1997; **24**: 653–71.

33 Ganem JP, Workman KR, Shaban SF. Testicular microlithiasis is associated with testicular pathology. *Urology* 1999; **53**: 209–13.

34 Renshaw AA. Testicular calcifications: incidence, histology and proposed pathological criteria for testicular microlithiasis. *J Urol* 1998; **160**: 1625–8.

35 Powell S, Hendry WF, Peckham MJ. Occult germ-cell testicular tumours. *Br J Urol* 1983; **55**: 440–4.

36 Azzopardi JG, Mostofi FK, Theiss EA. Lesions of testes observed in certain patients with widespread choriocarcinoma and related tumors. *Am J Path* 1961; **38**: 207–25.

37 Daugaard G, von der Maase H, Olsen J, Roith M, Skakkebaek NE. Carcinoma in situ testis in patients with assumed extragonadal germ cell tumours. *Lancet* 1987; **2**: 528–9.

38 Mason MD. Tumour markers. In: Horwich A, ed. *Testicular Cancer Investigation and Management*, 2. London: Chapman & Hall, 1996: 35–51.

39 Markland C, Kedia K, Fraley EE. Inadequate orchiectomy for patients with testicular tumours. *J Am Med Ass* 1973; **224**: 1025–6.

40 Boileau MA, Steers WD. Testis tumours: the clinical significance of the tumour-contaminated scrotum. *J Urol* 1984; **132**: 51–4.

41 Kennedy CL, Hendry WF, Peckham MJ. The significance of scrotal interference in stage I testicular cancer managed by orchiectomy and surveillance. *Br J Urol* 1986; **58**: 705–8.

42 Giguere JK, Stablein DM, Spaulding JT, McLeod DG, Paulson DF, Weiss RB. The clinical significance of unconventional orchiectomy approaches in testicular cancer: a report from the Testicular Cancer Intergroup Study. *J Urol* 1988; **139**: 1225–8.

43 Ozen H, Altug U, Bakkaloglu MA, Remzi D. Significance of scrotal violation in the prognosis of patients with testicular tumours. *Br J Urol* 1988; **62**: 267–70.

44 Capelouto CC, Clark PE, Ransil BJ, Loughlin KR. A review of scrotal violation in testicular cancer: is adjuvant local therapy necessary? *J Urol* 1995; **153**: 981–5.

45 Donat SM. Peri-operative care in patients treated for testicular cancer. *Semin Surg Oncol* 1999; **17**: 282–8.

46 Peckham MJ. Investigation and staging; General aspects and staging classification. In: Peckham MJ, ed. *The Management of Testicular Tumours*. London: Arnold, 1981: 89–101, 218–239.

47 Hoskin P, Dilly S, Easton D, Horwich A, Hendry WF, Peckham MJ. Prognostic factors in stage 1 non-seminomatous germ-cell testicular tumors managed by orchiectomy and surveillance: implications for adjuvant chemotherapy. *J Clin Oncol* 1986; **4**: 1031–6.

48 Albers P, Siener R, Hartmann M *et al.* Risk factors for relapse in stage I non-seminomatous germ-cell tumors: preliminary results of the German Multicenter Trial. (German Testicular Cancer Study Group.) *Int J Cancer* 1999; **83**: 828–30.

49 Moul JW, McCarthy WF, Fernandez EB, Sesterhenn IA. Percentage of embryonal carcinoma and of vascular invasion predicts pathological stage in clinical stage 1 non-seminomatous testicular cancer. *Cancer Res* 1994; **54**: 362–4.

50 Lee AHS, Mead GM, Theaker JM. The value of central histopathological review of testicular tumours before treatment. *Br J Urol* 1999; **84**: 75–8.

51 Sonneveld DJ, Koops HS, Sleijfer DT, Hoekstra HJ. Surgery versus surveillance in stage I non-seminoma testicular cancer. *Semin Surg Oncol* 1999; **17**: 230–9.

52 Gels ME, Hoekstra HJ, Sleijfer DT *et al.* Detection of recurrence in patients with clinical stage 1 nonseminomatous testicular germ cell tumors and consequences for further follow-up: a single-center 10-year experience. *J Clin Oncol* 1995; **13**: 1188–94.

53 Sogani PC, Perrotti M, Herr H, Fair WR, Bosl G. Clinical stage 1 testis cancer: long-term outcome of patients on surveillance. *J Urol* 1998; **159**: 855–8.

54 Sharir S, Jewett MAS, Sturgeon JFG *et al.* Progression detection of stage 1 nonseminomatous testis cancer on surveillance: implications for the follow up protocol. *J Urol* 1999; **161**: 472–6.

55 Colls BM, Harvey VJ, Skelton L *et al.* Late results of surveillance of clinical stage 1 nonseminoma germ cell testicular tumours: 17 years' experience in a national study in New Zealand. *Br J Urol* 1999; **83**: 76–82.

56 Hendry WF, Norman A, Nicholls J, Dearnaley DP, Pearson MJ, Horwich A. Abdominal relapse in Stage 1 nonseminomatous germ cell tumours of testis managed by surveillance or with adjuvant chemotherapy. *Br J Urol* 2000; **86**: 89–93.

57 Read G, Stenning SP, Cullen MH *et al.* Medical Research Council prospective study of surveillance for stage I testicular teratoma. *J Clin Oncol* 1992; **10**: 1762–8.

58 Sweeney CJ, Hermans BP, Heilman DK, Foster RS, Donohue JP, Einhorn LH. Results and outcome of retroperitoneal lymph node dissection for clinical stage I embryonal carcinoma-predominant testis cancer. *J Clin Oncol* 2000; **18**: 358–62.

59 Baniel J, Foster RS, Einhorn LH, Donohue JP. Late relapse of clinical stage 1 testicular cancer. *J Urol* 1995; **154**: 1370–2.

60 Cespedes RD, Peretsman SJ. Retroperitoneal recurrences after retroperitoneal lymph node dissection for low-stage nonseminomatous germ cell tumors. *Urology* 1999; **54**: 548–52.

61 Donohue JP, Thornhill JA, Foster RS, Bihrle R, Rowland RG, Einhorn LH. The role of retroperitoneal lymphadenectomy in clinical stage B testis cancer: the Indiana University experience (1965 to 1989). *J Urol* 1995; **153**: 85–9.

62 Horwich A, Norman A, Fisher C, Hendry WF, Nicholls J, Dearnaley DP. Primary chemotherapy for stage II nonseminomatous germ cell tumors of the testis. *J Urol* 1994; **151**: 72–8.

63 Tait D, Peckham MJ, Hendry WF, Goldstraw P. Post-chemotherapy surgery in advanced non-seminomatous germ-cell testicular tumours: the significance of histology with particular reference to differentiated (mature) teratoma. *Br J Cancer* 1984; **50**: 601–9.

64 Hendry WF, A'Hern RP, Hetherington JW, Peckham MJ, Dearnaley DP, Horwich A. Para-aortic lymphadenectomy after chemotherapy for metastatic non-seminomatous germ cell tumours: prognostic value and therapeutic benefit. *Br J Urol* 1993; **71**: 208–13.

65 Donohue JP, Rowland RG. The role of surgery in advanced testicular cancer. *Cancer* 1984; **54**: 2716–21.

66 Hendry WF, Goldstraw P, Husband JE, Barrett A, McElwain TJ, Peckham MJ. Elective delayed excision of bulky para-aortic lymph node metastases in advanced non-seminoma germ cell tumours of testis. *Br J Urol* 1981; **53**: 648–53.

67 Steyerberg EW, Keizer HJ, Habbema JD. Prediction models for the histology of residual masses after chemotherapy for metastatic testicular cancer. *Int J Cancer* 1999; **83**: 856–9.

68 Steyerberg EW, Marshall PB, Keizer HJ, Habbema JD. Resection of small, residual retroperitoneal masses after chemotherapy for nonseminomatous testicular cancer: a decision analysis. *Cancer* 1999; **85**: 1331–41.

69 Kuczyk M, Machtens S, Stief C, Jonas U. Management of the post-chemotherapy residual mass in patients with advanced stage non-seminomatous germ cell tumors (NSGCT). *Int J Cancer* 1999; **83**: 852–5.

70 Rabbani F, Goldenberg SL, Gleave ME, Paterson RF, Murray N, Sullivan LD. Retroperitoneal lymphadenectomy for post-chemotherapy residual masses: is a modified dissection and resection of residual masses sufficient? *Br J Urol* 1998; **81**: 295–300.

71 Christmas TJ, Doherty AP, Rustin GJ, Seckl MJ, Newlands ES. Excision of residual masses of metastatic germ cell tumours after chemotherapy: the role of extraperitoneal surgical approaches. *Br J Urol* 1998; **81**: 301–88.

72 Hahn TL, Jacobson L, Einhorn LH, Foster R, Goulet RJJ. Hepatic resection of metastatic testicular carcinoma: a further update. *Ann Surg Oncol* 1999; **6**: 640–4.

73 Weisberger EC, McBride LC. Modified neck dissection for metastatic nonseminomatous testicular carcinoma. *Laryngoscope* 1999; **109**: 1241–4.

74 Liu D, Abolhoda A, Burt ME *et al.* Pulmonary metastasectomy for testicular germ cell tumors: a 28-year experience. *Ann Thorac Surg* 1998; **66**: 1709–14.

75 Tognoni PG, Foster RS, McGraw P *et al.* Combined post-chemotherapy retroperitoneal lymph node dissection and resection of chest tumor under the same anesthetic is appropriate based on morbidity and tumor pathology. *J Urol* 1998; **159**: 1833–5.

76 Loehrer PJ, Williams SD, Clark SA. Teratoma following chemotherapy for non-seminomatous germ cell tumor: a clinicopathologic correlation. *Proc Am Soc Clin Oncol* 1983; **2**: 139.

77 Logothetis CJ, Samuels ML, Trindale A, Johnson DE. The growing teratoma syndrome. *Cancer* 1982; **50**: 1629–35.

78 Sonneveld DJ, Sleijfer DT, Koops HS, Keemers-Gels ME, Molenaar WM, Hoekstra HJ. Mature teratoma identified after postchemotherapy surgery in patients with disseminated nonseminomatous testicular germ cell tumors: a plea for an aggressive surgical approach. *Cancer* 1998; **82**: 1343–51.

79 Donohue JP, Leviovitch I, Foster RS, Baniel J, Tognoni P. Integration of surgery and systemic therapy: results and principles of integration. *Semin Urol Oncol* 1998; **16**: 65–71.

80 Baniel J, Foster RS, Rowland RG, Bihrle R, Donohue JP. Complications of post-chemotherapy retroperitoneal lymph node dissection. *J Urol* 1995; **153**: 976–80.

81 Skinner DG, Melamud A, Lieskovsky G. Complications of thoracoabdominal retroperitoneal lymph node dissection. *J Urol* 1982; **127**: 1107–10.

82 Ng CS, Husband JES, Padhani AR *et al.* Evaluation by magnetic resonance imaging of the inferior vena cava in patients with non-seminomatous germ cell tumours of the testis metastatic to the retroperitoneum. *Br J Urol* 1997; **79**: 942–51.

83 Ahlering T, Skinner DG. Vena caval resection in bulky metastatic germ cell tumours. *J Urol* 1989; **142**: 1497–9.

84 Donohue JP, Thornhill JA, Foster RS, Rowland RG, Bihrle R. Resection of the inferior vena cava or intraluminal vena caval tumor thrombectomy during retroperitoneal lymph node dissection for metastatic germ cell cancer: indications and results. *J Urol* 1991; **146**: 346–9.

85 Beck SD, Lalka SG. Long-term results after inferior vena caval resection during retroperitoneal lymphadenectomy for metastatic germ cell cancer. *J Vasc Surg* 1998; **28**: 808–14.

86 Christmas TJ, Smith GL, Kooner R. Vascular interventions during post-chemotherapy retroperitoneal lymph-node dissection for metastatic testis cancer. *Eur J Surg Oncol* 1998; **24**: 292–7.

87 Hartmann JT, Albrecht C, Schmoll HJ, Kuczyk MA, Kollmannsberger C, Bokemeyer C. Long-term effects on sexual function and fertility after treatment of testicular cancer. *Br J Cancer* 1999; **80**: 801–7.

88 Caffo O, Amichetti M. Evaluation of sexual life after orchidectomy followed by radiotherapy for early-stage seminoma of the testis. *BJU Int* 1999; **83**: 462–8.

89 Schilsky RL. Infertility in patients with testicular cancer: testis, tumour or treatment? *J Natl Cancer Inst* 1989; **81**: 1204–5.

90 Petersen PM, Skakkebaek NE, Vistisen K, Rorth M, Giwercman A. Semen quality and

reproductive hormones before orchiectomy in men with testicular cancer. *J Clin Oncol* 1999; **17**: 941–7.

91 Leiter E, Brendler H. Loss of ejaculation following bilateral retroperitoneal lymphadenectomy. *J Urol* 1967; **98**: 375–8.

92 Jewett MAS, Kong YSP, Goldberg SD *et al.* Retroperitoneal lymphadenectomy for testis tumour with nerve sparing for ejaculation. *J Urol* 1988; **139**: 1220–4.

93 Richie JP. Clinical stage 1 testicular cancer: the role of modified retroperitoneal lymphadenectomy. *J Urol* 1990; **144**: 1160–3.

94 Jones DR, Norman AR, Horwich A, Hendry WF. Ejaculatory dysfunction after retroperitoneal lymphadenectomy. *Eur Urol* 1993; **23**: 169–71.

95 Jacobsen KD, Ous S, Waehre H *et al.* Ejaculation in testicular cancer patients after post-chemotherapy retroperitoneal lymph node dissection. *Br J Cancer* 1999; **80**: 249–55.

96 Lynch JH, Maxted WC. Use of ephedrine in post-lymphadenectomy ejaculatory failure: a case report. *J Urol* 1983; **129**: 379.

97 Nijman JM, Jager S, Boer PW, Kremer J, Oldhoff J, Koops HS. The treatment of ejaculation disorders after retroperitoneal lymph node dissection. *Cancer* 1982; **50**: 2967–71.

98 Ochsenkuhn R, Kamischke A, Nieschlag E. Imipramine for successful treatment of retrograde ejaculation caused by retroperitoneal surgery. *Int J Androl* 1999; **22**: 173–7.

99 Ohl DA. Electroejaculation. *Urol Clin North Am* 1993; **20**: 181–8.

100 Hendry WF, Stedronska J, Jones CR, Blackmore CA, Barrett A, Peckham MJ. Semen analysis in testicular cancer and Hodgkin's disease: pre- and post-treatment findings and implications for cryopreservation. *Br J Urol* 1983; **55**: 769–73.

101 Herr HW, Bar-Chama N, O'Sullivan M, Sogani PC. Paternity in men with stage I testis tumors on surveillance. *J Clin Oncol* 1998; **16**: 733–4.

102 Rosenlund B, Sjoblom P, Tornblom M, Hultling C, Hillensjo T. In-vitro fertilization and intracytoplasmic sperm injection in the treatment of infertility after testicular cancer. *Hum Reprod* 1998; **13**: 414–18.

103 Hendry WF. Iatrogenic damage to male reproductive function. *J R Soc Med* 1995; **88**: 579–84.

104 Hendry WF. Cancer therapy and fertility. In: Horwich A, ed. *Oncology – a Multidisciplinary Textbook*. London: Chapman & Hall, 1995: 213–23.

Testicular Cancer: Commentary

J. Waxman

It may be paradigmatic to note that the successful treatment of testicular cancer has been one of the major developments in oncology in the last 30 years. The development of treatment algorithms has come as a result of a long series of clinical observations on the efficacy of treatment, and also from a detailing of the expectation for progression for patients with different histological variants and stages.

We now know how to manage testicular cancer and have a high expectation of cure for even the most advanced of testicular malignancies. The treatment of testicular cancer follows a logical pattern, a pattern that has evolved as a result of meticulous observation. In the year 2001 we seek the publication of survival figures for testicular cancer that show a reduction in mortality rates in England and Wales of 70% over the last 10 years, and this is a marvellous achievement.

In this part of the book we describe the management of localized disease, and the treatment of advanced tumours. Recommendations are made for optimal chemotherapy for patients at every stage of their illness in a series of excellent chapters from the Birmingham and Southampton groups. Bill Hendry has just retired from a most successful career, and is thought by many to be one of the finest urological surgeons in the world. In his precise and meticulous chapter, he details his enormous experience of the surgical management of patients with testicular cancer.

In step with this improvement in our understanding of how to treat patients with testicular cancer also comes a series of observations concerning the molecular biology of this tumour. Dr Houldsworth and her co-authors describe the significance of tumour suppressor genes and the genetics of differentiation and resistance in testicular malignancy.

Part 5
Penile Cancer

21: Viral Agents in the Development of Penile Cancer

P. H. Rajjayabun, T. R. L. Griffiths & J. K. Mellon

Introduction

Viruses account for a wide range of disease processes in both humans and animals. For more than a century, the role of viruses as protagonists in oncogenesis has received the attention of scientists and molecular biologists. Recently, there has been an explosion in the available data concerning the molecular interplay between viruses and genitourinary malignancy in both men and women. This reflects the development of powerful molecular biology techniques such as the polymerase chain reaction and *in situ* hybridization which are available for the analysis of tumour specimens. In this chapter, we aim to provide an overview of the terminology associated with viral cycling and tumorigenesis, with particular emphasis upon the role of viruses in the development of neoplastic lesions of the penis.

Characteristics of viruses

The majority of viral particles, with diameters ranging from 20 to 300 nm, are invisible without the aid of scanning electron microscopy. Although there is enormous variation in structure and complexity even within a single viral family, all viruses convey certain characteristics which distinguish them from other organisms. Each virus contains only a single nucleic acid (RNA or DNA) in its genome and this genetic filament is encased by a polypeptide shell of capsomeres termed the capsid. The proteins encoded by the viral genome are either involved in replicative processes or contribute to the formation of structural components. The term 'obligate intracellular parasite' refers to the fact that all viruses require host ribosomal function for the translation of their mRNA. Depending on the individual virus involved, further assistance may be required for genomic replication and transcription.

DNA virus transcription is a biphasic process. Using host-derived polymerase enzyme activity, 'early' transcription takes place within the nucleus of the affected cell. The resultant mRNA is translated by host cytoplasmic ribosomes into 'early' proteins. These then act as transcriptional activators for the synthesis of new viral DNA. 'Late' mRNA is transcribed, again within the nucleus, and the encoded proteins are utilized for capsomere construction.

Mature virions are subsequently assembled within the nucleus prior to their liberation.

By contrast, the majority of RNA viruses replicate within the host cell cytoplasm although variation exists in the precise mechanisms involved. Viral RNA can act as its own mRNA, which when translated can lead to RNA polymerase formation. The end product of this enzyme's activity is a double-stranded replicative intermediate which comprises parent RNA with its complementary strand. Single-stranded viral RNA molecules are then formed from the replicative intermediate which serves as mRNA for the formation of capsid proteins and templates for further viral RNA synthesis leading to the formation of mature virion particles. In the RNA virus group known as the retroviruses, the viral genome is incorporated into host genomic DNA. The conversion of viral RNA into a DNA replica (proviral DNA) is mediated by the enzyme reverse transcriptase. Once integration into the host cell DNA is complete, subsequent transcription is regulated by native RNA polymerase activity.

Viruses and their role in neoplasia

Epidemiological evidence linking a transmissible agent with cervical cancer in humans has been available for more than 150 years, yet early investigative studies of virus-induced tumour formation centred on animal systems. In 1903, Borrel hypothesized a role for infectious agents, including viruses, in the development of epithelial growths [1]. Five years later, Elleman and co-workers isolated a viral agent which induced erythroblastosis in chicken. In 1910, Peyton Rous demonstrated the experimental induction of chicken spindle-cell sarcoma by a transmissible agent [2]. While globally up to 20% of human malignancies are thought to involve viruses as part of the oncogenic process, the collection of definitive and supportive evidence has not been straightforward. It is well recognized that the event of viral infection may be far removed from the endpoint of tumour development and that the pathways involved implicate multiple co-factors. Three viruses have been closely scrutinized in the pursuit of understanding human viral carcinogenesis: Epstein–Barr virus (EBV), hepatitis B virus (HBV) and human papillomavirus (HPV).

In 1964, EBV, the large DNA virus responsible for infectious mononucleosis, was identified by electron microscopy in cultured Burkitt's lymphoma cells [3]. In addition, an association has also been observed between EBV and a lymphoepithelial neoplasm of the nasopharynx [4]. Interestingly, although EBV is widely prevalent, EBV-related tumours show distinctive geographical distribution, with Burkitt's lymphoma being common in West Africa and nasopharyngeal carcinoma frequently found in southern China.

Infectious hepatitis had been suspected as a factor in the development of hepatocellular carcinoma for many years, but firm evidence became available only following the discovery of the hepatitis B surface antigen (HBsAg) in the 1960s. Subsequent cloning studies of the HBV genome led to the development of hybridization probes which allowed the detection of viral DNA sequences in tumour tissue [5]. As a result of this technology it has been shown that, in certain populations, 80% of liver tumours from HBsAg positive patients contain integrated HBV-DNA [6].

For many years HPV has been implicated in the development of anogenital cancer, in particular pre-malignant and malignant lesions of the uterine cervix. In one study of cervical squamous cell carcinoma, 80–90% of biopsies demonstrated HPV-DNA [7]. Of the positive tumour samples, 80% were associated with either HPV-16 or HPV-18 [8]. Screening studies have also shown that 50–60% of men whose female partners exhibit HPV-associated intraepithelial neoplasia also have HPV lesions [9]. Conversely, epidemiological evidence has identified that the wives of men with penile cancer are prone to cervical and vulval neoplasia. This early information has helped to provide a framework for understanding the role for HPV in squamous neoplasia of the penis.

Unlike cervical carcinoma, which accounts for approximately 3300 cases in England and Wales per annum and is the second most common malignancy in females worldwide, penile cancer (300 cases p.a.) is relatively rare, accounting for less than 1% of adult male cancers in the developed world [10]. The phenomenon of geographical variation, however, also holds true for this disease, with higher levels seen in Asia, Africa and South America — in Puerto Rico penile cancer accounts for 20% of all cancers in men [11].

Initially, data collection for the assessment of the role of HPV in penile neoplasia was hampered by low clinical incidence and lack of investigative firepower. With ongoing developments in molecular biotechnology, the number of studies examining the role for this and other viral agents in the development of penile cancer has increased. As will be discussed, a number of key questions have been targeted.

The human papillomavirus

Papillomaviruses form part of the Papova subgroup of DNA viruses. Experimentally, exposure of traumatized mucosa to HPV results in basal epithelial cell infection. With most types of HPV this event usually gives rise to benign, self-limiting epithelial proliferation and wart formation. On electron microscopy, the 52–55 nm HPV appears as icosahedral particles, with 72 capsomeres per capsid.

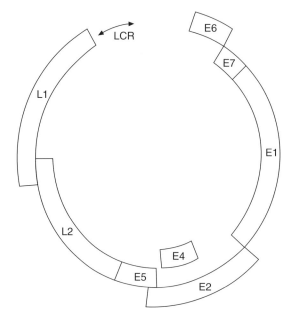

Figure 21.1 The structure of the HPV-16 genome. For details see text.

The molecular organization of all HPV genomes conforms to the same pattern [12]. The genome of the HPV-16 virus (see Fig. 21.1) comprises two functional groups called early (E) and late (L) open reading frames separated by a long control region (LCR). The LCR is necessary for control of normal virus replication; the E1 and E2 genes are involved in viral replication and transcriptional control; the E6 and E7 proteins inhibit the activity of negative regulators of the cell cycle (see below); the L1 and L2 genes encode structural proteins; the function of the E4 protein is unknown; the E5 gene encodes the major transforming protein of bovine papillomavirus type 1. Currently, the HPV group consists of more than 70 distinct types. The typing system is based on differences demonstrated by DNA hybridization, in particular, differences in the E6/E7 and L1 regions. A new HPV type is, by definition, less than 90% homologous with previously identified types with respect to these regions, as determined following complete viral cloning. A subtype shares 90–98% homology in these regions; a variant shares more than 98% homology.

Viral oncogenesis and HPV-associated transformation

Control of cell growth and differentiation results from a balance between growth promotion and restraint, with physiological demand dictating which of these two opposing forces is dominant. This interplay reflects the expression of growth promoting proto-oncogenes and growth inhibiting tumour-suppressor genes. Proto-oncogenes form part of the normal genome and encode for the machinery of cell division and proliferation, for example cell cycling enzymes, growth factors and their receptor molecules. Alteration in the normal patterns of activation of these genes, such as point mutation or overexpression, can result in the acquisition of malignant cellular characteristics—loss of contact inhibition, diminished growth factor requirements and anchorage-independent growth. Tumour-suppressor genes encode proteins which inhibit excessive cell proliferation. Mutation or deletion of these sequences can thus contribute to cellular oncogenesis. The p53 and retinoblastoma (Rb) tumour-suppressor genes have been studied extensively and both appear to be commonly implicated in the development of human tumours.

The ability of genes to extend the life span of cells in culture indefinitely is termed immortalization. By contrast, transformation requires the acquisition of at least some of the properties characteristic of malignant cells, in particular autonomous proliferation. Immortalizing activities of HPV-16 and HPV-18 DNA have been demonstrated in cultures of primary human keratinocytes, cells which resemble the normal target of the virus [13]. Although these cell lines do not display characteristics of transformed cells, alterations in differentiation have been demonstrated which are almost indistinguishable from those seen in low grade cervical intraepithelial neoplasia (CIN).

Other viruses, such as HPV-6 and HPV-11, have no immortalizing or transforming properties [14]. Analysis of the viral genome has revealed that only the E6 and E7 proteins are necessary for the immortalization of human genital keratinocytes [15]. In these immortalization assays, E7 can function alone when placed under the control of a powerful promoter, but E6 is required when E7 is under normal viral control. However, cell-specific factors are important in the outcome of these assays. For example, E6 alone is unable to immortalize primary human genital keratinocytes but can function alone in mammary-derived epithelial cells [16].

Function of HPV E7 viral oncoproteins

The protein product of the retinoblastoma tumour-suppressor gene and other Rb family members, including p107 and p130, can block cell cycle progression at the G1/S boundary. In its active state, Rb is hypophosphorylated and binds to a number of transcription factors, most notably the E2F family. Following cyclin-dependent kinase (CDK) phosphorylation of Rb, these transcription factors are released from Rb, allowing them to mediate transcriptional activation and progression through the G1/S boundary. The E7 protein blocks the negative regulation of Rb by binding to hypophosphorylated Rb and Rb-related proteins. E7 may also degrade Rb family members [17].

The E7 proteins of HPV-16 and HPV-18 bind hypophosphorylated Rb with higher affinity than do those of HPV-6 and HPV-11.

Function of HPV E6 viral oncoproteins

The p53 tumour-suppressor gene is located on chromosome 17p13.1 and functions as a negative regulator of cell growth. In response to DNA damage, it can induce G1 arrest and/or apoptosis. It is known that the p53 protein is a transcription factor which blocks cell proliferation and mediates G1 arrest via the induction of the p21 gene (WAF-1). The 21 kDa protein product of this gene encodes for an inhibitor of both CDK2 and CDK4 and thus, via hypo-phosphorylation of Rb and subsequent E2F binding, the cell cycle is pro-longed in the G1 phase. The E6 proteins of HPV-16 and HPV-18 target the p53 protein for degradation via a ubiquitin-dependent pathway [18]. Low risk HPV E6 protein binds to p53 protein less efficiently. In the general population, a polymorphism at codon 72 of the p53 gene results in translation to either arginine (p53Arg) or proline (p53Pro) [19]. One study has demonstrated that E6 from HPV-16 and HPV-18 is more effective at degrading p53Arg than p53Pro *in vivo*; HPV-11 E6 is less active towards p53Arg and inactive with p53Pro [20].

The same authors reported that white women, homozygous for the arginine allele, were seven times more likely to develop cervical cancer than Pro/Arg heterozygotes. However, not all studies agree with these findings: arginine homozygosity at codon 72 failed to be associated with an increased risk for cervical cancer in studies comprising white women from the UK [21] and Japanese women [22]. Finally, mutations in the p53 gene are very common in almost all solid tumours, with the exception of anogenital cancer [23]. This suggests that HPV targeting of p53 protein is an alternative to p53 gene mutation as a mechanism for p53 inactivation.

HPV and telomerase activity

More recently, the high risk HPV E6 oncoproteins have been implicated in activating the enzyme telomerase—a potential mechanism for HPV-induced immortalization [24]. Mammalian telomeres are structures at the chromosomal tips consisting of multiple repeats of TTAGG, which shorten as a function of division *in vivo* as a consequence of an intrinsic inability to replicate the 3′ end of DNA. Telomerase replaces the telomeric repeats and is not normally expressed in somatic cells. Activation of telomerase enables cells to escape from the senescence signalled by telomeric shortening. However, E6-induced telomerase activity alone cannot result in immortalization without co-expression of E7. E6 protein has also been shown to interact with cellular

MCM (minichromosome maintenance) proteins, which are believed to play a key role in regulating cellular DNA replication [25].

HPV and carcinoma of the penis

The development of carcinoma of the penis appears to be a multifactorial process which spans a period of many years. Known aetiological factors include smoking, phimosis and poor hygiene. Researchers have recently provided evidence to support a role for HPV in the pathogenic process. However, as previously mentioned, the low incidence of penile cancer in combination with the difficult *in vitro* characteristics of HPV, which is non-pathogenic in animals and not amenable to cell culture, have made the investigative process technically challenging. Initially non-specific histological features such as koilocytosis and cytoplasmic vacuolization were used as potential markers of HPV infection. Immunohistochemical techniques have also been used to detect HPV capsid antigens, and electron microscopy has detected HPV particles in tumour specimens [26].

Over the last decade, DNA hybridization and the polymerase chain reaction (PCR) have been used to detect specific viral genome sequences within the DNA of tumour cells. *In situ* hybridization, in particular, permits the localization of DNA at cellular level with the preservation of tissue architecture. However, despite the availability of these advanced molecular assays, highly variable frequencies of HPV detection in penile tumours have been reported. One possible explanation for this inconsistency is the high level of sensitivity associated with PCR. With this technique, detection of a specific DNA sequence does not necessarily correlate with pathological significance. In addition, contamination of paraffin-embedded tumour tissue during routine processing may occur, resulting in false-positive or misleading results. With the less sensitive *in situ* hybridization assays, cross-hybridization or non-specific binding of sequence probes to elements of the target tissue can occur, leading to discrepancies in laboratory findings.

HPV appears to have a role in the development of carcinoma of the penis and its clinical precursors. Three pre-malignant lesions of the penis have been described: erythroplasia of Queyrat, Bowen's disease and bowenoid papulosis. These lesions have also been referred to as high grade penile intraepithelial neoplasia (PIN) or carcinoma *in situ* (CIS) of the penis. However, the minor histological differences between bowenoid papulosis and Bowen's disease and erythroplasia of Queyrat do not allow for an accurate diagnosis on the basis of histological findings alone. Essentially, they are distinguished on the basis of clinical features.

Bowenoid papulosis and Bowen's disease both occur on the penile shaft whereas erythroplasia is found on the glans or prepuce. Characteristic features include papules in bowenoid papulosis, crusted and scaly plaques in Bowen's disease, and erythematous plaques in erythroplasia of Queyrat. Bowenoid papulosis usually presents in men in the age range 20–40 years, Bowen's disease in the range 30–50 years, and erythroplasia of Queyrat in the range 40–60 years. The incidence of progression to invasive squamous cell carcinoma is more common for erythroplasia of Queyrat than for Bowen's disease, with an incidence varying from 10% to 33% [27,28]. By contrast, the clinical course of bowenoid papulosis is invariably benign, despite being a CIS. In one study, the high risk HPV-16 was detected in 1 of 2 cases of Bowen's disease [29]; in another study HPV-16 DNA was detected in all 7 cases of Bowen's disease [30]. HPV has also been detected in a case of erythroplasia of Queyrat [31] and surprisingly HPV-16 has been detected in a case of bowenoid papulosis [32]. Recently, a case of bowenoid papulosis progressing to squamous cell carcinoma was described [33]. In this case, sequencing results revealed a heterogeneity of human papillomavirus DNA including HPV-6b, HPV-16, HPV-18 and HPV-33.

HPV has been detected in 15–80% of penile carcinoma specimens [30,34–39]. In a recent study of 156 patients, the presence of HPV-DNA was assessed in 42 cases of invasive penile carcinoma, 13 cases of CIS, 12 cases of PIN, 3 verrucous carcinomas, 25 cases of balanitis xerotica obliterans, 29 routine neonatal circumcision specimens and 32 adult circumcision specimens [34]. High risk subtypes of HPV, namely HPV-16 and HPV-18, were associated with penile carcinoma, as is seen in cervical cancer. The HPV-16 genetic sequence was identified in 80–90% of HPV positive lesions and HPV-18 in only 10%. In this study, HPV-DNA was detected in 55% of invasive penile carcinoma, 92% of CIS, 92% of PIN, 4% of balanitis xerotica obliterans, and 9% of adult circumcision specimens, but was undetectable in verrucous carcinomas, which are a well-differentiated subtype of penile carcinoma with low potential for progression, and neonatal circumcision specimens.

In another study of 117 patients with carcinoma of the penis, HPV-DNA (mainly type 16) was detected in 26 (22%) and was significantly associated with penile carcinomas exhibiting basaloid changes, high grade tumours and those localized to the glans penis [35]. In a study of 18 Brazilian patients using single strand conformational polymorphism analysis (SSCP), HPV-18 was detected in 39% of penile carcinoma specimens but HPV-16 was not found [39]. These different results may reflect a unique epidemiology in Brazil. HPV-11, which was previously considered non-carcinogenic, has also been detected in a case of an invasive verrucous carcinoma of the penis [40] and HPV-33 in a well-differentiated squamous carcinoma of the penis [41]. There have also been case reports of HPV-16 in a verrucous carcinoma [42] and HPV-6 in an invasive penile carcinoma [43].

Twenty years ago, a case of concurrent penile and cervical carcinoma in a married couple was reported [44]. Since then, a number of studies have described an increased incidence of cervical carcinoma in the partners or ex-partners of men with penile cancer [45,46]. In the latter study, 423 wives of 671 men with penile cancer in Norway were compared with 444 wives of 569 men who did not have this disease. The relative risk for the development of cervical cancer amongst the wives of men with penile cancer was 1.75. By contrast, in an earlier Finnish study of 239 patients with penile carcinoma and their 224 wives, the relative risk of developing cervical carcinoma was only 1.05 [47]. Epidemiological studies assessing the risk of developing penile carcinoma in the partners of women who have cervical carcinoma have also been performed. In a large French study, 1000 male partners of women with genital condylomata or intraepithelial neoplasia were screened for evidence of PIN—92 had lesions meriting biopsy of which 93% were positive for PIN. In addition, oncogenic HPV was detected in 75% of grade I, 93% of grade II and 10% of grade III PIN [9]. In this study, circumcised and uncircumcised males had similar rates of HPV-associated lesions, whereas the rate of PIN was higher in uncircumcised males. In a more recent study, peoscopy was used to assess penile lesions in the male sexual partners of 326 women with CIN or flat condylomata. Naked eye examination revealed abnormal lesions in 39/233 males, whereas peoscopic examination revealed abnormal lesions in 233/326 (71%)—37 had PIN I–III and 7 had HPV [48].

The long latency of HPV-induced neoplasia suggests that other genetic changes are important as well. An activating c-ras^{Ha} mutation has been detected in an inguinal lymph node metastasis in a patient with HPV-18 penile carcinoma [49]. Positive p53 immunoreactivity is found in approximately 40% of genital warts and bowenoid papulosis but p53 mutations assessed by SSCP and sequencing are rarely detected in these lesions or in other forms of CIS of the penis [50]. On account of the possible interaction between HPV viral oncoproteins and p53 as a mechanism of p53 inactivation a number of groups have studied these two factors in penile cancer. Pilotti and colleagues studied 5 cases of verrucous penile carcinoma but failed to detect either HPV-DNA or alteration in p53 [51]. Subsequently, HPV-DNA (subtypes 16, 31, 33) was detected in 7/13 (54%) penile tumours but without evidence of p53 mutations [52].

More recent studies, however, do suggest that alterations in expression of p53 and p53 gene mutations do occur in penile carcinoma. Lam *et al.* [53] have reported p53 immunoreactivity in 17/42 (40%) penile carcinomas with lack of immunostaining in cases of verrucous carcinoma and penile warts. They also reported that all HPV positive cases showed p53 immunoreactivity in contradistinction to the theory suggesting an inverse correlation between these two factors in penile cancer. Detection of p53 in penile carcinoma has been confirmed by the most recent study of p53 and HPV in penile cancer, in which p53 immunopositivity was reported in 26% of 64 penile cancers studied, with results corroborated by SSCP and direct p53 gene sequencing [54]. This study also reported a higher incidence of HPV-DNA detection in fresh compared with paraffin-embedded material (HPV-DNA in 26% of paraffin sections compared with in 56% of fresh samples). Further work is needed with regard to the interplay between HPV and genetic alterations in penile cancer. In summary, although high risk HPV types 16 and 18 are associated with penile carcinoma, a causal relationship remains to be established.

Herpes simplex virus

Herpes simplex virus (HSV) is a 100 nm, spherical, double-stranded DNA virus which is responsible for a wide spectrum of clinical syndromes. HSV type-2 is the main cause of the vesicular lesions associated with genital herpes, but up to one-third of cases are related to HSV type-1. HSV-2 has been implicated in cervical neoplasia, but it does not appear to be a main aetiological factor. Studies have shown that up to 30% of cervical carcinoma biopsies contain HSV-2 specific binding proteins ICSP 11/12 and ICSP 34/35. The role of this virus in penile cancer appears to be even less convincing. McCance and colleagues [55], using monoclonal antibodies to ICSP 11/12, failed to identify the presence of HSV-2 antigens in 10 penile carcinoma specimens. Similarly, in another immunohistochemical study of 20 penile squamous carcinomas, no tumours were found to contain HSV-2 antigenic material [56].

Conclusion

The development of penile cancer appears to follow a complex stepwise progression, which spans a latent period of years and involves multiple co-factors. The available data suggest that two distinct aetiological groups exist—those in which viral agents are partly implicated and those where tumours evolve via other mechanisms. Functional analysis of the E6 and E7 HPV viral oncoproteins has highlighted how viruses can interact with and influence elements of cell cycle control and potentially contribute to cell transformation and tumorigenesis. The current body of evidence suggests that the high risk HPV subtypes 16 and 18 are associated with pre-invasive and invasive penile tumours, but a direct causal relationship has not been established. Further work is therefore needed to evaluate in more detail the downstream subcellular and genetic sequelae of HPV-induced neoplasia.

References

1   Borrel A. Epithelioses infectieuses et epitheliomas. *Ann Inst Pasteur* 1903; **17**: 81–112.
2   Rous P. A transmissible avian neoplasm (Sarcoma of the common fowl). *Exp Med* 1910; **12**: 696–705.
3   Yamaguchi J, Hinuma Y, Grace JT Jr. Structure of virus particles extracted from a Burkitt lymphoma cell line. *J Virol* 1967; **1**: 640–2.
4   Schryver A, Friberg S Jr, Klein G *et al.* Epstein-Barr virus-associated antibody patterns in carcinoma of the post-nasal space. *Clin Exp Immunol* 1969; **5**: 443–59.
5   Brechot C, Pourcel C, Louise A, Rain B, Tiollais P. Presence of integrated hepatitis B virus DNA sequences in cellular DNA of human hepatocellular carcinoma. *Nature* 1980; **286**: 533–5.
6   Chen JY, Harrison TJ, Lee CS, Chen DS, Zuckerman AJ. Detection of hepatitis B virus DNA in hepatocellular carcinoma. *Br J Exp Pathol* 1986; **67**: 279–88.
7   Alani RM, Munger K. Human papillomaviruses and associated malignancies. *J Clin Oncol* 1998; **16**: 330–7.
8   Evander M, Frazer IH, Payne E *et al.* Identification of the alpha-6 integrin as a candidate receptor for papillomaviruses. *J Virol* 1997; **71**: 2449–56.
9   Aynaud O, Ionesco M, Barrasso R. Penile intraepithelial neoplasia: specific clinical features correlate with histologic and virologic findings. *Cancer* 1994; **74**: 1762–7.
10 Hanash KA, Furlow WI, Utz DC, Harrison EG. Carcinoma of the penis: a clinicopathological study. *J Urol* 1970; **104**: 291–7.
11 Persky L. Epidemiology of cancer of the penis: recent results. *Cancer Res* 1997; **60**: 97–109.
12 Sonnex C. Human papillomavirus infection with particular reference to genital disease. *J Clin Pathol* 1998; **51**: 643–8.
13 Durst M, Dzarlieva-Petrusevska RT, Boukamp P, Fusenig NE, Gissman L. Molecular and cytogenetic analysis of immortalised human primary keratinocytes obtained after transfection with human papillomavirus type 16 DNA. *Oncogene* 1987; **1**: 251–6.
14 Schlegel R, Phelps WC, Zhang Y-L, Barbosa M. Quantitative keratinocyte assay detects two biological activities of human papillomavirus DNA and identifies viral types associated with cervical carcinoma. *EMBO J* 1988; **7**: 3181–7.
15 Hawley-Nelson P, Vousden KH, Hubbert NL, Lowy DR, Schiller JT. HPV 16 E6 and E7 proteins cooperate to immortalise human foreskin keratinocytes. *EMBO J* 1989; **8**: 3905–10.
16 Band V, DeCaprio JA, Delmolino L, Kulesa V, Sager R. Loss of p53 protein in human papillomavirus type 16 E6 immortalized human mammary epithelial cells. *J Virol* 1991; **65**: 6671–6.
17 Boyer SN, Wazer DE, Band V. E7 protein of human papilloma virus 16 induces degradation of retinoblastoma protein through the ubiquitin-proteasome pathway. *Cancer Res* 1996; **56**: 4620–4.
18 Scheffner M, Werness BA, Huibregtse JM, Levine AJ, Howley PM. The E6 oncoprotein encoded by human papillomavirus 16 and 18 promotes the degradation of p53. *Cell* 1990; **63**: 1129–36.
19 Matlashewski GJ, Tuck S, Pim D, Lamb P, Schneider J, Crawford LV. Primary structure polymorphism at amino acid residue 72 of human p53. *Mol Cell Biol* 1987; **7**: 961–3.
20 Storey A, Thomas M, Kalita A *et al.* Role of a p53 polymorphism in the development of human papillomavirus-associated cancer. *Nature* 1998; **393**: 229–34.
21 Rosenthal AN, Ryan A, Al-Jehani RM, Storey A, Harwood CA, Jacobs IJ. P53 codon 72 polymorphism and risk of cervical cancer in UK. *Lancet* 1998; **352**: 871–2.
22 Minaguchi T, Kanamori Y, Matsushima M, Yoshikawa H, Taketani Y, Nakamura Y. No evidence of correlation between polymorphism at codon 72 of p53 and risk of cervical

cancer in Japanese patients with papillomavirus 16/18 infection. *Cancer Res* 1987; **58**: 4585–6.

23   Scheffner M, Munger K, Byrne JC, Howley PM. The state of the p53 and retinoblastoma genes in human cervical carcinoma cell lines. *Proc Natl Acad Sci USA* 1991; **88**: 5523–7.

24   Klingelhutz AJ, Foster SA, McDougall JK. Telomerase activation by the E6 gene product of human papillomavirus type 16. *Nature* 1996; **380**: 79–82.

25   Kuhne C, Banks L. E3-ubiquitin ligase/E6-AP links multicopy maintenance protein 7 to the ubiquination pathway by a novel motif, the L2G box. *J Biol Chem* 1998; **273**: 34302–9.

26   Thomas JA. Penile carcinoma and viruses. *J Urol* 1982; **128**: 307–8.

27   Graham JH, Helwig EB. Erythroplasia of Queyrat: a clinicopathologic and histological study. *Cancer* 1973; **32**: 1396–414.

28   Mikhail GR. Cancers, precancers, and pseudocancers on the male genitalia: a review of clinical appearances, histopathology, and management. *J Dermatol Surg Oncol* 1980; **6**: 1027–35.

29   Wiener JS, Effert PJ, Humphrey PA, Yu L, Liu ET, Walther PJ. Prevalence of human papillomavirus types 16 and 18 in squamous-cell carcinoma of the penis: a retrospective analysis of primary and metastatic lesions by differential polymerase chain reaction. *Int J Cancer* 1992; **12**: 694–701.

30   Sarkar FH, Miles BJ, Plieth DH, Crissman JD. Detection of human papillomavirus in squamous neoplasm of penis. *J Urol* 1992; **147**: 389–92.

31   Mitsuishi T, Sata T, Iwasaki T *et al*. The detection of human papillomavirus 16 DNA in erythroplasia of Queyrat invading the urethra. *Br J Dermatol* 1998; **138**: 188–9.

32   Hauser B, Gross G, Schneider A, de Villiers EM, Gissman L, Wagner D. HPV-16-related Bowenoid papulosis. *Lancet* 1985; **2**: 106.

33   Park KC, Kim KH, Youn SW *et al*. Heterogeneity of human papillomavirus DNA in a patient with Bowenoid papulosis that progressed to squamous cell carcinoma. *Br J Dermatol* 1998; **139**: 1087–91.

34   Cupp MR, Malek RS, Goellner JR, Smith TF, Espy MJ. The detection of human papillomavirus deoxyribonucleic acid in intraepithelial, in situ, verrucous and invasive carcinoma of the penis. *J Urol* 1995; **154**: 1024–9.

35   Higgins GD, Uzelin DM, Phillips GE, Villa LL, Burrell CJ. Differing prevalence of human papillomavirus RNA in penile dysplasias and carcinomas may reflect differing aetiologies. *Am J Clin Pathol* 1992; **97**: 272–8.

36   Gregoire L, Cubilla AL, Reuter VE, Haas GP, Lancaster WD. Preferential association of human papillomavirus with high-grade histologic variants of penile-invasive squamous cell carcinoma. *J Natl Cancer Inst USA* 1995; **87**: 1705–9.

37   Chan KW, Lam KY, Chan AC, Lau P, Srivastava G. Prevalence of human papillomavirus types 16 and 18 in penile carcinoma: a study of 41 cases using PCR. *J Clin Pathol* 1994; **47**: 823–6.

38   Ding Q, Zhang Y, Sun S. Role of PCR and dot blot hybridisation in the detection of human papillomavirus of the penile cancer. *Chinese J Surg* 1996; **34**: 19–21.

39   Villa LL, Lopes A. HPV DNA sequences in penile carcinomas in Brazil. *Int J Cancer* 1986; **37**: 853–5.

40   Dianzani C, Bucci M, Pierangeli A, Calveri S, Degener AM. Association of human papillomavirus type 11 with carcinoma of the penis. *Urology* 1998; **51**: 1046–8.

41   Amerio P, Offidani A, Cellini A, Bossi G. Well-differentiated squamous cell carcinoma of the penis associated with HPV type 33. *Int J Dermatol* 1998; **37**: 128–30.

42   Nishikawa T, Kobayashi H, Shindoh M, Yamashita T, Fujinaga K, Ohkawara A. A case of verrucous carcinoma associated with human papillomavirus type 16 DNA. *J Dermatol* 1993; **20**: 483–8.

43 Turazza E, Lapena A, Sprovieri O *et al.* Low-risk human papillomavirus types 6 and 11 associated with carcinomas of the genital and upper aero-digestive tract. *Acta Obstet Gynecol Scand* 1997; **76**: 271–6.

44 Goldberg HM, Pell-Ilderton R, Daw E, Saleh N. Concurrent squamous cell carcinoma of the cervix and penis in a married couple. *Br J Obstet Gynaecol* 1979; **86**: 585–6.

45 Graham S, Priore R, Graham M, Browne R, Burnett W, West D. Genital cancer in wives of penile cancer patients. *Cancer* 1979; **44**: 1870–4.

46 Iversen T, Tretli S, Johansen A, Holte T. Squamous cell carcinoma of the penis and of the cervix, vulva and vagina in spouses: is there any relationship? An epidemiological study from Norway, 1960–92. *Br J Cancer* 1997; **76**: 658–60.

47 Maiche AG, Pyrhonen S. Risk of cervical cancer among wives of men with carcinoma of the penis. *Acta Oncol* 1990; **29**: 569–71.

48 Cardamakis E, Kotoulas IG, Relakis K. Peoscopic diagnosis of flat condyloma and penile intraepithelial neoplasia: clinical manifestation. *Gynecol Obstet Invest* 1997; **43**: 255–60.

49 Leis PF, Stevens KR, Baer SC, Kadmon D, Goldberg LH, Wang X-J. A c-ras^{Ha} mutation in the metastasis of a human papillomavirus (HPV)-18 positive penile squamous cell carcinoma suggests a cooperative effect between HPV-18 and c-ras^{Ha} activation in malignant progression. *Cancer* 1998; **83**: 122–9.

50 Castren K, Vahakanga K, Heikkinen E, Ranki A. Absence of p53 mutations in benign and pre-malignant male genital lesions with over-expressed p53 protein. *Int J Cancer* 1998; **77**: 674–8.

51 Pilotti S, Donghi R, D'Amato L *et al.* HPV detection and p53 alteration in squamous cell verrucous malignancies of the lower genital tract. *Diagnostic Mol Pathol* 1993; **2**: 248–56.

52 Suzuki H, Sato N, Kodama T *et al.* Detection of human papillomavirus DNA and state of p53 gene in Japanese penile cancer. *Jap J Clin Oncol* 1994; **24**: 1–6.

53 Lam KY, Chan AC, Chan KW, Leung ML, Srivastava G. Expression of p53 and its relationship with human papillomavirus in penile carcinomas. *Eur J Surg Oncol* 1995; **21**: 613–16.

54 Levi JE, Rahal P, Sarkis AS, Villa L. Human papillomavirus DNA and p53 status in penile carcinomas. *Int J Cancer* 1998; **76**: 779–83.

55 McCance DJ, Kalache A, Ashdown K *et al.* Human papillomavirus types 16 and 18 in carcinomas of the penis from Brazil. *Int J Cancer* 1986; **37**: 55–9.

56 Raju GC, Lee YS. Role of herpes simplex virus type-2 and human papillomavirus in penile cancers in Singapore. *Ann Acad Med Singapore* 1987; **16**: 550–1.

22: Current Concepts in the Management of Penile Cancer

R. Sarin & H. B. Tongaonkar

Introduction

Cancer of the penis is a rare disease with considerable geographical variation. Age adjusted incidence rates vary from 1 per 100 000 in Europe to 3 per 100 000 in Madras, India [1]. Single institution reports have shown either a rise [2], fall [3] or no change [4] in the incidence of new penile cancers referred over the past 30–50 years. The rise or fall in the circumcision rate has been postulated as the reason for these conflicting trends but this could well be due to the change in the referral pattern as these are not population based studies. A history of phimosis was noted in a quarter of the 102 men treated for penile cancer at the Institut Gustave-Roussy [5]. The role of human papillomavirus in the pathogenesis of this disease is discussed in the previous chapter of this book.

Natural history, histology and clinical presentation

The median age at presentation is around 60 years, and the disease is confined to the glans in most cases [4,6]. The vast majority of these invasive cancers are squamous carcinomas or their variants such as verrucous or basaloid carcinoma. Other rare histological types are the spindle cell or metaplastic carcinoma, melanoma, mucoepidermoid carcinoma of the distal urethra and metastatic carcinoma. We do not know enough about the natural history of *in situ* penile carcinoma, unlike cervical intraepithelial neoplasia. However, *in situ* penile carcinoma at resection margin generally progresses to histologically proven clinical recurrence within 5 years [7]. In a large study from Institut Gustave-Roussy it was found that one-quarter of patients with invasive penile carcinoma had associated *in situ* carcinoma or dysplasia [5].

Penile carcinomas arise from the mucosa of the glans or coronal sulcus and sometimes from the foreskin of uncircumcised men. The initial lesion may be ulcerative, proliferative, ulceroproliferative or sometimes like a plaque over the glans. The tumour then invades deeply to involve the corpus cavernosum and spongiosum, the skin of the shaft and the urethra and, at very late stages, the perineum or prostate.

Cubilla *et al.* [7] described the following clinico-pathological variants on whole organ sections of 66 penile resections for epidermoid carcinoma:

1 *Superficially spreading carcinoma.* This commonest variety presented with centrifugal or radial growth to large areas of the epithelial compartments such as the glans, coronal sulcus and the foreskin.

2 *Vertical growth carcinoma.* These unifocal tumours have a tendency towards earlier vertical growth. They are characteristically aggressive, with infiltration of deep anatomic structures, higher histological grade and a higher propensity for lymph node metastases.

3 *Verrucous carcinoma.* These papillary exophytic tumours have a low histological grade. While they are locally aggressive, vascular or perineural invasion is rare and lymph node metastases are infrequent.

4 *Multicentric carcinoma.* In this uncommon variety there is normal epithelium in between the multiple foci of carcinoma.

The pattern of spread of the superficially spreading carcinoma and multicentric carcinomas would suggest that anatomical structures such as the glans mucosa, coronal sulcus and foreskin may be considered, from diagnostic, therapeutic and biological viewpoints, as a single field susceptible to malignant transformation.

Penile cancers spread via lymphatic pathways to the superficial and deep inguinal nodes and later to the iliac chain. The involvement of iliac nodes in the absence of inguinal node involvement is very unusual [8,9]. The risk of nodal metastases increases with increasing depth of invasion [7,10,11], higher 'T' stage and histological grade [4,9,12,13]. Lymphatic spread is very uncommon in the verrucous variety [5,7]. Solsona *et al.* [10] in a study of 66 patients observed three prognostic groups with increasing risk of nodal metastases. Nodal metastases were observed in none of the 19 patients in the T1 G1 low-risk group, in 8/22 (36%) patients in the T1 G2/3 or T2/3 G1 intermediate-risk group and in 20/25 (80%) patients in the T2/3 G3 high-risk group. In contrast to the above reports, no significant relationship was observed between lymph node status and pathologically proved infiltration of the corpora cavernosa, urethra and adjacent structures (stages T2, T3 and T4, respectively, of the 1992 UICC TNM classification) in a multivariate analysis of 145 Brazilian patients treated by amputation and lymphadenectomy [14]. Venous and lymphatic embolization was the only significant predictor of lymph node metastasis in this study.

Haematogenous spread is rare at presentation but during follow-up 5–10% of patients may develop distant metastases, generally in the setting of uncontrolled loco-regional disease [4,6].

Table 22.1 Staging for carcinoma of the penis

UICC TNM staging, 1992 (Spiessl *et al.* [57])

Primary tumour	*Regional nodes*
T1: Subepithelial connective tissue	N0: Uninvolved
T2: Corpus spongiosum or cavernosum	N1: One superficial inguinal node
T3: Urethra, prostate	N2: Multiple or bilateral superficial inguinal nodes
T4: Other adjacent structures	N3: Deep inguinal or pelvic nodes

Jackson staging (Jackson [15])
Stage 1: Limited to glans and/or prepuce
Stage 2: Extending into the shaft or corpora but without nodal metastases
Stage 3: Confined to the shaft with malignant but operable inguinal nodes
Stage 4: Invasion beyond shaft, inoperable regional nodes or distant metastases

---

Staging

The two most commonly used staging systems for penile carcinoma are the Jackson [15] and the UICC TNM ones (Table 22.1). The Jackson staging is now going out of favour as it groups together tumours with different size and infiltration without considering the prognostic and therapeutic implication of these groupings.

Horenblas *et al.* [8], in a clinico-pathological study of 98 cases, reported that the primary tumour was clinically under staged in 10% of cases, due to unsuspected infiltration, and over staged in 16%, due to oedema and infection mimicking infiltration and masking the actual size. Even ultrasound is not accurate enough for staging small penile tumours as it fails to distinguish between invasion of subepithelial connective tissue and invasion into the corpus spongiosum [16].

It is well known that the clinical examination of the groin may be fallacious. Palpable nodes may not be involved pathologically in up to 60% of cases if the clinical node size is less than 2 cm and in 10% of cases if they measure more than 2 cm [9]. By contrast, 15–20% of patients with clinically uninvolved groin nodes may have nodal metastases on pathological examination following groin dissection [17]. Horenblas *et al.* [8] found that the easiest way to confirm clinically suspicious nodes was through fine needle aspiration cytology (FNAC) and showed a sensitivity of 71% and specificity of 100% in 18 patients. The sensitivity and specificity of computerized tomography in 14 patients was 36% and 100%, respectively, and for lymphangiography in 23 patients was, respectively, 31% and 100%.

Biopsy

Histological confirmation of malignancy is mandatory before planning definitive treatment. Patients with small lesions restricted to the prepuce or the penile skin may undergo wide excision, and provided there have been clear margins this will be both diagnostic and therapeutic. Lesions involving the glans, however, require a deep punch or incision biopsy to prove the diagnosis of malignancy, its histological subtype, grade and invasiveness.

Treatment options, techniques, results and sequelae

The management of this uncommon disease has gradually evolved. Surgery and radiotherapy have evolved as treatments and may be given, either as a single modality or in combination, depending upon the extent of the primary and metastases if any. Because of the disease's rarity, therapeutic approaches have evolved empirically and have not been defined by prospective studies.

While there are no randomized trials, most literature reviews conclude that initial local control rates with amputative surgery are superior to external radiotherapy in all stages [4,18] and comparable to brachytherapy in selected early stage tumours [6].

Despite high initial local failure rates of about 35–40% observed in the two largest external beam radiotherapy series, reported by Ravi *et al*. [18] and Sarin *et al*. [4], it was possible to salvage surgically the vast majority of these penile recurrences, thus achieving 90–98% local control rates eventually (Table 22.2). These results support a policy of initial treatment with radical radiotherapy, with surgery reserved for salvage in the absence of metastases. The aim of modern treatment should therefore be organ and function preservation whenever possible, without compromising the chances of survival. In fact the European Board of Urology has endorsed this treatment strategy of organ conserving therapy and watchful waiting for early stage disease [19].

In more advanced tumours the results of radiotherapy alone are poor [4,18], and for this reason penectomy is the treatment of choice for such tumours.

The radiotherapeutic management of the primary

As discussed earlier, the policy of radical radiotherapy with surgery reserved for salvage would allow a half to two-thirds of men with early stage disease to retain a functioning penis. There are a variety of different ways of delivering radiotherapy, including a surface mould [20], an interstitial implant [6] and external beam radiotherapy (EBRT) [4]. The type of radiotherapy best suited for an individual depends upon the size, site and thickness of the tumour, and its proximity to the urethra. Thus superficial small tumours at any site on the glans can be treated with surface mould therapy, localized small tumours away from the urethra can be treated with an interstitial implant whilst a

Table 22.2 Treatment results of major radiotherapy studies

Reference	Institute	Mean follow-up (years)	Study period	Treatment modality	Median radiation dose	No. of patients	Initial local control	Eventual local control after salvage	Penectomy for necrosis	Urethral stricture
6	French multicentre	11.7	1959–89	Implant alone Implant + surgery or EBRT (40 Gy)	63 Gy 50 Gy	184 75	218/259 (85%)	243/259 (94%)	19/259 (7%)	79/259 (30%)
53	Toulouse, France	6.9	1971–89	Implants	60 Gy	51	42/51 (82%)	48/51 (94%)	8/51 (16%)	21/51 (41%)
18	Cancer Institute, Adyar, India	11.6	1959–88	EBRT Implants/moulds	50–60 Gy 60–70 Gy	128 28	101/156 (65%)	152/156 (97%)	10/156 (6%)	37/156 (24%)
4	Royal Marsden, UK	5.2	1960–90	EBRT Implants	60 Gy 60 Gy	56 13	39/69 (57%)	62/69 (90%)	2/69 (3%)	10/69 (14%)
54	Tata Memorial, India	2.0	1988–96	Implant	50 Gy	23	18/23 (78%)	22/23 (96%)	0	2/23 (9%)

tumour in any location is suitable for treatment with EBRT. Other factors such as the facilities and expertise available, patient's choice and compliance have to be taken into account when planning treatment. Thus, even for a small localized tumour, it may be preferable to give EBRT if the expertise and facilities for interstitial implantation are unavailable or poor patient compliance is expected.

Treatment outcome in terms of initial local control, eventual local control after surgical salvage, urethral stricture and penectomy for radionecrosis in the important studies of the last 10 years is shown in Table 22.2. A superior initial control rate in the implant series compared with the predominantly EBRT series is seen. However, this could well have been due to strong selection bias in favour of the implant series, as the small superficial tumours are preferentially selected for implant. Moreover, the eventual local control rates after salvage surgery are comparable between the implant and EBRT series. Another important fact to note is that higher initial local control rates in the large implant series are accompanied by a much higher complication rate compared with EBRT. Thus it may be possible to achieve similar results by escalating the EBRT dose.

A few important findings relevant to technique have emerged from these large retrospective reviews. In the French multicentre survey [6], 259 men were treated, mostly with a two plane iridium implant. They observed that limiting the implant volume to $30\,cm^3$ could substantially reduce the complication rates. This would correspond to a gross tumour volume of $8\,cm^3$. A dose of 55–60 Gy was recommended for such implant volumes. They also observed a significantly higher incidence of phimosis due to foreskin fibrosis in men who were not circumcised before the implant.

In the Royal Marsden study [4], treatment interruptions during the course of EBRT and prolongation of the overall treatment time beyond the planned 6–6.5 weeks was common. Incorporating the time factor in the linear quadratic model, it was seen that the local recurrence rate was doubled from 24% to 52% ($P = 0.052$) if the biologically effective dose (BED) was <60 Gy. This BED of 60 Gy is equivalent to 60 Gy with 2 Gy daily fractions given over 45 days assuming a α/β of 10 and a time factor (K) of 0.5 Gy per day starting after a lag period of 21 days.

These treatment interruptions were primarily due to the problems of treating a painful, oedematous and exudative penis in a wax block after 3–4 weeks of EBRT. Conservative management of these acute reactions has now been recommended, while continuing with the EBRT. This is possible by changing the size of the block. The use of transparent perspex material allows the visualization of the penis and maximum sparing of the penile shaft in tumours confined to the glans. This technique of EBRT thus seems to be superior to other techniques involving the use of wooden jigs [18] or wax blocks [20].

A variety of fractionation schedules have been described in the literature, including 50–57.5 Gy in 16 daily fractions over 3 weeks [21], 50–55 Gy in 20–22 daily fractions over 4 weeks [20] and 60 Gy in 30 daily fractions over 6 weeks [4]. It is difficult to compare the results of these different fractionation regimens. The shorter fractionation allows the completion of treatment before the manifestation of inevitable severe acute reactions, thus avoiding treatment interruptions. The use of a high dose per fraction in such schedules is likely to result in enhanced late sequelae.

We have started a prospective study evaluating the effect of radiotherapy on quality of life issues in early stage disease (T1, T2, N0) at the Tata Memorial Hospital. Ten patients have been enrolled since 1996. Using a water-filled Perspex block and bilateral telecobalt portals, a midplane dose of 55 Gy in 16 daily fractions was given in six patients and between 50 and 60 Gy in 16–24 fractions in the remaining four patients. At a median follow-up of 22 months, one patient failed at the primary site, which was salvaged with penectomy, and two patients who developed nodal metastases were salvaged with groin dissection. All the patients had severe acute reactions over the glans and the distal penile shaft lasting for 1–4 months. Acute urethral reactions were surprisingly minimal and no patient required catheterization. All the six patients with more than 18 months of follow-up have developed hypochromia of the glans and mild to moderate telangiectasia over the treated shaft. In two patients the urethral meatus appears to be slightly narrowed following radiation but none of these 10 patients has any urinary symptoms. Apart from these cosmetic changes none of these patients has experienced any symptom related to late radiation sequelae. Sexual function in these patients is described later on in this chapter.

Surgical management of the primary

Surgical excision of the primary lesion with adequate margins is essential to ensure local control and cure from penile cancer. Various factors need to be considered while planning optimum treatment, including location, extent, size and type of lesion, its relation with the external urethral meatus, status of the inguinal lymph nodes, age of the patient and the desire to retain an intact penis. With the selection of a proper surgical procedure, local relapses should be rare.

Conservative surgical procedures like circumcision or wide excision should be adequate for lesions involving the prepuce or for small, non-invasive or minimally invasive lesions away from the urethra. The margins of excision must be confirmed to be disease free by intraoperative frozen section examination. Improper selection of patients for conservative procedures may lead to high local recurrence rates, as have been reported by many authors [3,22–24].

In a study from Heidelberg, excessive local recurrence rates of 56% for T1 and 100% for T2 tumours were seen after organ preserving surgical procedures vs. 0% and 20% for T1 and T2, respectively, after amputative procedures in 51 patients [25].

Partial penectomy is indicated for lesions involving the glans, corona and distal shaft, where after adequate surgical excision the residual penile stump should be serviceable for upright micturition without scrotal soiling and for sexual function. Penile augmentation surgery using reconstructive techniques may be done at a later date in patients who are cured and desire to have the normal length of penis restored.

Total penectomy with perineal urethrostomy is indicated when the lesion extends to involve the proximal shaft or the base of the penis. Limited extension to scrotum or skin overlying the pubis may also be included in the surgical excision if involved by the disease. Urethra sparing total or subtotal penectomy followed by subsequent delayed penile reconstruction has been reported for invasive penile lesions involving only the dorsum of the penis [26].

The risk of local recurrence after partial or total penectomy should be negligible [23,27–30].

Mohs micrographic surgery

Mohs micrographic surgery (MMS) represents a penile tissue sparing surgical technique which essentially employs removal of diseased tissue in thin layers, accurate construction and mapping of excised tissue and confirmation of negative margins by frozen section examination of horizontal tissue sections. This technique can trace out silent tumour extensions that can be completely excised, with cure rates equivalent to more radical surgical procedures, allowing at the same time preservation of maximum normal penile tissue. This procedure is best suited for small lesions involving the distal portion of the glans [31]. Mohs reported a 100% local control rate for lesions less than 1 cm but only a 50% local control rate for >3 cm tumours. This procedure has the disadvantages of being quite time consuming, and for larger lesions leads to a misshapen glans and the occasional need for reconstruction of the glans or correction of meatal stenosis.

Laser therapy

Laser therapy has been tried in the treatment of preinvasive and small invasive penile cancers. Although it has the potential for preservation of normal penile tissue and function, it should be used judiciously. Laser treatment leads to local control rates comparable with more radical procedures. Bandiermonte *et al.* [32] reported a 15% relapse rate in T1 tumours following CO_2 laser therapy. The Nd:YAG laser has also been used for complete destruction of the lesion or for laser coagulation of the base after partial excision of the tumour with good results [33]. In a Mayo Clinic study it was reported that aggressive laser therapy of the visible lesions and the entire dysplastic epithelium produced good cosmetic results and local control [34]. However, laser therapy has the disadvantages of an uncontrolled depth of excision and of not providing adequate tissue for pathological examination. Close follow-up of these laser treated patients is mandatory because of the relatively high rate of local failure.

The management of ilio-inguinal lymph nodes

Certain important facts need to be kept in mind before deciding on a treatment policy for ilio-inguinal nodes. These are as follows:
1   35–60% of patients with penile cancer have palpable inguinal nodes at presentation;
2   approximately 50% of these palpable inguinal nodes have no metastases on pathological examination [27,35–37];
3   approximately 20% of patients with non-palpable inguinal nodes will have occult lymph node metastasis.

The management of patients with clinically uninvolved groin examinations has undoubtedly aroused a great amount of interest and controversy. The controversies mainly involve the indication, timing and extent of lymphadenectomy. Since the curative benefit of lymphadenectomy in the presence of palpable metastatic nodes is well established, it seems logical that lymphadenectomy performed in the setting of microscopic nodal disease would confer an even greater advantage. However, no significant adverse effect on survival was found in patients undergoing delayed therapeutic groin dissection for metastatic nodes detected at follow-up [27,35], with survival rates equivalent to initial therapeutic groin dissection for palpable metastatic nodes at presentation [38]. But all these studies report on lymph node dissection being done for clinically palpable nodal disease and do not exclude the possibility that lymphadenectomy for clinically non-palpable occult microscopic disease may yield better results. Other authors have reported a significant reduction in survival in patients undergoing delayed therapeutic rather than prophylactic lymphadenectomy, thereby suggesting that best results can be obtained in the presence of a low tumour load [39,40] and that delayed surgery may be inappropriate [23,28,40,41]. However, the lack of prospective randomized trials indicating the benefit of prophylactic over delayed therapeutic lymphadenectomy, the morbidity of the lymphadenectomy and the lack of therapeutic benefit in nearly 75% of patients undergoing this procedure have prevented prophylactic lymphadenectomy from becoming the standard practice for patients with non-palpable nodes.

Early prophylactic lymphadenectomy may be considered for those at a high risk of harbouring metastases while those at a lesser risk may be kept on surveillance. Data from various retrospective reviews suggest that lymph node metastases are more common in patients with deeply invasive [23,36] or poorly differentiated tumours [4,40]. Cabanas [37] described sentinel node biopsy and advocated formal lymph node dissection if the node was infiltrated. He hypothesized that it was impossible to get lymph node metastases in the inguinofemoral or iliac regions without sentinel node metastases. Aspiration cytology under lymphangiographic guidance was suggested by Scappini *et al.* [42] as an alternative to node biopsy. Both these procedures may have significant false negative rates [30,42,43]. Superficial inguinal lymphadenectomy has been proposed by deKernion *et al.* [36] followed by total lymphadenectomy if superficial nodes are positive. This has the advantage of providing the complete superficial lymphatic tissue for pathological examination, thereby avoiding error in sentinel node identification, and is associated with minimal morbidity.

The incidence of false negative nodes is 10–20% in T1–T2 tumours. It is very difficult to justify routine lymphadenectomy, with its consequent morbidity, in these patients and they should be kept under close surveillance. Delayed lymphadenectomy for nodal metastases detected during active surveillance does not seem to jeopardize long-term survival [6,44]. Because most inguinal node metastases occur within 2–3 years following initial therapy, the surveillance must cover this period with repeated examinations at 2- to 3-monthly intervals. Poorly differentiated T1–T2 tumours have a marginally higher incidence of inguinal node metastases and should be considered for early adjunctive lymphadenectomy if there is any question of lymph node enlargement.

In T3–T4 tumours, the incidence of occult nodal metastases may be more than 50%, thus prophylactic lymphadenectomy is advocated notwithstanding its morbidity, and may result in improved survival.

There is consensus that surgical treatment is recommended for patients who have palpable or cytologically positive operable ilio-inguinal nodal metastases at presentation. Most patients with inguinal node metastasis succumb to their disease within 2 years, if untreated. By contrast, 20–67% of patients with clinically palpable metastatic inguinal lymph nodes will be disease free at 5 years after undergoing lymphadenectomy [23,27,28,35,36,39,45]. Single or limited inguinal nodal metastases lead to 82–88% 5-year disease-free survival rates after lymphadenectomy [39].

EXTENT OF LYMPHADENECTOMY

Bilateral inguinal lymph node metastases warrant a bilateral lymphadenectomy. Bilateral lymphadenectomy is also recommended for patients presenting with unilateral palpable lymphadenopathy occurring synchronously with the primary lesion, because the incidence of clinically unsuspected contralateral node metastases is greater than 50% [27]. The contralateral node dissection may be limited to superficial node dissection if no histological evidence of metastasis is found in the contralateral superficial nodes. In patients who develop unilateral lymph node metastasis while on surveillance, it may not be necessary to perform a bilateral lymph node dissection especially if the metastasis-free interval is longer than 1 year.

The therapeutic benefit of extending the dissection to iliac nodes is as yet undetermined. Iliac lymph node metastases are found in approximately 15–30% of patients with metastatic inguinal lymph nodes, their frequency being dependent on the positivity and number of positive inguinal lymph nodes, the presence of perinodal extension and bilaterality of disease [17,39]. While Srinivas *et al.* [39] reported that none of their 11 patients with iliac lymph node metastasis survived 3 years, with most dying within 7 months, others have reported survival with positive pelvic nodes [36,37] and improved survival after iliac node dissection [22]. In view of this, iliac node dissection seems to be reasonable.

COMPLICATIONS OF INGUINOPELVIC LYMPHADENECTOMY

The perioperative mortality of the procedure is less than 1%, but the morbidity of the procedure is very high. Skin flap or edge necrosis and wound breakdown along with persistent lymphorrhoea are the commonest early complications, occurring in up to 80% of patients [28,41] and leading to prolonged hospitalization and secondary reconstruction with skin grafts or pedicled flaps in a significant number of patients. The dreaded complication of femoral vessel blowout is seldom encountered in recent times because of routine transposition of the rectus muscle to cover the femoral vessels. Debilitating limb lymphoedema is seen in nearly one-third of patients and is the commonest complication in most reports. In view of this, a lot of attention in recent times has focused on modifying the surgical procedure to reduce morbidity.

Fraley & Hutchens [46] described a technique employing two parallel incisions in the groin, one above and one below the inguinal ligament, to reduce the skin flap or edge necrosis. Similarly, a technique of a transverse incision below the inguinal ligament for the inguinal node dissection and a midline infra-umbilical incision for pelvic node dissection has been described with significant reduction in the skin loss. However, the choice of incision had no bearing on reduction of lower extremity oedema.

Catalona [47] described his technique of saphenous vein preserving modified inguinal lymphadenectomy, which reportedly reduced the incidence of debilitating limb oedema. He also redefined the lateral boundary of the dissection as the femoral artery and dispensed with mobilization and transposition of sartorius muscle. Iliac node dissection was also not carried out in the absence of inguinal nodal metastases. This resulted in reduction of the rate of wound breakdown and skin loss to less than 20%. However, metastatic lymphadenopathy in the inguinal region warrants a complete dissection and this modified procedure may not be suitable for this situation.

We have been removing the skin overlying the inguinal nodal area routinely in all patients undergoing inguinal lymphadenectomy, even when it is not infiltrated by the nodal disease, and have been doing immediate reconstruction using a tensor fascia lata myocutaneous flap or anterolateral thigh flap [48,49]. We have had no problems of skin loss or wound breakdown since the time we began employing this procedure. In addition, the incidence of lower extremity lymphoedema has significantly reduced with a long follow-up in these patients. In our opinion, this may represent a significant advance in the reduction of morbidity of ilio-inguinal lymphadenectomy.

Chemotherapy

Chemotherapy has been evaluated for *in situ* carcinoma as well as advanced stage disease but has no role in early stage invasive cancer. Topical 5-fluorouracil creams have been successfully used in selected patients with carcinoma *in situ* [50]. In a Southwest Oncology Group study, 45 patients with locally advanced or metastatic penile carcinoma were treated with cisplatin 75 mg/m^2 on day 1, methotrexate 25 mg/m^2 on days 1 and 8 and bleomycin 10 units/m^2 on days 1 and 8 with a cycle length of 21 days. While the response rate was only 32%, five toxic deaths and six life-threatening toxic episodes were seen [51].

Pizzocaro *et al*. [12] reported the treatment results of 26 patients with fixed inguinal nodes. One of the first 10 patients treated with radiotherapy, with or without methotrexate or bleomycin, was downstaged to operable disease, but all died of cancer within 3 years. By contrast, nine (56%) of the subsequent 16 patients treated with neoadjuvant chemotherapy could undergo subsequent surgery and five (31%) were disease free after 5 years.

Prognosis

The long-term overall survival rates are significantly lower than the cause specific survival rates in several large studies from Europe [4,6,52] and the USA [3]. This is not surprising, as a substantial proportion of patients would naturally die of causes other than penile cancer because of their age at diagnosis. Depending upon the proportion of cases in different stages, 66–88% 5-year penile cancer specific survival rates have been reported [4,6,52,53]. In the few large studies with multivariate analysis of prognostic factors, nodal metastases [4,5,14], high T stage or invasion [4,5,19] and high histological grade [4,19] were identified as independent adverse prognostic factors for survival. Substratification of nodal status into groups with >3 nodes, bilateral disease, extranodal extension and iliac node metastases shows these to portend an especially poor prognosis [17,22,30,39,41].

Quality of life and psychosexual issues

It is surprising that while the emphasis is now on organ and function preservation [54], there are only a few small, mostly retrospective studies evaluating quality of life and psychosexual issues. In a Norwegian study [55], moderate to severe sexual dysfunction was observed in only 2/10 patients after radiotherapy compared with 4/5 after wide excision, 7/9 after partial penectomy and 4/4 after total penectomy. We have previously reported [4] that of the 29 patients treated with penectomy, one committed suicide and another had a failed suicide attempt. In an Italian study [56], of the 17 patients treated with amputative surgery, anxiety was evident in 30% and depression in 6%, and global sexual function was compromised in 76%.

All 10 patients treated in our prospective study at the Tata Memorial have maintained normal penile erection following radiotherapy. Eight men were sexually active before the treatment, with the median frequency of coitus being three times per month. Of these eight men, one underwent penectomy for residual disease and another patient has not resumed sexual activity, as it is only 3 months following radiotherapy. All the remaining six men have fully regained their pretreatment sexual interest, ability and satisfaction. The coital frequency has also remained unchanged.

Conclusion

The aim of modern treatment should be organ and function preservation whenever possible, without compromising the chances of survival. Thus patients with small tumours confined to the glans should be considered for conservative treatment in the form of primary radiotherapy, with surgery reserved for salvage or wide excision with clear margins in very select cases. More advanced tumours are difficult to control with radiotherapy hence initial penectomy is the treatment of choice. The indication, timing and extent of lymphadenectomy remain controversial. However, the consensus seems to be emerging for surveillance of clinically negative groin in patients with early stage disease and lymphadenectomy for the remaining patients. There is also an urgent need for more detailed prospective studies of the psychosexual aspects of treatment.

References

1   Parkin DM, Whelan SL, Ferlay G, Raymond L, Young J. *Cancer Incidence in Five Continents*, Vol. VII. IARC Scientific Publication No. 143. Lyon: IARC, 1997.

2   Sandeman TF. Carcinoma of the penis. *Australas Radiol* 1990; **34**: 12–16.

3   Narayana AS, Olney LE, Loening SA, Weimar G, Culp DA. Carcinoma of the penis: analysis of 219 cases. *Cancer* 1982; **49**: 2185–91.

4   Sarin R, Norman AR, Steel GG, Horwich A. Treatment results and prognostic factors in 101 men treated for squamous carcinoma of the penis. *Int J Radiat Oncol Biol Phys* 1997; **38**: 713–22.

5   Soria JC, Fizazi K, Piron D *et al*. Squamous cell carcinoma of the penis: multivariate analysis of prognostic factors and natural history in monocentric study with a conservative policy. *Ann Oncol* 1997; **8**: 1089–98.

6   Rozan R, Albuisson E, Giraud B *et al*. Interstitial brachytherapy for penile carcinoma: a multicentric survey (259 patients). *Radiother Oncol* 1995; **36**: 83–93.

7   Cubilla AL, Barreto J, Caballero C, Ayala G, Riveros G. Pathological features of epidermoid carcinoma of the penis. *Am J Surg Pathol* 1993; **17**: 753–63.

8   Horenblas S, Van Tinteren H, Delemarre JFM, Moonen LMF, Lustig V, Kroger R. Squamous cell carcinoma of the penis: accuracy of tumour, node and metastases classification system, and role of lymphangiography, computerized tomography scan and fine needle aspiration cytology. *J Urol* 1991; **146**: 1279–83.

9   Ayappan K, Ananthakrishnan N, Sankaran V. Can regional lymph node involvement be predicted in patients with carcinoma of the penis? *Br J Urol* 1994; **73**: 549–53.

10 Solsona E, Iborra I, Ricos JV *et al*. Corpus cavernosum invasion and tumour grade in the prediction of lymph node condition of penile carcinoma. *Eur Urol* 1992; **22**: 115–18.

11 Villavicencio H, Rubio-Briones J, Regalado R, Chechile G, Algaba F, Palou J. Grade, local stage and growth pattern as prognostic factors in carcinoma of the penis. *Eur Urol* 1997; **32**: 442–7.

12 Pizzocaro G, Piva L, Nicolai N. Treatment of lymphatic metastasis of squamous cell carcinoma of the penis: experience at the National Tumor Institute of Milan. *Arch Ital Urol Androl* 1996; **68**: 169–72.

13 Demkow T. The treatment of penile carcinoma: experience in 64 cases. *Int Urol Nephrol* 1999; **31**: 525–31.

14 Lopes A, Hidalgo GS, Kowalski LP, Torloni H, Rossi BM, Fonseca FP. Prognostic factors in carcinoma of the penis: multivariate analysis of 145 patients treated with amputation and lymphadenectomy. *J Urol* 1996; **156**: 1637–42.

15 Jackson SM. The treatment of carcinoma of the penis. *Br J Surg* 1966; **53**: 33–5.

16 Horenblas S, Kroger R, Gallee MPW, Newling DWW, Van Tinteren H. Ultrasound in squamous cell carcinoma of the penis: a useful addition to clinical staging? A comparison of ultrasound with histopathology. *Urology* 1994; **43**: 702–7.

17 Ravi R. Correlation between the extent of nodal involvement and survival following groin dissection for carcinoma of the penis. *Br J Urol* 1993; **72**: 817–19.

18 Ravi R, Chaturvedi HK, Sastry DVLN. Role of radiation therapy in the treatment of carcinoma of the penis. *Br J Urol* 1994; **74**: 646–51.

19 Lindegaard JC, Nielsen OS, Lundbeck FA, Mamsen A, Studstrup HN, von der Maase H. A retrospective analysis of 82 cases of cancer of the penis. *Br J Urol* 1996; **77**: 883–90.

20 Neave F, Neal AJ, Hoskin PJ, Hope-Stone HF. Carcinoma of the penis: a retrospective review of treatment with iridium mould and external beam irradiation. *Clin Oncol* 1993; **5**: 207–10.

21 Duncan W, Jackson SM. Treatment of early cancer of penis with megavoltage X-rays. *Clin Radiol* 1972; **23**: 246–8.

22 Hardner GJ, Bhanalaph T, Murphy GP, Albert DJ, Moore RH. Carcinoma of the penis: analysis of therapy in 100 consecutive cases. *J Urol* 1972; **108**: 428–30.

23 McDougal WS, Kirchner FK Jr, Edwards RH, Killon LT. Treatment of carcinoma of the penis: the case of primary lymphadenectomy. *J Urol* 1986; **136**: 38–41.

24 Jensen MS. Cancer of the penis in Denmark 1942 to 1962 (511 cases). *Dan Med Bull* 1977; **24**: 66–72.

25 Brkovic D, Kalble T, Dorsam J *et al*. Surgical treatment of invasive penile cancer—the Heidelberg experience from 1968 to 1994. *Eur Urol* 1997; **31**: 339–42.

26 Bissada NK, Morcos RR, El-Senoussi M. Post-circumcision carcinoma of the penis. I. Clinical aspects. *J Urol* 1986; **135**: 283–5.

27 Ekstrom T, Edsmyr F. Cancer of the penis: a clinical study of 229 cases. *Acta Chir Scand* 1958; **115**: 25–45.

28 Johnson DE, Lo RK. Management of regional lymph nodes in penile carcinoma: five year results following therapeutic groin dissections. *Urology* 1984; **24**: 308–11.

29 Horenblas S, Van Tinteren H, Delemare JFM. Squamous cell carcinoma of the penis: treatment of the primary tumour. *J Urol* 1992; **147**: 1533–8.

30 Kamat MR, Kulkarni JN, Tongaonkar HB. Carcinoma of the penis: the Indian experience. *J Surg Oncol* 1993; **52**: 50–5.

31 Mohs FE, Snow SN, Messing EM, Kuglitsch ME. Microscopically controlled surgery in the treatment of carcinoma of the penis. *J Urol* 1985; **133**: 961–6.

32 Bandiermonte Santoro O, Boracchi P, Piva L, Pizzocaro G, DePalo G. Total resection of glans penis surface by CO_2 laser microsurgery. *Acta Oncol* 1988; **27**: 575–8.

33 Rothenberger KH. Value of the neodymium YAG laser in the therapy of penile carcinoma. *Eur Urol* 1986; **12** (Suppl. 1): 34–6.

34 Tietjen DN, Malek RS. Laser therapy of squamous cell dysplasia and carcinoma of the penis. *Urology* 1998; **52**: 559–65.

35 Beggs JH, Spratt JS. Epidermoid carcinoma of the penis. *J Urol* 1961; **91**: 166–72.

36 deKernion JB, Tynbery P, Persky L, Fegen JP. Carcinoma of the penis. *Cancer* 1973; **32**: 1256–62.

37 Cabanas RM. An approach for the treatment of penile carcinoma. *Cancer* 1977; **39**: 456–66.

38 Baker BH, Spratt JS, Perez-Mesa C. Carcinoma of the penis. *J Urol* 1976; **116**: 458–61.

39 Srinivas V, Morse MJ, Herr HW, Sogani PC, Whitmore WF Jr. Penile cancer: relation of extent of nodal metastasis to survival. *J Urol* 1987; **137**: 880–2.

40 Fraley EE, Zhang G, Manivel C, Niehans GA. The role of ilioinguinal lymphadenectomy and significance of histological differentiation in treatment of carcinoma of the penis. *J Urol* 1989; **142**: 1478–82.

41 Ornellas AA, Seixas LC, Marota A. Surgical treatment of invasive squamous cell carcinoma of the penis: retrospective analysis of 350 cases. *J Urol* 1994; **151**: 1244–9.

42 Scappini P, Piscioli F, Pusiol T, Hofstetter A, Rothenberger KH, Luciani L. Penile cancer: aspiration biopsy cytology for staging. *Cancer* 1986; **58**: 1526–33.

43 Perinetti EP, Crane DC, Catalona WJ. Unreliability of sentinel node biopsy for staging penile carcinoma. *J Urol* 1980; **124**: 734–5.

44 Theodorescu D, Russo P, Zhang ZF, Morash C, Fair WR. Outcomes of initial surveillance of invasive squamous cell carcinoma of the penis and negative nodes. *J Urol* 1996; **155**: 1626–31.

45 Horenblas S, Van Tinteren H. Squamous cell carcinoma of the penis. IV. Prognostic factors of survival: analysis of tumor, nodes and metastasis classification system. *J Urol* 1994; **151**: 1239–43.

46 Fraley E, Hutchens H. Radical ilio-inguinal node dissection: the skin bridge technique — a new procedure. *J Urol* 1972; **108**: 279–81.

47 Catalona WJ. Modified inguinal lymphadenectomy for carcinoma of the penis with preservation of saphenous veins: technique and preliminary results. *J Urol* 1988; **140**: 306–10.

48 Tongaonkar HB, Kulkarni JN, Kamat MR. Carcinoma of the penis: relationship of nodal metastases to survival. *Indian J Urol* 1993; **9**: 54–7.

49 Savant DN, Dalal AV, Patel SG, Bhathena HM, Kavarana NM. Tensor fasciae lata myocutaneous flap reconstruction following ilioinguinal node dissection. *Eur J Plast Surg* 1996; **19**: 174–7.

50 Goette DK, Carson TE. Erythroplasia of Queyrat: treatment with topical 5-Fluorouracil. *Cancer* 1976; **38**: 1498–502.

51 Haas GP, Blumenstein BA, Gagliano RG *et al.* Cisplatin, methotrexate and bleomycin for the treatment of carcinoma of the penis: a Southwest Oncology Group study. *J Urol* 1999; **161**: 1823–5.

52 Rozan R, Albuisson E, Giraud B, Boiteux JP, Dauplat J. Epithelioma of the penis treated with surgery. (Study Group on Urogenital Tumors of the National Federation of the Centers for Cancer Control.) *Prog Urol* 1996; **6**: 926–35.

53 Delannes M, Malavaud B, Douchez J, Bonnet J, Daly NJ. Iridium-192 interstitial therapy for squamous cell carcinoma of the penis. *Int J Radiat Oncol Biol Phys* 1992; **24**: 479–83.

54 Chaudhary AJ, Ghosh S, Bhalavat RL, Kulkarni JN, Sequeira BV. Interstitial brachytherapy in carcinoma of the penis. *Strahlenther Onkol* 1999; **175**: 17–20.

55 Opjordsmoen S, Waehre H, Aass N, Fossa SD. Sexuality in patients treated for penile cancer: patient's experience and doctor's judgement. *Br J Urol* 1994; **73**: 554–60.

56 Ficarra V, Mofferdin A, D'Amico A *et al.* Comparison of the quality of life of patients treated by surgery or radiotherapy in epidermoid cancer of the penis. *Prog Urol* 1999; **9**: 715–20.

57 Spiessl B, Beahrs OH, Hermanek P *et al.* (eds) *TNM Atlas: Illustrated Guide to the TNM/pTNM Classification of Malignant Tumours (UICC)*, 3rd edn, 2nd revision. Heidelberg: Springer-Verlag, 1992.

Penile Cancer: Commentary

J. Waxman

Penile cancer is a rare tumour whose incidence varies geographically. India has one of the highest incidences of this condition, and the experience of Indian clinicians provides a significant lead for the rest of the world.

The rarity of this tumour has meant that our experience of management has not evolved through the same logical evidence-based trial work as we have seen in, for example, testicular cancer. In their chapter, Drs Sarin and Tongaonkar describe a vast experience of the management of penile cancer and make recommendations for the management of this tumour, providing a guide for the practising clinician.

The history of viral oncogenesis is very long, dating back to beyond the original observations of Rous and the demonstration of a transmissible agent for the development of malignancy. Theories of viral oncogenesis have fallen in and out of fashion over the years. However, there has been a renaissance of interest in viral oncogenesis in the last two decades with the observations of the significance of the herpes virus family in the development of cervical cancer, the Epstein–Barr virus in lymphoma, and the hepatitis virus in the development of hepatoma. Similarly, for penile cancer the significance of the herpes virus family has emerged, although its role as an aetiological factor in all patients with this tumour has not been confirmed. We hope that the next decade will bring us vaccines to prevent the development of penile cancer.

Index

Bold text marks references to tables, *italic* text marks references to figures

abl oncogene 144
acid phosphatase 264
adjuvant chemotherapy 104–5, **105**
   trials of **105**
adjuvant hormone therapy 196–7
adrenocorticotrophin-releasing hormone
      (ACTH) 221
adriamycin, in bladder cancer 100–1, **107**
AG3340 44
Agency for Health Care Policy and Research
      (AHCPR) 226
alpha-fetoprotein, in testicular cancer 331
alprostadil 260
American Brachytherapy Society,
      recommendations for prostate cancer
      200
American Joint Committee on Cancer (AJCC)
      173
American Society for Therapeutic Radiology
      and Oncology (ASTRO) 190
American staging system 174
American Urological Association 174
aminoglutethimide 226, 227
androgen ablation *167*
androgen blockade
   combined 228
   intermittent 228–9
androgen deprivation therapy 168–9, 221
   sequential 229
androgen inhibitors 226–7
androgen receptors 146–51
   and androgen synthesis 146–8, *146*, *147*
   differentiation 148
   treatment resistance 148–50, *149*
   trinucleotide repeats 150
androgens, circulating 220–1
angiogenesis
   bladder cancer 77–8
   renal cancer 41

angiogenesis inhibitors 41–4
   bladder cancer 77–8
   renal cancer 42–4
   thalidomide 42–3
   TNP-470 42
angiogenic switch 41
angiostatin 41, 44
anthracyclines
   bladder cancer 124
   prostate cancer 240
anti-androgens 225–6
apoptosis 63, *64*, 181–2
   derangement of 182
apoptotic markers 180–2
   apoptotic bodies 181–2
   Ki-67 and MIB-1 181
   mitotic figures 180
   proliferating cell nuclear antigen 180–1
apoptotic bodies 181–2
artificial neural network analysis 78
Australasian Germ Cell Trial Group 306
autologous bone marrow transplantation
      322
autologous stem cell transplantation 318

BAY 12-9566 44
BCG, in superficial bladder cancer 124,
      125–8
bcl-2 oncogene 143–4
Beckwith–Weidemann syndrome 13, 15
beta-human chorionic gonadotrophin, in
      testicular cancer 311, 331
bicalutamide 220, 226
biochemotherapy 39, **40**
biopsy
   penile cancer 370–1
   prostate cancer 164–7, *167*, 170
bladder cancer 137
   basic science 59

cell cycle control 61–74, *62*
  apoptosis 63, *64*
  p14ARF and p16 73
  p21/WAF1 73–4
  p53 tumour-suppressor gene 65–72,
    67–9
  retinoblastoma 72–3
chemotherapy 98–117
  adjuvant 104–6, **105**
  metastatic disease 107–12, **107**
  neoadjuvant 99–104, **100**, **103**
cytogenetic studies 59–61
  comparative genomic hybridization 60,
    61
  loss of heterozygosity **60**
molecular biology 59–83
prognostic markers 74–8, **75**
  angiogenesis and angiogenesis inhibitors
    77–8
  combinations of 78
  epidermal growth factor receptor 76–7
  MDM2 74–6
  proliferation antigens 77
staging 85–6
superficial *see* superficial bladder cancer
surgery 84–97
  partial cystectomy 86–7
  radical cystectomy 87–96
  transurethral resection 84–6
transitional cell carcinoma 98
transurethral surveillance 123
tumour classification 118–19
tumour recurrence 95
bleomycin
  germ cell tumours 296
  penile cancer 379
  testicular cancer 305, 306, 309, 312
  omission **307**
Bloom syndrome 13
bowenoid papulosis 361–2
Bowen's disease 358–60
brachytherapy, prostate 197–201, *199*, **200**,
  270–1
complications **200**
BRCA-1 mutations **145**
buserelin 220

Canadian National Cancer Institute, bladder
  cancer trials 102
Cancer and Leukemia Group B, prostate
  cancer trials 242

Cancer Research Campaign (CRC), renal
  cancer trials 40
captopril 43
carboplatin
  bladder cancer **107**
  testicular cancer 300–1, 308–9, **309**, 312,
    323
carcinoma *in situ* 121–2, 280
castration 222
CCND2 gene 281
CD8+ marker 37
CD44 marker 16–17
cell cycle control 61, *62*
cervical cancer, viral aetiology 354, 355
cervical intraepithelial neoplasia 357
CGS27023a 44
chemotherapy
  bladder cancer 98–117
    adjuvant 104–6, **105**
    metastatic disease 107–12, **107**
    neoadjuvant 99–104, **100**, **103**
  germ cell tumours 296–8
  nephrectomy improving response to 51
  penile cancer 379
  prostate cancer 232, 237–51
  testicular cancer 300–1
chromosome alterations, renal tumours **17**
CISCA chemotherapy 105, 108
cisplatin 87
  bladder cancer 101, 105, **107**, 108
  germ cell tumours 296
  penile cancer 377
  prostate cancer 243
  testicular cancer 305, 306, **307**, 308–9,
    309
    dose escalation 310
    salvage chemotherapy 318, 321, 322
colony stimulating factors, in testicular cancer
  311
corticosteroids, in hormone refractory
  prostate cancer 238
cryptorchidism 329
Cullin-2 6
cyclin-dependent kinases 62, 359
cyclophosphamide
  bladder cancer 105, **107**, 108
  prostate cancer 240, 248
  testicular cancer 306, **307**, 323
cyproterone acetate 220, 223
cystectomy
  partial 86–7

radical 87–96
  early complications 93–5
  late complications 95–6
  lymph node dissection **89**
  in men 88–92, *90, 91*
  preoperative management 87–8
  urethrectomy 92
  urinary diversion 93
  in women 92, *93, 94*
cytokines 32–9, 55
  interferons 33–5, **34**, 37–8
  interleukin 2 35–7, **36**, 37–8
  interleukin 12 37
cytotoxic T lymphocytes 33

dactinomycin, in testicular cancer 306, **307**
Damocles syndrome 295
Denys–Drash syndrome 13
diethylstilboestrol 222
DNA polymerase 246
docetaxel
  bladder cancer 110, **111**
  prostate cancer **244**, 245
doxorubicin
  bladder cancer 105, 108
  prostate cancer 240
  superficial bladder cancer 124

E-cadherin 154
Eastern Cooperative Oncology Group (ECOG)
  renal cancer trials 31
  testicular cancer trials 307, 323
elongin B 6
elongin C 6
endostatin 44
epidermal growth factor receptor (EGFR) 76–7
epirubicin 87
  bladder cancer **107**
  superficial bladder cancer 124
epithelial growth factor **153**
Epstein–Barr virus 356
erb-B2/HER-2/neu oncogene 143
erectile dysfunction 259
erythroplasia of Queyrat 359, 360
estramustine 223, 243–6, *243*, **244**
etoposide, in testicular cancer 296, 297, 305, 306, **307**, 309, 312
  salvage chemotherapy 319, 322, 323

European Organization for Research and Treatment of Cancer (EORTC)
  bladder cancer trials 87, **100**, 101
  Genitourinary Group 109, 174
  prostate cancer trials 208, 211, 241
  renal cancer trials 40
  testicular cancer trials 307, 308, 310, 321

fibroblast growth factors 42, 152–4, **153**
fibroblast-derived growth factor 246
fibronectin 8
filgrastim, in testicular cancer 311
finasteride 220, 229, 230
fine needle aspiration cytology 370
fluorescence *in situ* hybridization (FISH) 61, **62**, 281
5-fluorouracil
  bladder cancer **107**
  metastatic renal cancer 39, **40**
  penile cancer 377
  prostate cancer 240
flutamide 220, 226
fms oncogene 144
follicle-stimulating hormone 284
fos oncogene 144
fosfesterol 223
French Federation of Cancer Centres 308
fumigillin 42

gallium nitrate, in bladder cancer **107**
GAP proteins 10
gemcitabine
  bladder cancer **107, 109**, 110
  testicular cancer 320–1
gene loci, in transitional cell carcinoma 60
genetics
  of bladder cancer 59–61
  of testicular cancer 281–9, *281, 284, 287, 288, 289*
germ cell tumours *see* testicular cancer
German Testicular Cancer Study Group 308–9
Gleason score 161, **162**, *164*, 266–9
gonadotrophin releasing hormone analogues 220, 224–5
goserelin 220, 224
growth factors 151–4, **153**

hepatitis B virus 356
hereditary papillary renal cell carcinoma 12

hereditary renal clear cell carcinoma 9
  chromosomal alterations **17**
herpes simplex virus, and penile cancer 362
Hoosier Oncology Group, prostatic cancer
      trials 244
hormone therapy
  nephrectomy improving response to 51
  prostate cancer 209–10, *209*, 213–14,
      220–36
    adrenal androgen inhibitors 226–7
    anti-androgens 225–6
    chemoprevention 230
    combined androgen blockade 228
    early versus deferred therapy 229–30
    GnRH analogues 224–5
    intermittent androgen blockade 228–9
    neoadjuvant and adjuvant 230–2
    oestrogens 222–3
    orchiectomy 222
    progestational agents 223–4
    radical prostatectomy 230–1
    rationale for 220–2
    5α-reductase inhibitors 227
    relapsed disease 232–3
    sequential androgen deprivation 229
hormone refractory prostate cancer 237–52
  definition of 237–8
  estramustine 243–6, *243*, **244**
  evaluation of response/benefits of therapy
      238–9
  mitoxantrone plus prednisolone 240–3,
      241, *242*
  novel targets for therapy 247–8
  older studies of chemotherapy 239–40
  supportive treatments 238
  suramin 246–7
HPV E6 viral oncoproteins 360
HPV E7 viral oncoproteins 357–9
HPV-6 genome 357
HPV-11 genome 357
HPV-16 genome *356*
human papillomavirus 355, 356–62
  and carcinoma of penis 359–62
  HPV E6 viral oncoproteins 358
  HPV E7 viral oncoproteins 357–8
  HPV-16 genome *356*
  and telomerase activity 359–60
  viral oncogenesis and HPV-associated
      transformation 356–7
Huntington's chorea 150
hydrocele 332

hypothalamic–pituitary–gonadal endocrine
      axis *146*

ifosfamide
  bladder cancer **107**
  testicular cancer 310–11, 313
    salvage chemotherapy 319–20, 323
ilio-inguinal lymph nodes, management of
      374–7
  complications of lymphadenectomy
      376–7
  extent of lymphadenectomy 376
immunomodulators, in superficial bladder
      cancer 130
immunotherapy
  bladder cancer 126–7
  nephrectomy improving response to 51
inferior vena cava, metastases 51–2
insulin-like growth factor-1 147, **153**
intensity modulated radiation therapy 203
interferons 33–5, **34**, 37–8
interferon-alpha 33–5, **34**, 37–8
  and interleukin 2 37–8
  metastatic renal cancer 39, **40**
  and survival in renal cancer **34**
interferon-gamma 35
interleukin 2 35–7, **36**, 37–8
  and interferon-alpha 37–8
  metastatic renal cancer 39, **40**
  and survival in renal cancer **36**
interleukin 12 37
International Germ Cell Consensus
      Classification 305, **306**
International Union Against Cancer, tumour
      classification 118–19
intratubular germ cell neoplasia 280
intravesical therapy, in bladder cancer
      124–8

KAI1 gene 154
keratinocyte growth factor 147, **153**
ketoconazole 226–7
keyhole limpet haemocyanin 130
Ki-67 181
kidney cancer *see* renal cancer

laparoscopic radical prostatectomy 257–8
laser therapy, penile cancer 373–4
leucovorin 248
leuporelin 220, 224
lobaplatin, in bladder cancer **107**

loss of heterozygosity
   bladder cancer 60
   renal cancer 5
low molecular weight heparin 43
luteinizing hormone 220
luteinizing hormone-releasing hormone
      analogues 264
lymph nodes
   dissection
      following orchidectomy 334–5, **335**
      radical cystectomy **89**
      retroperitoneal 293, 295
   irradiation of 193, *194*
   penile cancer 374–7
   prostate cancer 178
lymphadenectomy
   complications of 376–7
   extent of 376
lymphocytes
   cytotoxic T 33
   tumour infiltrating 37
lymphokine-activated killer (LAK) cells
      36–7, 127

M-VAC regimen 108
marimastat 43
Massachusetts General Hospital, bladder
      cancer trials 102, **103**
matrix metalloproteinases 44
MDM2 oncogene 74–6
Medical Research Council
   bladder cancer trials 87, 101
   germ cell tumour trials 293–4
   prostate cancer trials 208, *209*, *212*, **213**,
      230
   testicular cancer trials 308, 312, 313
medicated urethral system for erection
      (MUSE) 260
medroxyprogesterone acetate 31, 223, 224
megesterol acetate 223, 224
Memorial Hospital, bladder cancer trials
      107–8
men, radical cystectomy in 88–92, *90*, *91*
MET proto-oncogene 11–13
metalloproteinases 155
metanephric adenoma 16
   chromosomal alterations **17**
metastatic cancer
   bladder 107–12, **107**
   penile 369
   prostate 214–15

renal 49–54
testicular 305–12, 322–4
methotrexate 87
   bladder cancer 101, **107**
   prostate cancer 240, 243
   testicular cancer 320, 322
MIB-1 181
microtubule-associated proteins 243
microvessel density analysis 182–5
   prediction of cancer recurrence and survival
      183–4
   prediction of pathological stage 183
   vascular endothelial growth
      factors/receptors 184–5
mitomycin 87
   bladder cancer **107**
   prostate cancer 240, 243
   superficial bladder cancer 124, 125–6
mitotic figures 180
mitoxantrone 240–3, *241*, **242**
MMC, in superficial bladder cancer 124–5,
      130
Mohs micrographic surgery 375
molecular markers 16–18, **17**
myb oncogene 144
myc proto-oncogene 143

National Bladder Cancer Collaborative
      Group 119
National Cancer Institute of Canada, prostate
      cancer trials 238
National Prostate Cancer Project 239–40
natural killer cells 38, 130
neoadjuvant chemotherapy 99–104, **100**,
      103
   and bladder preservation 103–4, **103**
   randomised trials of **100**
neoadjuvant hormone therapy 196–7
neovascularization 41
nephrectomy 49–51
   improved response to treatment 51
   palliation of local symptoms 50
   psychological support 50
   spontaneous regression of metastases
      49–50
nephrogenic rests 14
nilutamide 226
NME1 gene 285
NME2 gene 285
Nordic Cystectomy I trial **100**
Nordic Cystectomy II trial 101

oestrogens, in prostate cancer 222–3
oncogenes
  abl 144
  bcl-2 143–4
  Erb-B2/HER-2/neu 143
  myc 143
  prostate cancer 142–4
  ras 143
  transitional cell carcinoma **61**
orchidectomy 222, 328–50
  excision of residual masses *336–41*
  investigations preceding 331–2
  lymph node dissection following 334–5,
    335
  staging after 333–4, **333**
  technique 332–3
orchidopexy 329

p14ARF 73
p16 73
p21/WAF1 73–4
p53 tumour-suppressor gene 65–72, 144,
    360
  interpretation of expression 66–72, *67–9*
  prognostic value *67–9*
p53-induced genes 63
p53-mediated apoptosis 63, *64*
paclitaxel
  bladder cancer **111**, 112
  prostate cancer **244**, 245
  testicular cancer 312, 320–1, 322
papillary adenoma 16
  chromosomal alterations **17**
papillary renal cell carcinoma 10–13, *11*
  chromosomal alterations **17**
  hereditary 12
pelvic node irradiation 193, *194*
penile cancer
  biopsy 369–71
  natural history, histology and presentation
    366–7
  prognosis 377–8
  quality of life and psychosexual issues 378
  staging 368–9, **368**
  treatment 369–77
    chemotherapy 377
    of ilio-inguinal lymph nodes 374–7
    laser therapy 373–4
    Mohs micrographic surgery 373
    radiotherapy 369–72, **370**
    surgery 372–3

viruses and 353–65
  characteristics of viruses 353–4
  herpes simplex virus 362
  human papillomavirus 355–62, *356*
  role of viruses in neoplasia 355–6
perineal prostatectomy 257
perineural invasion 177
peripheral blood stem cells 323
Perlman syndrome 13
photofrin-mediated photodynamic therapy
    130–1
piritrexim, in bladder cancer **107**
platelet-derived growth factor 246
platinum compounds 240
polymerase chain reaction 361
polyoestradiol phosphate (PEP) 223
prednisone 240–3, *241*, **242**
progestational agents, in prostate cancer
    223–4
prognostic markers 74–8, **75**
  angiogenesis and angiogenesis inhibitors
    77–8
  epidermal growth factor receptor 76–7
  MDM2 74–6
  proliferation antigens 77
proliferating cell nuclear antigen 70, 180–1
proliferation antigens 77
proliferation markers 180–2
  apoptotic bodies 181–2
  Ki-67 and MIB-1 181
  mitotic figures 180
  proliferating cell nuclear antigen 180–1
prostate cancer
  androgen receptors 146–51
    and androgen synthesis 146–8, *146*, *147*
    in differentiation 148
    5α-reductase activity 150–1
    treatment resistance 148–50, *149*
    trinucleotide repeats 150
  biochemical control **191**
  biopsy 164–7, *167*, 170
  cellular–matrix interactions 154–6, **155**
  chemoprevention 230
  chemotherapy 232, 237–52
    earlier stage prostate cancer 248–9
    estramustine 243–6, *243*, **244**
    evaluation of response/benefit 238–9
    mitoxantrone plus prednisone 240–3,
      241, **242**
    older studies 239–40
    supportive 238

suramin 246–7
epidemiology 141–2, **142**
Gleason scores 161, **162**, *164*
  and survival 266–9, **267**, **268**
grading 161–9
  after androgen deprivation therapy
    168–9
  after radiation therapy 167–8, *167*
  prior to radical prostatectomy 161–4,
    162, *163*, *164*
  transrectal needle biopsy 164–7, *167*
growth factors 151–4, **153**
hormone refractory 237–52
hormone therapy 209–10, *209*, 213–14,
  220–36
  adrenal androgen inhibitors 226–7
  anti-androgens 225–6
  chemoprevention 230
  combined androgen blockade 228
  early versus deferred therapy 229–30
  GnRH analogues 224–5
  intermittent androgen blockage 228–9
  neoadjuvant and adjuvant 230–2
  oestrogens 222–3
  orchiectomy 222
  progestational agents 223–4
  radical prostatectomy 230–1
  rationale for 220–2
  5α-reductase inhibitors 227
  relapsed disease 232–3
  sequential androgen deprivation 229
immediate versus deferred treatment
  206–19
  hormone treatment and disease outcome
    209–10, *209*
  patients dying without treatment
    210–14, *212*, **213**, *214*
  reasons for deferral 206–8, **207**, **208**
location of 169
microvessel density 182–5
  and prediction of cancer recurrence and
    survival 183–4
  and prediction of pathological stage 183
  vascular endothelial growth
    factors/receptors 184–5
molecular biology 141–59
morphometric markers 178–80, **179**
natural history 265–6
oncogenes 142–4
  bcl-2 143–4
  erb-B2/HER-2/neu 143

myc 143
ras 143
pathogenesis and progression *155*
pathological stage 173–7
  American staging system 174
  limitations of current staging systems
    174–7
  TNM staging system 173–4
practical management 214–17
  localized disease 215–16
  locally advanced disease 216–17
  metastatic disease 214–15
progression in **208**
proliferation and apoptotic markers 180–2
  apoptosis and apoptotic bodies 181–2
  Ki-67 and MIB-1 181
  mitotic figures 180
  proliferating cell nuclear antigen 180–1
radical prostatectomy *see* radical
  prostatectomy
radiotherapy *see* prostatic radiotherapy
relapse 232–3
reporting **184**
risk factors **142**
surgical margins 171–3, *172*
surgical pathology 160–88
  cancer grade 161–9, **162**, *163*, *164*, *167*
  cancer volume 169–71
  location of cancer 169
  microvessel density 182–5, **184**
  morphometric markers 178–80, **179**
  pathological stage 173–7
  perineural invasion 177
  surgical margins 171–3, *172*
  vascular/lymphatic invasion 178
survival **191**, 266–9, **267**, **268**
tumour-environment interactions 151–4,
  153
tumour-suppressor genes 144–6
  BRCA-1 145
  loss of heterozygosity 145–6
  p53 144
  retinoblastoma 144–5
vascular/lymphatic invasion 178
volume of 169–71
  radical prostatectomies 170–1
  small biopsies 170
Prostate Cancer Trialists' Collaborative
  Group 228
prostate-specific antigen 168, 246, 253
  adenocarcinoma detection 175–6

failure 201–2
as indicator of persistent disease 258
Prostate-Specific Antigen Working Group
    239
prostatic acid phosphatase 168
prostatic radiotherapy 189–205, 231–2,
    270–1
    brachytherapy 197–201, *199*, **200**
    comparison with radical prostatectomy
        189–91, **191**
    grade after 167–8, *167*
    irradiation of pelvic lymph nodes 193, *194*
    management of PSA failure 201–2
    neoadjuvant and adjuvant hormones
        196–7
    new developments 203
    palliative 202
    radiation dose 195
    radiation morbidity 195–6
    seminal vesicle irradiation 194–5
    survival **191**
    target volume 193–6
    techniques 192–3, *192*
protein kinase C 7, 246
proto-oncogenes 11
PSA *see* prostate-specific antigen
PTEN/MMAC1 gene 154–5

Radiation Therapy Oncology Group (RTOG)
    bladder cancer trials 102, **103**
    prostate cancer trials 194, 208, 248
radical prostatectomy 161–4, **162**, *163*, *164*,
        170–1, 230–1, 253–63, 269–70
    case against 264–74
    comparison with radiotherapy 189–91,
        191
    complications 259–61
    laparoscopic 257–8
    patient selection 253–4
    perineal 257
    results 258–9
    retropubic 254–7
    selection bias 270
radiotherapy
    dose 195
    morbidity 195–6
    penile cancer 369–72, **370**
    prostate cancer *see* prostatic radiotherapy
    testicular cancer 299–300
ras oncogene 143
5α-reductase activity 150–1

5α-reductase inhibitors 227–8
renal cancer
    aetiology 3
    incidence 3
    metastatic 49–54
        nephrectomy 49–51
        renal vein and inferior vena cava 51–2
        surgery 52
    molecular biology 3–30
    prognostic factors 31, **32**
    survival **32**
    TNM staging system 49, **50**
    treatment
        angiogenesis inhibitors 42–4
        biochemotherapy 39–40, **40**
        interferon 33–5, **34**, 37–8
        interleukin 2 35–7, **36**, 37–8
    see also individual tumours
renal clear cell carcinoma *4*
    chromosomal alterations **17**
    hereditary 9
    sporadic 8–9
renal oncocytoma 15
    chromosomal alterations **17**
renal vein, metastases 51–2
reproductive function, testicular cancer
        effects 341–4, *340*, *341*, *343*, *344*
restriction fragment length polymorphism
    282
retinoblastoma gene product 72–3, 144–5
retroperitoneal lymph node dissection 293,
    295
retropubic prostatectomy 254–7
    post-operative care 257
    surgical technique 254–6
rhabdomyosarcoma of bladder 98
Royal Marsden Hospital
    penile cancer study 371
    staging classification **333**

S-phase fraction 76
Scottish International Guidelines Network
    313
seminal vesicle irradiation 194–5
seminoma *see* testicular cancer
sildenafil 260
sis oncogene 144
Southeastern Cancer Study Group
    bladder cancer trials 108
    testicular cancer trials 306, 310
Southwest Oncology Group

bladder cancer trials 87, 101, 126
  prostate cancer trials 240, 245, 248
  testicular cancer trials 310
sporadic renal clear cell carcinoma 8–9
  chromosomal alterations **17**
squamous cell carcinoma of bladder 98
staging
  American (Whitmore–Jewett) system 174
  bladder cancer 85–6
  limitations of 174–7
    clinical understaging with digital rectal
      examination 175
    PSA-detected adenocarcinoma 175–6
  penile cancer **368**
  Royal Marsden Hospital staging
    classification **333**
  testicular cancer **333**
  TNM system
    penile cancer **370**
    prostate cancer 173–4
    renal cancer 49, **50**
  transurethral resection 85–6
SU416 44
superficial bladder cancer 118–36
  alternative therapies 130–1
    immunomodulators 130
    photofrin-mediated photodynamic
      therapy 130–1
  G2pT1 disease 129
  intravesical therapy 124–8
    in CIS treatment 128
    intravesical cytotoxic chemotherapy
      124–6
    intravesical immunotherapy 126–7
    in prevention of tumour progression 128
  natural history 119–22
    carcinoma *in situ* 121–2
    pTa/pT1 disease 119–21, *120*
  risk factors and prognosis 122, **123**
  transurethral surveillance and tumour
    resection 123–4
  tumour classification 118–19
suramin 246–7
surgery
  bladder cancer 84–97
  Mohs micrographic 373
  penile cancer 372–3
  prostate cancer *see* radical prostatectomy
  renal metastases 52
    contralateral kidney 52
  testicular cancer 328–50

surveillance, of germ cell tumours 293–6,
    294

tamoxifen 40
tandem therapy 323
taxoids, in bladder cancer 110–12, **111**
taxol, in bladder cancer **107, 111**
taxotere, bladder cancer **111**
telomerase 358–9
testicular cancer
  adjuvant chemotherapy 296–8
  chemotherapy 305–16
    metastatic non-seminoma 305–12, 335
    post-orchidectomy 334–5
    seminoma 312–13
  clinical diagnosis 329–31, *331*
  desperation surgery 318
  genetics
    of differentiation 285–6
    of resistance 286–9, *287, 288, 289*
    of transformation 281–5, *281, 284*
  impact on reproductive function 341–4,
    342, 343, 344
  late relapse 324
  management preferences 298–301
  pathobiology 280
  prognosis 317–19, **319**
  refractory 317
  relapsing 317
  Royal Marsden Hospital staging
    classification **333**
  salvage chemotherapy 317–27
    drug combinations 321–2
    high dose 322–4
    new drugs 320–1
    single agents 319–20, **320**
  seminoma 280
    adjuvant chemotherapy 300–1
    radiotherapy 299–300
    surveillance 299
  surgery *see* orchidectomy
  surveillance 293–6, *294*
    post-orchidectomy 334–5, **335**
  ultrasound examination 330
tetrasomy 7 16
thalidomide 42–3
thiotepa, in testicular cancer 323, 324
TNM staging system
  problems of 176–7
  prostate cancer 173–4
  renal cancer **50**, 59

TNP-470 42
topoisomerase II 246
topotecan, in bladder cancer **107**
transcription factor TEF3 11
transforming growth factor-β 7–8, 246
transitional cell carcinoma of the bladder 98
transrectal needle biopsy 164–7, *167*
transrectal ultrasound (TRUS) 216
transurethral resection of bladder (TURB)
      84–6
   staging 85–6
   for superficial bladder cancer 123–4
   therapeutic, for invasive tumours 86
transurethral resection of prostate (TURP)
      209, 215, 255
treatment deferral in prostatic cancer 206–19
   clinical trials 208
   hazards of **207**
   hormone treatment and disease outcome
      209–10, *209*
   patients dying without treatment 210–14,
      212, **213**, *214*
   reasons for 206–8
trimetrexate, in bladder cancer **107**
trinucleotide repeats 150
trisomy 7 16
trisomy 17 11, 16
tuberous sclerosis 10
   chromosomal alterations **17**
tuberous sclerosis complex 1 (TSC1) 10
tuberous sclerosis complex 2 (TSC2) 10
tumour growth factor 151–2, **153**
tumour infiltrating lymphocytes 37
tumour necrosis factor-α, inhibition by
      thalidomide 43
tumour-suppressor genes
   apoptosis 63, *64*
   bladder cancer 59, **60**, 61–74, *65*
   BRCA-1 145
   p14ARF and p16 73
   p21/WAF1 73–4
   p53 65–72, **67–9**, 144
   prostate cancer 144–6, **145**
   retinoblastoma 72–3, 144–5

ubiquitin 6
Union Internationale Contre le Cancer 173
ureteric obstruction 95

urethrectomy 92
urinary diversion 93
   complications of 93–5
urinary incontinence 259, 261

vascular endothelial growth factor (VEGF) 7,
      44, 77, 147, 184–5
vascular leak syndrome 35
Veterans Administration Cooperative
      Research Group (VACURG), prostate
      cancer trials 207, 208, 212, 222, 224,
      229, 271
Viagra 260
vinblastine 39, 87
   bladder cancer 101, **107**
   prostate cancer **244**
   renal cancer 39
vinca alkaloids
   germ cell tumours 296
   prostate cancer 240, 243
   testicular cancer 306, **307**, 321, 322
   see also vinblastine; vincristine
vincristine, in testicular cancer 296, 322
vinorelbine **244**, 245
viruses, and penile cancer 353–65
   characteristics of viruses 355–6
   herpes simplex virus 362
   human papillomavirus 355–62, *356*
      and carcinoma of penis 359–62
      HPV E6 viral oncoproteins 358
      HPV E7 viral oncoproteins 357–68
      and telomerase activity 358–9
      viral oncogenesis and HPV-associated
         transformation 356–7
   role of viruses in neoplasia 355–6
vitaxin 44
von Hippel–Lindau disease 3, 4, 5, 6–8
   chromosomal alterations **17**
   epidemiology 4
   VHL gene 5–6, 8, 9

WAF1 73–4
Whitmore–Jewett staging system 174
WHO grading system **163**
Wilms' tumour 13–15
   chromosomal alterations **17**
women, radical cystectomy in 92, *93*, *94*
WT1 gene 14